Family Nurse Practitioner Certification

Intensive Review

About the Author

Maria T. Codina Leik (MSN, ARNP, BC, NP-C [GNP, ANP, FNP]), developed materials for the nurse practitioner review courses that she has presented nationally since 1997 through her company, National ARNP Services, Inc. She received her advanced practice nursing licensure in 1991 and certification as an Adult Nurse Practitioner. She was certified as a Gerontological Nurse Practitioner in 1995 and as a Family Nurse Practitioner in 1999. She maintains an NP practice for students on a per diem basis at Florida International University and a primary care practice at the Plantation Medical Clinic.

Family Nurse Practitioner Certification

Intensive Review

Maria T. Codina Leik, MSN, APRN, BC, FNP-C

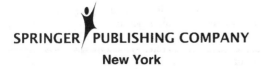

SPRINGER PUBLISHING COMPANY
New York

Special discounts on bulk quantities of our books are available to corporations, professional associations, pharmaceutical companies, health care organizations, and other qualified groups. If you are interested in a custom book, including chapters from more than one of our titles, we can provide that service as well.

For details, please contact:
Special Sales Department, Springer Publishing Company, LLC
11 West 42nd Street, 15th Floor, New York, NY 10036-8002
Phone: 877-687-7476 or 212-431-4370; Fax: 212-941-7842
Email: sales@springerpub.com

Springer Publishing Company, LLC
11 West 42nd Street
New York, NY 10036–8002
www.springerpub.com

Acquisitions Editor: Sally J. Barhydt
Managing Editor: Mary Ann McLaughlin
Production Editor: Tenea Johnson
Cover Design: Joanne E. Honigman
Composition: Aptara, Inc

15 14 13 12 / 7 8 9 10

Library of Congress Cataloging-in-Publication Data

Codina Leik, Maria T.
   Family nurse practitioner certification : intensive review / Maria T.
  Codina Leik.
     p. cm.
   Includes bibliographical references and index.
    ISBN-13: 978–0–8261–0296–6 (pbk.)
  1. Nurse practitioners—Examinations, questions, etc. I. Title.
[DNLM: 1. Nurse Practitioners–Problems and Exercises. 2. Family
Practice—Problems and Exercises. WY 18.2 C669f 2007]

RT82.8.C63 2007
610.73076—dc22

2007017431

Printed in United States by Bang Printing.

Notice: The author and the publisher of this work have made every effort to use sources believed to be reliable to provide information that is accurate and compatible with the standards generally accepted at the time of publication. Because medical science and the science of pharmacology are continually advancing, our knowledge base continues to expand. Therefore, as new information becomes available, changes in treatments and in the use of drugs become necessary. We recommend that the reader always refer to the manufacturer's product information, especially in the case of drug dosages, contraindications, and administration guidelines before giving any medication. This is particularly important with new or rarely used drugs. The author and publisher shall not be liable for any special, consequential, or exemplary damages resulting, in whole or in part, from the readers' use of, or reliance on, the information contained in this book.

Writing this book taught me many things.
Most important, how blessed and lucky I am
to have E.J.L., my wonderful husband,
and my daughters, Maryfaye and Christina.
I am truly grateful for your love and support.
Many heartfelt thanks to my talented and patient editor,
Sally J. Barhydt, who helped make a dream into reality.
And to all my review course students,
May your salary hit the stratosphere.
Of course, good dark chocolate is an absolute necessity
when one is writing review books way past midnight.
And most of all, thank you dear God.

Preface

The purpose of this family nurse practitioner (FNP) review book is simple. It is designed to save you valuable time reviewing for the FNP certification exam. The content is applicable for both exams from the American Nurses Credentialing Center (ANCC) and the American Academy of Nurse Practitioners (AANP).

A special effort has been made to cut down as much extraneous information as possible without sacrificing the quality of the book's contents. The end result is a review guide that will not only help to cut down your total review time, but will also give you a more productive and less frustrating experience.

The guiding principle that I kept in mind when writing this review guide is that most of you have a limited amount of time to study. Your review time is valuable. Ultimately, I designed this book to assist you to thoroughly study for the family nurse practitioner certification exam in an efficient manner. The end result of this idea is the format that I used when writing this book. I call it the "Fast Facts" method. Information is delivered in a brief, yet concise manner. It is easier to comprehend. It is also more realistic.

The entire lifespan, ranging from pediatrics, adolescence, adulthood (including pregnancy), into geriatrics, is reviewed. In addition, nonclinical content, such as ethics, medico-legal issues, advanced practice law, reimbursement and others, is included. For the adult nurse practitioner (ANP) who wants to use this book to study, simply skip the pediatric and obstetrics sections. Your review should start with the adolescence section and continue until the geriatrics section, including the nonclinical content.

I have combined five resources into one "Mega Review" study guide. It contains (1) specific certification exam information which includes instructions on speeding up the application process, (2) test-taking techniques that are highly relevant for both the ANCC and AANP exam, (3) a question dissection and analysis section where you learn to pick out the "Best Clues" to solve problems, along with the necessary clinical knowledge, (4) a review of primary care disorders including specific "Exam Tips" with advice on some current exam topics, and finally, (5) a total of 500 sample questions and answers to practice your new skills.

Included in this review guide are many pictures and tables. Physical exam maneuvers (i.e., the Drawer sign, McMurrays sign, etc.) are beautifully illustrated by photographs and notes. In addition, unlike the other nurse practitioner review books out in the market today, this book approaches the organ systems review in an unusual manner.

This review guide does not follow the usual head-to-toe order in the systems review section. The first section is on dermatology. I have chosen to do this because of feedback from new nurse practitioner graduates, many of whom report that they felt deficient in their knowledge of skin disorders.

I have been teaching and designing review courses for 10 years. I am also in active clinical practice. If you would like an ANP, FNP, pediatric (PNP) review course at your school or have comments and suggestions about this book, please contact me by email from my company's web site at *www.NPreview.com*.

Contributors

The following Nurse Practitioners have graciously contributed questions for this review book.

Ivette Baker, MSN, ARNP, BC
Adult Nurse Practitioner and Pediatric
  Nurse Practitioner
Adjunct Faculty
Florida International University
Graduate School of Nursing
Adult and Family Nurse Practitioner
  Track
Miami, Florida

Therese A. Boyd, EdD, ARNP, BC
Adult Nurse Practitioner
Florida International University
Health Care & Wellness Center
Biscayne Bay Campus
North Miami, Florida

Nancy Gonzalez, MSN, ARNP, BC, CLNC
Pediatric Nurse Practitioner
Private Practice
Medical Legal Consulting Service
Pembroke Pines, Florida

Mayra Lima, MSN, ARNP, BC
Family Nurse Practitioner
Memorial Cancer Institute
Breast Cancer Center
Hollywood, Florida

Lourdes Lizardo, MSN, ARNP, EdD
Clinical Professor
Florida International University
Graduate School of Nursing
Family and Adult Nurse Practitioner
  Track
Miami, Florida

Susanne Pavlovich-Danis, MSN, ARNP, BC, CDE
Adult Nurse Practitioner
Plantation Medical Clinic
University of Phoenix
Area Chair, Nursing Program
Plantation, Florida

Contents

Preface vii

Contributors ix

Chapter 1 Certification Exam Information 1

Chapter 2 Question Dissection and Analysis 15

Chapter 3 Health Screening and Systems Review 59
       Health Screening Recommendations: U.S. Preventative
       Task Force   59
       United States Health Statistics   61
       Dermatology   62
          Danger Signals   62
          Normal Findings   63
          Benign Variants   64
          Topical Steroids   65
          Disease Review   66
       Head, Eyes, Ears, Nose, and Throat   79
          Danger Signals   79
          Normal Findings   80
          Benign Variants   81
          Abnormal Findings   81
          Disease Review   83
       Cardiovascular System   92
          Danger Signals   92
          Normal Findings   93

Benign Variants 95

Abnormal Findings 96

Disease Review 98

Pulmonary System 113

Danger Signals 113

Normal Findings 113

Disease Review 114

Endocrine System 125

Danger Signals 125

Normal Findings 126

Disease Review 127

Gastrointestinal System 135

Danger Signals 135

Normal Findings 136

Benign Variants 136

Disease Review 137

Disease Review 142

Renal System 144

Danger Signals 144

Normal Findings 145

Laboratory Testing 145

Disease Review 146

Hematology/Blood Disorders 150

Danger Signals 150

Laboratory Testing 151

Benign Variants 153

Disease Review 153

Nervous System 158

Danger Signals 158

Neurological Testing 159

Benign Variants 162

Disease Review 162

Sexually Transmitted Diseases (STDs) 170

Danger Signals 170

Disease Review 170

Women's Health: Gynecology 179

Danger Signals 179

Normal Findings 180

Menopausal Body Changes 181

Laboratory Procedures 182

Oral Contraceptives 183

Benign Variants   187
Disease Review   187
Women's Health: Pregnancy and Childbirth   192
Danger Signals   192
Laboratory Testing   193
Drugs and Vaccines During Pregnancy   194
Health Education for Pregnancy   197
Signs of Pregnancy   198
Fundal Heights   199
Physiologic Changes During Pregnancy   199
Naegele's Rule   201
Disease Review   201
Pediatrics   205
Danger Signals   205
Pediatric Skin Lesions   207
Screening Tests   208
Normal Findings   210
Immunizations   212
Growth and Development   215
Disease Review   218
Adolescence   224
Danger Signals   224
Normal Findings   225
Laboratory Tests   227
Legal Issues   228
Disease Review   228
Geriatrics   232
Danger Signals   232
Normal Findings   233
Screening for Dementia   236
Disease Review   237
Men's Health   239
Danger Signals   239
Normal Findings   240
Disease Review   241
Musculoskeletal System   246
Danger Signals   246
Normal Findings   247
Exercise and Injuries   247
Orthopedic Maneuvers   248
Disease Review   250

Mental Health   255
   Danger Signals   255
   Disease Review   256
   Psychotropic Drugs   258
Professional Issues   262
   Nursing Practice   262
   Nurse Practitioner Role   263
   Case and Risk Management   264
   Legal Health Issues   264
   Public Health Policy   266
   Theoretical Concepts   266
   Health Care Organizations   267

Chapter 4 Practice Questions 269

Answers to Questions 371

References 391

Index 395

Family Nurse Practitioner Certification

Intensive Review

Certification Exam Information

CREDENTIALING ORGANIZATIONS

American Nurses Credentialing Center (ANCC)

www.nursingworld.org/ancc
Phone: 800-284-2378
The ANCC is the credentialing body of the American Nurses Association (ANA). The credentialing exams currently being offered to nurse practitioners are for the following specialties: adult, family, pediatric, gerontologic, acute care, adult or family psychiatric and mental health, and advanced diabetes management.

American Academy of Nurse Practitioners (AANP)

www.aanp.org
Phone: 512-442-5202
Fax: 512-442-5221
Email: certification@aanp.org
The AANP is a specialty organization that serves only nurse practitioners. It is currently offering three specialty exams: adult, family, and geriatric nurse practitioner.

Thomson Prometric Computer Testing Centers

www.2Test.com
Both the ANCC and the AANP use this company to administer their computer-based certification exams. Their testing centers are located in most major cities in the United States and in some international sites. All of the testing centers are open Monday to Friday. Some are also open on weekends.

For the ANCC, the AANP acceptance letter includes a toll-free number to schedule for their exam. You can register, schedule, reschedule, confirm or cancel your appointment online at the Thomson Prometric Web site. In order to register for the exam, you must have a candidate eligibility number. The number is mailed to you directly from Thomson Prometric within 2 weeks after you have received your authorization-to-test letter from the credentialing agency.

BACKGROUND INFORMATION

American Nurses Credentialing Center

Generally, the ANCC updates their nurse practitioner exams every 2 to 3 years.

The questions in the exam are all referenced from major textbooks, national expert panel guidelines, papers, and official governmental reports and statistics. Do not assume that because these are exams for nurse practitioners, the references used are written mostly by nurse practitioner authors. The opposite is true. Currently, a large number of the clinical references are obtained from medical textbooks.

American Academy of Nurse Practitioners

The reference sources for AANP exams are not publicly known. The content of their exams is based on the results of a role delineation study that was conducted by both the AANP and the Professional Examination Service.

Exam Format

Nurse practitioner certification exams from both the ANCC and the AANP are now all computer-based tests (CBT). The computer will give you the entire 3.5 hours to take the test. It will not shut down automatically like the RN NCLEX exams do after enough points have been earned to pass the exam.

Total Number of Questions

The ANCC exam comprises 175 total questions. Of these, 25 sample questions are not graded because they are being evaluated statistically. Therefore, the actual number of scored questions is 150. Unfortunately, there is no way to tell the questions apart so it is best to assume that all are scored.

The AANP exam comprises 150 total questions. Some of the questions are also sample questions and are not worth any points. As in the ANCC, it is best to assume that all the questions are being graded in the exam because there is no way to tell them apart from each other.

Total Time

The actual testing time that is counted is 3.5 hours. An additional 30 minutes of "free" time is allotted for the computer tutorial; this time period does not count.

When the 30-minute tutorial period expires, the test automatically starts on the computer screen. There are no breaks. Most students generally finish the exam within 2.5 hours.

Certification Exam Questions

Because the AANP certification exam has fewer questions, more time is available to solve the test questions compared with those on the ANCC exam.

In general, each question is allotted about 1 minute. Sometimes, the first few questions seem more difficult. This is a common test design.

Each question is worth one point no matter how long it takes to solve or how difficult it may be.

Fast Facts | The ANCC and AANP Exams

Which board certification is better?

Both certifications are equally recognized as national specialty organizations, and credentials awarded by them are acceptable to governmental entities such as Medicare, local state agencies such as the state boards of nursing (BON), and private corportations. For new graduates, it is a good idea to speak to nurse practitioners and faculty in your area of practice to find out whether one certification is preferred over the other.

What is an official transcript?

A transcript is considered "official" only if it remains inside the sealed envelope in which it was mailed from the college registrar's office. Ask to have the transcripts mailed directly to your residence and not to the certifying organization. If you are planning to take both the ANCC and AANP exams at the same time, then you will need at least three copies of your final transcripts. Open one copy (yours) and check it for accuracy and keep the other two unopened to mail with your applications.

What is the ANCC's "Form E" and how is it used?

The AANP does not use this form. It is only used by the ANCC. Another name for it is the "Nurse Practitioner Educational Preparation" form. It is part of the application packet that can be downloaded from the ANCC Web site at www.nursingworld.org/ancc.

The Form E must be signed by the current director of the program you attended even if you are not a recent graduate.

What is the difference between the testing dates for the AANP and the ANCC?

The ANCC exams can be taken almost anytime of the year (except major holidays), whenever the Thomson Prometric Testing Centers are open. The ANCC has no application deadlines, and their applications can be sent in at anytime of the year.

The AANP exams can only be taken three times a year during a specified time period known as the testing "window." Each window lasts 10 weeks and has an application deadline. Therefore, there are three deadlines per year to watch for when applying for the AANP exam. There are also "late deadlines" for which you are charged an extra fee of $50.00 in addition to the normal testing fees.

The testing windows are generally around the dates listed here. Window #1 is from January to April (deadline is December; late deadline is in January). Window #2 is May to August (deadline is April; late deadline is in May). Window #3 is September to December (deadline is July; late deadline is usually in August). These dates may change. Check the AANP Web site at www.aanp.org for the most current dates.

When can I apply for the certification exams?

According to the ANCC staff to whom I have spoken (by phone), their organization prefers that the test takers apply only when the final transcripts are available. They want the entire application with the official final transcript and the check together in one large envelope. Sending them separately can delay the processing of an application.

For both, you may apply as early as the last semester before you graduate. If you apply before you graduate, include an official copy of your current transcript (even if it is not the final one). When the final transcript is released, mail an official copy as soon as possible to complete your application. Do not forget to photocopy the application forms and the check before mailing them. Your authorization-to-test letter usually arrives within 4 to 6 weeks afterward if there are no problems with your application.

For those who want to take the AANP exam, it is a good idea to apply early, during the last semester before you graduate, because of the testing window deadlines.

For example, if you plan to graduate during the fall semester, you will be graduating in the month of December. Unfortunately, the deadline for the first testing window of the year (January to April) is also in December. Therefore, if you miss the deadline, you will have to wait 5 months (after you graduate) to take the AANP test because the second testing window of the year doesn't start until June.

It is easy to miss this deadline (and the late deadline) if you decide to wait for your final transcripts before applying.

Your early application will be acceptable as long as you include an official copy of your most current transcript and have paid the testing fee. When the final transcripts are released, send an official copy as soon as possible to complete your application. Call the AANP to follow up and check that they did receive the final transcript.

Are there special instructions for AANP applicants?

Be warned that the AANP applications must be filled out very carefully. Do not leave any of their questions unanswered or leave any blanks on their forms. Avoid answering the questions with notes such as *"refer to enclosed transcript"* or *"not applicable."*

Doing any of these things will cause your application to be rejected. It will delay the processing. Keep in mind that you must provide the course numbers, credit hours, and dates on the application forms.

After receiving an acceptance letter, how much time do I have before it expires?

For the ANCC, you have up to 90 days from the date stamped in the acceptance letter to take your exam.

In contrast, the AANP's acceptance letter is valid only for the testing window for which you applied. If you miss taking your exam within the dates assigned for that window, then your acceptance letter will no longer be valid. A memo must be faxed to the AANP certification department with a request to sit for another testing window. For more information and instructions, call their office at 512-442-4262.

When can I schedule for the exam?

You may schedule yourself for the exam only after you have been assigned a Thomson Prometric eligibility ID number. To schedule an appointment, go to the Thomson Prometric Web site at www.2Test.com.

If you cancel an appointment online, you must give them at least 48 hours notice. If you have less than 48 hours, call the local testing center to cancel your appointment. When you reschedule, a rescheduling fee will be charged.

What should I do if the morning time slot I want is no longer available?

Morning time slots tend to be filled quickly. If you are unable to find a morning slot, some testing centers have a waiting list. This option is not available online; you must call the local center to find out if a waiting list is available. Another idea is to look for an alternate testing center that still has the times or dates that you want.

Apply as early as you can after receiving the acceptance letter. You can always change the date and/or time later. Some testing centers are very busy and get booked very fast. I had a student from one of my review courses who had to take her exam on the last day before her letter expired because the testing center she wanted was so full.

In addition, avoid scheduling yourself at the time of the day when you tend to feel the most tired or sleepy. For most, this is usually after lunchtime. Simply picking the "wrong" time of the day to take your exam may cause you to make careless errors. It can take as few as one to two points to fail the exam.

When do I receive my test scores?

Scores from the ANCC exam are usually mailed within 7 days of completing the exam.

Test takers of the AANP exam find out immediately whether they have passed or failed. The unofficial score is shown on the computer screen only after you have finished and shut down the exam. You will not get a paper printout of your scores from the testing center. The official letter with your scores are mailed within 1 to 2 weeks after the exam.

What are the passing rates for each exam?

Historically, the passing rates for the certification exams have ranged between the 70th and the 80th percentile.

What are the passing scores?

The ANCC passing score is 350 points or higher with a range of 100 to 500 points.

The AANP passing score is 500 points or higher with a range of 100 to 800 points.

How are the official scores listed?

The scores for each domain (ANCC term) or category (AANP term) are listed individually in addition to the total scores. The lower scores indicate your weakest areas; devote more study time to these areas if you do not pass on your first attempt. If you have not yet taken a review course, I recommend that you find one or buy their tapes. My review courses are listed at my Web site *www.npreview. com.*

How does the board of nursing (BON) from my state receive my scores?

There are two ways for the BON to get your scores. One way is for the ANCC or the AANP to mail your scores directly to them. You must sign the special form in the application packet giving them permission to mail out your scores. Another method is for you to mail a copy of the official letter with your scores to your state's BON.

What happens if I fail to pass my certification exam?

A permission-to-retest application form is mailed to you along with a retest fee charge.

The ANCC exam may be retaken as early as 90 days after the date of the last exam you took as long as you have reapplied and paid the retest fee.

Test takers of the AANP exam are required to take 15 contact hours of continuing education credits that address their "area of weakness." For example, someone whose scores are low under the "diagnosis" category must choose courses that address this area or the continuing education credits may be rejected.

Mail or fax your certificates of completion as proof. After your continuing education credits have been approved, an application-to-retest form will be mailed to you.

What if I fail the AANP or ANCC exam the second time?
You must resubmit a full application (like the first time) along with all the required documentation and pay the full test fee.

What is the professional designation used by each organization?
The ANCC now uses the initials "FNP-BC" (Family Nurse Practitioner-Board Certified). No periods or spaces are necessary when writing these initials.

The AANP uses the designation of "NP-C" (Nurse Practitioner-Certified). Do not use a comma before the "C" (certified). Use only a hyphen.

How long is my certification valid?
Board certification from both the ANCC and AANP is valid for 5 years.

What do I need to do to for recertification?
According to the ANCC, recertification for adult nurse practitioners (ANPs) and family nurse practitioners (FNPs) requires 1,000 hours of clinical practice (over a 5-year period). In addition professional development credits are required. These categories are continuing education credits, graduate courses, lectures, presentations, publications, research, and preceptorships.

The AANP requires a mandatory minimum of 1,000 hours of clinical practice as a nurse practitioner (in your area of specialty) along with 75 contact hours of continuing education credits in order to recertify.

Another method of recertification for both ANCC and AANP is to retake (and pass) the board certification exam.

Is there any reciprocity between the ANCC and AANP?
Yes, both the AANP and ANCC have a reciprocity program. Family, adult, and geriatric nurse practitioners who are certified by other approved national certification bodies that meet their criteria are eligible to apply. To request information and applications, contact the AANP by the following methods:

1) Email: certification@aanp.org
2) Fax: 512-442-5221
3) Phone: 512-442-5202

Contact the ANCC by calling their Customer Care Center at 1-800-284-2378.

Statistical Information

ANCC Scoring Classification
This is the breakdown of the domains used in the ANCC exam. These numbers have gradually changed over time, but what has remained consistent in their exam is that a large percentage of the questions are on the clinical management and the assessment/diagnosis of illness.

Table 1.1 | ANCC Domains of Practice

Domain of Practice	Percent
I. Clinical management	34
II. Professional role and policy	6
III. Nurse practitioner and patient relationship	11
IV. Assessment of acute and chronic illness	26
V. Research	2
VI. Health promotion and disease prevention	21
Total	100

*Adapted from the ANCC Adult Nurse Practitioner Board Certification Exam Content Outline; October 9, 2006. http://www.nursingworld.org/ancc/cert/

Summary

These are the top three domains in the ANCC certification exam:

■ Clinical management (34%)
■ Assessment of acute and chronic illness (26%)
■ Health promotion and disease prevention (21%)

Test takers who score low in any two of the domains previously listed usually fail the exam because these account for the majority of questions (81% or 121) on the exam.

The percentage of nonclinical questions has recently been increased from 10% to 19%. The nonclinical domains (29 questions) are:

■ Nurse practitioner and patient relationship (11%)
■ Professional role and policy (6%)
■ Research (2%)

AANP Scoring Classification

The AANP does not currently release any of their statistics. The percentage makeup of their exam questions for each of the categories listed in the following is not public knowledge:

■ Health promotion
■ Disease prevention
■ Diagnosis
■ Management of acute disease
■ Management of chronic disease

Summary

A larger number of questions on this exam are clinically based. This conclusion is based on personal experience and on feedback from former review course students.

TIPS FOR THE ANCC AND AANP EXAMS

- The most current treatment guidelines and protocols that have been released within the past 1 to 2 years before you sit for the exam will not be included. It takes at least 2 years for these changes to appear as questions on the exams.
- The nurse practitioner certification tests are national exams concentrating mainly on primary care disorders. These are not tests on specialty disorders. Keep this in mind when you are reading the answer options. In general, avoid picking exotic diseases as answers.
- The AANP exams list the normal lab results of the pertinent lab in a test question. The ANCC does not do this. A list of suggested lab values to memorize is in chapter 2.
- No asymptomatic or borderline cases of disease states are presented in the test. For example, in real life, most patients with iron-deficiency anemia are asymptomatic and do not have either pica or spoon-shaped nails. In the exam, they will have both.
- Disease states are given in their classic textbook presentation. For example, if a case of acute mononucleosis is being presented, the patient will most likely be a teenager with the classic triad of sore throat, fatigue, and enlarged cervical nodes.
- Learn the disorders for which examination maneuvers are used. For example, Tinel's and/or Phalen's is used to assess for carpal tunnel syndrome.
- Learn what a positive result means for a physical exam maneuver. For example, a positive anterior or posterior drawer test means that a knee is unstable. A positive finding of either the Ortolani or Barlow maneuver signifies an abnormal hip due to congenital hip dysplasia or a hypoplastic hip.
- Be knowledgeable about normal results of a physical exam. There will be very few questions on benign variants. Some examples are torus palatinus and fishtail uvula (listed under the HEENT system review).
- Learn what a lab result means and what it is used for. It is very rare to get a question asking for an actual numeric value. Instead a question may ask about the clinical significance of an abnormal test result.
- Medications are listed in both generic and brand name forms. Most of the drugs mentioned in the exam are the older, well-recognized drugs and may include Macrolide: erythromycin or clarithromycin (Biaxin); Cephalosporins: first generation (Keflex), second generation (Ceftin/Cefzil), third generation (Rocephin); Quinolones: Cipro, Floxin, and the newer quinolones: levaquinolone (Levaquin); Sulfa: Bactrim, Pediazole; Tetracyclines: tetracycline, doxycycline; Nonsteroidal anti-inflammatories (NSAIDs): ibuprofen, naproxen

(Anaprox); and cough suppressants: dextromorphan (Robitussin). Other examples are in the chapter 3 systems review section.

■ Some answer options for drugs list only the drug class instead of the generic and brand names.

■ When memorizing drugs, learn the drug class, generic or brand name, the action, major drug interactions, major contraindications and other safety issues, and the common side effects. There is no need to memorize drug doses. For example, a common side effect of ACE inhibitors is a dry cough (up to 10%).

■ The ANCC exam is more likely to have answer options written as declarative statements in questions in which a case scenario addressing mental health is used. You should keep these communication tips in mind: ask open-ended questions, avoid judgmental statements, do not reassure, do not give abrupt responses, respect the patient's culture, and do not confront a patient.

■ One or two questions on bioterrorism topics have appeared in the AANP exam. Remember that the best method for spreading a virus or bacterium is to make it airborne or nebulize it. Also, ciprofloxacin (Cipro) is used to treat anthrax.

■ Questions about nursing theory have not been seen on any exams from either the ANCC or AANP for several years.

■ Other health theorists (not nurses) and theories that have been included on the exams in the past are (not inclusive): Erickson, Freud, Piaget, Elizabeth Kübler-Ross's theory on bereavement, health belief model, self-efficacy model, System's theory, etc.

■ The ANCC has increased the number of questions on nonclinical issues (19%) in the past 2 years. These include health policy, nurse practice act, nurse practitioner role, living wills, durable power of attorney, advanced directives, privacy laws, documentation, quality assurance, risk management, etc.

■ Keep in mind that the majority of questions in the AANP and 81% of the questions (2005 stats) on the ANCC exams are clinically based.

■ Follow national treatment guidelines for certain disorders. The following is a list of treatment guidelines used as references by the ANCC (AANP does not publish a list):

Hypertension
Joint National Committee on Prevention, Detection, and Treatment of High Blood Pressure (JNC) 7th Report

Community-Acquired Pneumonia (CAP)
American Thoracic Society or the ATS Treatment Guidelines

Hyperlipidemia
National Cholesterol Education Panel (2002). Third Report of the Expert Panel on Detection, Evaluation, and Treatment of High Cholesterol in Adults

Asthma
Guidelines for the Diagnosis and Management of Asthma. Expert Panel Report. National Asthma Education and Prevention Program (2003)

Sexually Transmitted Diseases (or sexually transmitted infections)
Sexually Transmitted Disease Treatment Guidelines (2002). Centers for Disease Control and Prevention

Bacterial Endocarditis
Prevention of Bacterial Endocarditis (1997). American Heart Association

Health Prevention
The Guide to Clinical Preventative Services (2002). US Preventative Task Force

TIPS FOR MAXIMIZING YOUR SCORES

- You can save yourself more time by learning the computer commands before taking the exam. Go to the ANCC web site: www.nursingworld/ancc/. Click the *Computer Tutorial* link and practice.
- Before the test plan ahead of time at home what you want to write on the scratch paper.
- If you are taking the computer tutorial for the first time in the center, it usually takes about 10 to 15 minutes to learn the system.
- Use the remaining "free" time to write your notes on the scratch paper provided by the test proctor. Do not waste actual testing time to start writing your notes.
- There is no penalty for guessing. If you run out of time, quickly fill out the remaining questions at random.
- Never leave any question unanswered. It only takes one point to fail the test.
- Do not read questions too rapidly. You will go into "autopilot" mode. Frequently remind yourself to "read slowly and read carefully."
- The first few questions are usually "harder" to solve. This is a common test design. Do not let it shake your confidence.
- Remember, no matter how hard a question is to solve, it is still worth only one point.
- If you are having problems understanding the answer options, read them again from the bottom up (from option D to A).
- Save yourself time (and mental strain) with the longer questions by *first* reading the last sentence (or stem). Then read the question again from the beginning. The advantage of this "backward reading" technique is that you know ahead of time what the question is asking. When you read it again "normally," it becomes easier to recognize important clues that will help you answer the question faster.
- One method of guessing is to look for a pattern. Pick the one answer that does not fit the pattern.
- Another method is to pick the answer that most "attracts" you. Go with your gut feeling and do not change the answer unless you are sure it is the correct one.
- In general, it is not a good idea to change too many answers on any exam.

- Wear an analog watch so that you can check to see if you are spending too much time answering questions.
- Each question is allotted approximately 60 seconds to solve. Most test takers finish the exam within 2.5 hours.
- If you need more than 1.5 minutes to answer a question, you are wasting time.
- On questions that you are spending too much time on, guess or pick an answer at random and "mark" it.
- "Marking" a question allows you to return to it later and change an answer.
- Return to all your "marked" questions only after you have answered all questions on the exam.
- If you have failed the test before, try not to memorize what you did on the previous one you took. The answers you remember may be wrong.
- Regarding the above advice, "pretend" that you have never seen the test before so that you can begin fresh mentally when you retake the test.
- Small pieces of hard candy are allowed inside the testing area – they have to be unwrapped before they can be taken in. Wear clothes with pockets to store the candy. If you are mentally exhausted, eat some of the unwrapped hard candy you brought with you.
- If you still feel fatigued and have enough time left, consider a quick bathroom break. Drink and splash cold water on your face. Jump in place or do jumping jacks to wake up.
- The clock in the computer keeps counting down and does not stop for breaks.

MORE EXAM TIPS: REVIEW TIMELINE

- The amount of time you need to study depends on how well you are prepared.
- Look over the table of contents of your primary care textbook and plan the time you want to allocate to each organ system.
- Start reviewing your weakest areas first and assign more time to them. Save the areas you know well for the last.
- Try to study daily even if you can only afford 10 to 15 minutes. You can break up your study sessions over the day. You will retain information better this way than by doing one large cram session per week.
- Take some notes or photocopy material that you want to learn and place it in your purse or wallet. If you are in a line or waiting, read and study them.
- Use all the senses you can when studying. Be familiar with how you learn best.
- Read not only visually, but also read out loud to yourself. You will be using both your visual and auditory senses and will retain information better.
- Pick an area to study where you will not be disturbed. For some with small children, this may mean studying outside the home in places such as libraries, bookstores, or even in a car!

■ If you learn better in a group, organize one. Decide ahead of time what to cover so that you do not waste time.

TIPS ON OTHER TEST-TAKING ISSUES

Emotional Readiness

Studies show that high levels of "stress hormones" such as adrenaline interfere with memory and actually kill neurons. Your internal beliefs about the exam are very important and should not be minimized. Try the following exercises if you feel too anxious or fearful about passing the exam. This is especially true for test takers who have failed the exam before.

Make yourself a tape or write down positive affirmations on sticky notes. Post them on your bathroom mirror, the refrigerator, the car dashboard, and other places where you can see them often. Some examples:

■ I know *deep inside me* that I will pass this test. I always do well on multiple-choice tests. I have passed many other tests before. I will also pass the certification exam.

Read it at least 10 times a day. Even if you don't feel it, your subconscious will start believing it. The week before the test, do this exercise as often as you can.

Your Panic Button

If you find yourself starting to panic, try the following calming technique:

■ Close your eyes. Tell yourself to "stop." Keep repeating the word until you calm down. At this time, concentrate on your breathing as much as you can.
■ Take three deep breaths through your nose and exhale slowly through pursed lips.
■ Tell yourself "I feel more confident" (inhalation) "and relaxed" when exhaling.

Testing Center Details

To help ease your anxiety, know in advance the details involved with the testing center.

■ Call the testing center 2 days before to verify your appointment.
■ Locate the testing center before taking the exam so that you do not get lost.
■ Arrive early, at least 20 minutes before your scheduled time.
■ Know the required documents: the authorization-to-test letter and two types of "positive" ID. You will not be allowed to take the test if your ID is not accepted.
■ You are assigned a small locker to store your bag, backpack, or jacket inside.

▓ Each test-taker is assigned one small cubicle with one computer.
▓ You can request earplugs; consider this option if you are sensitive to noise.
▓ Do not forget your computer reading glasses.
▓ The test-taking area is monitored closely by videotape and microphones.

Identification Issues

One ID should be from an official governmental body (driver's license or passport). Both IDs should have your picture and signature. Expired IDs are not acceptable.

The Night Before the Exam

The following are suggested activities the night before you take the exam:

▓ Avoid eating a heavy meal or drinking alcohol.
▓ Get enough sleep. Aim for 7 to 8 hours. Lack of sleep affects memory.
▓ Set two alarms to wake you up the next morning if you are taking your exam early.

The Day of the Exam

The following activities are suggested the day of the exam:

▓ Avoid eating a heavy or fatty breakfast (causes heartburn).
▓ The best meals are a combination of protein (i.e., cheese, eggs, peanut butter, and nuts) with a complex or high-fiber carbohydrate (i.e., whole wheat bread, oatmeal).
▓ Do not forget to bring some unwrapped hard candy inside your clothes pocket.
▓ Wear comfortable shoes and clothes and dress in layers.
▓ Consider limiting the amount of fluid you drink 1 to 2 hours before the test.

Notice: The aforementioned are only suggestions. Use your judgment and choose what works for you. The food suggestions are not meant to be taken as medical advice. If doing any of these things is contraindicated for you, please do not do them. Consult your health provider for food advice if you have dietary and/or health restrictions.

Question Dissection & Analysis

2

EMERGENT CASES

Discussion

The ability to recognize emergent conditions that may present in the primary care area is an important skill that will definitely be tested on the exam. Questions will also address the clinical decision-making skills necessary to manage them correctly in the primary care setting such as a physician's office.

Depending on the emergent condition, answer options can range from giving a patient an injection of epinephrine (i.e., anaphylaxis, status asthmaticus) to referring the patient to the local emergency room or to calling 911.

Memorize not only the presenting signs and symptoms of the emergent condition, but also how it is initially managed in primary care. Learn how these conditions present so that you can recognize them in the exam. The following is an alphabetical list of emergent conditions. They are discussed in detail in the "Danger Signals" section under the appropriate organ system.

- acute appendicitis/acute abdomen (GI)
- anaphylaxis (pulmonary)
- asthmatic exacerbation or status asthmaticus (pulmonary)
- cauda equina syndrome (neurology)
- epiglottitis (pediatrics)
- meningococcemia (dermatology)
- placenta abruptio (obstetrics)
- pulmonary emboli (pulmonary)
- Rocky Mountain spotted fever (dermatology)

- ruptured tubal ectopic pregnancy (obstetrics)
- testicular torsion (pediatrics)

Example

During an episodic visit, a middle-aged man with asthma complains of the sudden onset of itching and coughing after taking two aspirin tablets for a headache in the waiting room. The patient's lips are starting to swell. Which of the following is the best initial intervention to follow?

a) Initiate a prescription of a potent topical steroid and Medrol Dose Pack.
b) Ask the patient if he wants to lie down on an examining table until he feels much better before being examined by the NP.
c) Immediately give an intramuscular injection of epinephrine 1:10,000.
d) Immediately administer intramuscular injections of prednisone and cimetidine (Tagamet).

The correct answer is option c: Immediately give a subcutaneous injection of epinephrine 1:10,000.

Question Dissection

Best Clues
- The patient's signs and symptoms are classic for anaphylaxis (diagnostic skill).
- The acute onset of the signs and symptoms.

Notes
Severe anaphylactic episodes occur almost immediately or within 1 hour after exposure (acute timing). Look carefully at the "time factor" involved in this question. A quick onset of symptoms or sudden change in symptoms signals a possible emergent condition. In the outpatient setting, anaphylaxis should be managed as follows:

- If only one clinician is present, give an injection of epinephrine 1:1000 stat (immediately) and then call 911.
- If two clinicians are present, one gives the epinephrine and the other clinician calls 911.

In the emergency room (ER) setting, anaphylaxis is treated as follows:

- 100% oxygen by nasal cannula, epinephrine, diphenhydramine (Benadryl), a B2 agonist such as cimetidine (Tagamet), a short-acting B2 agonist such as albuterol (Ventolin), and a systemic steroid such as prednisone.

OTHER EMERGENT CONDITIONS

Discussion

During life-threatening situations, managing the airway, breathing, and circulation (the ABCs) is always the top priority. If the question does not describe conditions requiring the ABCs, but you are asked to pick the top priority or most emergent situation, the next level of priorities to consider is listed in the following. The mnemonic device is "MS. SPAIN."

- Acute *Mental Status* changes or "MS"
- Acute onset of *Severe Pain* or "SP"
- *Acute Infection Now* or "AIN"

Example

A 3-month-old infant who has a high fever is being evaluated by the nurse practitioner. The mother of the infant wants to know what signs to watch for that indicate a serious condition. Which of the following is considered a serious sign to watch for in this infant?

a) The posterior fontanel is closed.
b) The infant voids more than 6 times in a 24-hour period.
c) The infant is sleeping more and is not easily aroused.
d) Lack of skin tenting.

The correct answer is option c: The infant is sleeping and is not easily aroused.

Question Dissection

Best Clues
- The phrase in option c "is not easily aroused" is very important.

Notes
Any recent changes in level of consciousness such as lethargy or excessive sleepiness in an infant or small child should ring a bell in your head.

- Notice the word "more" in Option b. If read carelessly, you may automatically assume that it is the emergent condition because the cutoff limit for dehydration in infants is "6 or *less* wet diapers in a 24-hour period."
- Read answer options slowly and carefully. This helps avoid "automatic" reading.
- The mnemonic "MS. SPAIN" is a good reminder that acute changes in the level of consciousness (LOC) is considered emergent not only in infants, but also in adults.

- A closed posterior fontanel is normal in a 3-month-old. Some infants are born with their posterior fontanels already closed.
- Skin tenting is a sign of decreased skin turgor (i.e., severe dehydration).

COMPLEX SENTENCES

Discussion

Another problematic area for most test takers are answer options written as complex sentences. Complex sentences have two "halves" and both parts are joined together by words such as "and" and "but." Both halves of the sentence must be in agreement for the sentence to make sense. Otherwise, the sentence is incorrect and can easily be ruled out as the answer.

When a complex sentence is written in the negative as is seen in the following example ("The toddler *has not* lost weight ..."), it becomes even harder to comprehend and must be read carefully several times to make sense. Keep in mind that even if both halves of a sentence are in agreement and true, it does not mean that it is the correct answer, as illustrated by the following example.

Example

A 2-year-old toddler in whom acute bronchiolitis has recently been diagnosed is brought in by his father for a follow-up exam. The toddler's blood pressure (BP) is 90/60, his pulse is 100 beats per minute (BPM), and his respiratory rate is 20. Which of the following statements is indicative of an emergent condition?

First Part of Sentence	Second Part of Sentence
a) The toddler is crying more frequently	*but* is not lethargic.
b) The toddler is more lethargic	*and* has been sleeping most of the day.
c) The toddler is not eating solids	*but* is drinking fluids.
d) The toddler has not lost weight	*and* is starting to eat solids.

The correct answer is option b: The toddler is more lethargic and has been sleeping most of the day.

Question Dissection

Best Clues
- The toddler has become "more lethargic," indicating an acute change in LOC.

Notes
The content of the sentences should be viewed as follows:

a) crying more frequently (negative); not lethargic (positive)
b) *more lethargic (negative); has been sleeping most of the day (negative)*
c) not eating solids (negative); drinking fluids (positive)
d) not lost weight (positive); drinking fluids (positive)

In option d, even though both portions of the sentence may be in agreement, it is still incorrect because it does not indicate an emergent condition.

Options a and c both have both positive and negative portions within one statement and are therefore not an emergent condition.

Notes on toddler behavior:

- Toddlers are normally very active and curious. They like to mimic behaviors.
- Toddlers understand simple one-step commands and can speak in two-word sentences that are understood by family (but not by strangers).
- Toddlers are "picky" eaters and like to have their foods separated and not mixed together.
- The rapid growth spurt seen during infancy has slowed down by toddlerhood.

CHOOSING THE BEST INITIAL INTERVENTION

Discussion

Failure to recognize the importance of taking a history during a new patient encounter is a common mistake that is easily avoided. Obtaining the history (or subjective information) can be as simple as asking patients about their current medications or about their signs and symptoms.

Students who "skip" steps during the patient encounter may find it helpful to use the SOAPE mnemonic (Subjective, Objective, Assessment, Planning, and Evaluation) to help guide them with the correct order of actions to follow during a patient encounter. Other questions about initial interventions may ask about laboratory tests (pick screening or low-tech tests), best initial intervention (think of SOAPE), or the most appropriate initial statement (open-ended statements).

The following are examples of using the SOAPE process as a guide.

Subjective: Look for subjective evidence by taking a verbal history of the illness.
- Interview the patient and/or family.
- Ask about the patient's current medications, signs and symptoms, duration of illness, medical history, diet, lifestyle, and so forth.

Objective: Look for objective evidence of the patient's condition.
- Perform a physical exam (general or targeted such as a cardiac exam).
- Order lab tests or perform other exams/procedures.
- If given an option, choose a "manual method" of testing a patient such as checking the pulse before a laboratory test such as blood work or procedures.

*A*ssessment: Make a diagnosis or assessment.
- What is the most likely diagnosis based on the presenting signs and/or symptoms?
- Is the condition emergent or not (if applicable)?

*P*lanning: Initiate a treatment plan.
- Prescribe an appropriate medication regime.
- Educate the patient about the condition.
- Make lifestyle recommendations about areas such as diet and exercise.

*E*valuation: Evaluate the patient's response to the treatment/intervention or evaluate the situation.
- If the patient has a poor or no response to treatment or if worse, make a referral to a specialist.
- If the condition is emergent, refer the patient to the ER.

Example

A 30-year-old woman with a history of mild intermittent asthma complains of a new onset of cough that has been waking her up very early in the morning for the past 2 weeks. She reports a viral upper respiratory infection 1 week before the onset of her current symptoms. Her last office visit was 8 months ago. Which of the following is the best initial course of action?

a) Initiate a prescription for a short-acting B2 agonist.
b) Refer the patient for a scratch test.
c) Interview the patient and find out more about her symptoms.
d) Perform a thorough physical examination concentrating on the lungs.

The correct answer is option c: Interview the patient and find out more about her symptoms.

Question Dissection

Best Clues
- The patient has a history of asthma.
- The symptoms started 1 week after a viral URI.

Notes
All four answer options are correct interventions in this case. But, which one should be done first?

The correct order of actions in this case scenario is the following:

- Interview the patient to find out more about her illness.
- Perform a thorough physical examination.

- Prescribe a short-acting B2 agonist.
- Refer the patient to an allergist for a scratch test (if necessary).

The case scenario is that of an acute asthmatic exacerbation. If it is not treated appropriately, it can worsen and may progress into status asthmaticus, a life-threatening condition.

Regarding an early morning cough, some of the common differential diagnoses also include postnasal drip, sinusitis, allergic rhinitis, and GERD (gastroesophageal reflux disease).

QUESTIONS ASKING FOR A DIAGNOSIS

Discussion

There are numerous questions on the exam in which the test taker is asked to make a diagnosis. According to recent American Nurses Credentialing Center (ANCC) data, this area accounts for 26% of the total questions in their family nurse practitioner (FNP) exam (data from the American Academy of Nurse Practitioners [AANP] is unknown at present).

The stem of the questions may ask for the diagnosis based on the description of the disease's classic signs and/or symptoms or may ask about the best intervention or test (based on the signs and/or symptoms) presented.

Test takers who are weak in diagnostic skills are more likely to fail the certification exam. Some of the questions will ask for the sign and/or symptoms of a given disease, as shown in the following example.

Example

Which of the following is most likely to be found in patients with a long-standing, severe iron deficiency anemia?

a) pica
b) fatigue
c) pallor
d) irritability

The correct answer is option a: pica.

Question Dissection

Best Clue
- The description of the iron deficiency anemia indicates that it is "severe."
- Knowledge that fatigue, pallor, and irritability are also seen in many other conditions.

Notes

- ▨ Fatigue is found in many disease states (i.e., autoimmune disorders, chronic fatigue, cancer chemotherapy, etc.) but also with poor lifestyle choices (i.e., chronic lack of sleep) and is a side effect of certain drugs (i.e., beta blockers).
- ▨ Irritability is a state of mood and is not a specific finding.
- ▨ Pallor is also found in other conditions such hypoxia, anemia, and chronic illness.

Pica is also found in pregnancy, but compared with the other options, it is the best choice.

CLASSIC FINDINGS

Discussion

The classic textbook presentation of disease is always the rule in the exams. This is true not only in the nurse practitioner exams, but in exams from other health professions as well. The reason this is done is to provide consistency and statistical validity for the exams.

It is rare for a disease process to be presented at its early preclinical stages. The majority of the cases on the exams are presented with the classic signs and symptoms of the disease as written in the textbooks.

One does not need clinical experience to sit for the exam; most of the test takers are new graduates. For experienced nurse practitioners, clinical experience may actually interfere with doing well on the test. What is done in "real life" and what the textbooks and national guidelines recommend do not always go together. Therefore, experienced NPs taking the test should keep in mind that the test is based on classic textbook cases, and national guidelines must be strictly followed. Currently, almost all the states mandate board certification as a requirement for initial licensure and clinical practice.

Example

An 8-year-old boy is complaining of pruritic rashes that have been disturbing his sleep at night for the past few weeks. On physical examination, the FNP notices several excoriated rashes on the child's axilla and penis. The rashes are also present on the interdigital webs of both hands. Which of the following conditions is most likely?

a) scarlatina
b) impetigo
c) erythema migrans
d) scabies

The correct answer is option d: scabies.

Question Dissection

Best Clue
■ Pruritic rashes located in the interdigital webs of the fingers and on the penis indicate scabies until proven otherwise (classic presentation).

Notes
■ The rash of scarlatina has a sandpaper-like texture and is accompanied by a strawberry tongue and skin desquamation (peeling) of the palms and soles. It is not pruritic.

■ Impetigo rashes are pruritic and appear as papules, bullae, and superficial bright weeping rashes with honey-colored exudate crusts. The rashes are located on areas that are easily traumatized such as the face, arms, or legs.

■ Chicken pox lesions are also pruritic but the location is all over the body. They may also become secondarily infected, resulting in impetigo.

■ Larva migrans rashes are very pruritic, but are located as a lone rash on areas of the body exposed to contaminated soil or sand such as the sole of the foot and the buttocks. The rash is caused by hookworm larvae that have burrowed under the skin; the larvae come from dog or cat feces infested with hookworms.

■ Larva migrans rashes are shaped like raised wavy snakelike lines (or serpiginous).

CHOOSING THE CORRECT DRUG

Discussion

Test takers are expected to know not only the drug's generic and/or brand name, but also its drug class. If you are familiar only with the drug's brand or generic name you can recognize the drug on the test because both names are listed together. Some questions pertaining to drugs only list drug classes instead of generic and brand names. The drug's action, its indication(s), common side effects, serious drug interactions, contraindications, and serious side effects are also addressed on the test. Good examples of serious side effects are found with the statins and isoniazid, both of which can be hepatotoxic.

Example

Which of the following drugs is indicated as first line treatment for community-acquired atypical pneumonia in patients younger than 60 years of age with no comorbid condition?

a) macrolides
b) penicillins
c) fluoroquinolones (quinolones)
d) sulfas

The correct answer is option a: macrolides.

Question Dissection

Best Clues
- The patient has community-acquired atypical pneumonia (diagnosis).
- The patient is younger than 60 years of age (demographics).
- The patient has no comorbid condition (lack of risk factors).

Notes
- Be familiar with the guidelines for community-acquired pneumonia from the American Thoracic Society (ATS).
- ATS Guidelines recommend macrolides for persons 65 years or less who have no comorbitiy. For those older than 65 years or who have a comorbid condition (i.e., heart disease, COPD, diabetes), β-lactum and a macrolide or the new quinolones with gram positive activity (i.e., levaquinolone) are preferred.
- The guidelines used for the exams are listed in chapter 1 and are detailed in the pertinent organ system section.

Example

A 17-year-old college student complains of pain and fullness of her left ear, which is getting steadily worse. She has a history of allergic rhinitis and is allergic to dust mites. On physical exam, the left tympanic membrane is red with cloudy fluid inside. The landmarks are displaced in the same ear. The student denies frequent ear infections and the last antibiotic she took was 1 year ago for a urinary tract infection. She is allergic to sulfa and tells the NP that she will not take any erythromycin because it makes her very nauseous. Which of the following is the best choice of treatment for this patient?

a) Prescribe a course of amoxicillin/clavulanic acid (Augmentin) in 875-mg tablets, one to be taken PO (by mouth) twice a day (BID) for 14 days.
b) Prescribe pseudoephedrine (Sudafed) in 20-mg tablets, one to be taken PO as needed every 4 to 6 hours.
c) Prescribe amoxicillin in 500-mg tablets, one to be taken PO three times a day (TID) for 14 days.
d) Prescribe Biaxin (clarithromycin) in 500-mg tablets, one to be taken PO BID for 10 days.

The correct answer is option c: Prescribe amoxicillin in 500-mg tablets, one to be taken PO TID for 14 days.

Question Dissection

Best Clues
- A red tympanic membrane with cloudy fluid inside and displaced landmarks are classic signs of acute otitis media (AOM).
- Because the patient's last antibiotic taken was 1 year ago and she has infrequent ear infections, there are no apparent risk factors for beta-lactam–resistant bacteria.
- You can rule out clarithromycin Biaxin; the patient has said she will not take erythromycin because it makes her nauseous.

Notes
This question is more complicated compared with the first example. Although the question is regarding the correct drug treatment, it is also listing the signs and symptoms of the illness. To answer this question correctly, you must first have arrived at the correct diagnosis, which is AOM.

- Amoxicillin is the preferred first line antibiotic for both AOM and acute sinusitis in areas with low beta-lactam resistance.
- The ideal patient is someone who has not taken any antibiotics in the previous 3 months and/or does not live in an area with high rates of beta-lactam–resistant bacteria.
- If the patient is younger than 2 years of age, attends nursery school, is a treatment failure, or has taken an antibiotic in the previous 3 months, then a second line antibiotic such as Augmentin, Ceftin, or Rocephin injection (up to three separate injections) is indicated.
- Biaxin is a good choice for penicillin-allergic patients, but this patient's adverse reaction of severe nausea to erythromycin rules it out.
- Pseudoephedrine (Sudafed) is useful for symptoms only. Also, avoid decongestants in patients with hypertension.

LABORATORY RESULTS AND DIAGNOSTIC TESTS

Discussion

The ANCC exam does not list all of the normal results of laboratory tests. Laboratory tests such as the hemoglobin, hematocrit, MCV (mean corpuscular volume), platelets, percentage of neutrophils in the white blood cell (WBC) differential, serum creatinine and the international normalized ratio (INR) are some of the tests that are most commonly encountered. It's essential to learn the meaning of an abnormal result and its clinical significance. In contrast to the ANCC, the AANP exam does list the normal results of pertinent laboratory tests. For both exams, learn what the necessary tests are to further evaluate abnormal laboratory test results. For example, an MCV of 110 means that the patient has macrocytic RBCs and needs to be evaluated for both B12 and folate deficiency anemia. Some of the follow-up laboratory tests are the B12 and folate levels and/or the Shilling test. In addition, don't be surprised if extraneous laboratory test results are included in some questions.

Example

An elderly man of Mediterranean descent undergoes a routine complete blood count (CBC) for an annual physical. The following are his lab test results: hemoglobin 11.0 g/dL, hematocrit 38%, and mean corpuscular volume (MCV) 72 fL. His prostate specific antigen (PSA) result is 3.1 ng/mL. The urinalysis (UA) shows few epithelial cells. Which of the following laboratory tests are indicated next?

a) serum B12 and folate levels and a peripheral smear
b) a CBC with white cell differential and a urinalysis
c) a peripheral smear and urine for culture and sensitivity
d) serum iron, serum ferritin, and total iron binding capacity (TIBC)

The correct answer is option d: serum iron, serum ferritin, and TIBC.

Question Dissection

Best Clues
- Low hemoglobin and hematocrit levels indicate anemia.
- An MCV of 72 fL is indicative of microcytic anemia.
- The demographics (i.e., ethnic background).
- Ignore the urinalysis and PSA tests because they are not necessary to solve the problem.

Notes
To answer this question correctly, you must go through "four stages" of thinking through the question. The first stage is that you must be familiar with the normal results of the hemoglobin, hematocrit, and the MCV. The second stage is knowledge of what the abnormal results mean. The third stage is knowledge of the correct follow-up laboratory test. The fourth and final stage is the knowledge of the differential diagnosis of microcytic anemia (iron deficiency or thalassemia minor/trait).

- The MCV is indicative of microcytic anemia but does not indicate the type of anemia.
- The differential diagnosis for microcytic anemia is either iron deficiency or thalassemia trait. In high risk young children such as toddlers living in older homes, lead poisoning can manifest as a microcytic, hypochromic anemia.
- In iron deficiency anemia, the following results are found: low serum ferritin, low serum iron, and elevated TIBC levels.

| Table 2.1 | Laboratory Tests |

Laboratory Test	Reference Ranges
Hemoglobin	
Males	13.5 to 17.5 g/dL
Females	12.0 to 15.5 g/dL
Hematocrit	
Males	41% to 53%
Females	36% to 46%
MCV (size of RBC)	80 to100 fL
	>100 fl (macrocytic anemia) such as B12 deficiency (due to pernicious anemia) or folate deficiency
	<80 (microcytic anemia) such as iron deficiency or thalassemia trait
Platelet count	$140 - 415 \times 10^3$/mL
	Thrombocytopenia increased risk of bleeding
	Thrombocytosis increased risk of clotting, emboli
Total WBC count	$4.0 - 10.5 \times 10^3$/mL
	Elevation usually due to bacterial infection
Neutrophils (or segs)	56%–62%
	>70% usually due to bacterial infections
Bands	Also called "shift to the left"
	Elevation due to serious bacterial infection
	Bands are immature neutrophils
Lymphocytes	Elevation due to viral infections
Eosinophils	Elevation in allergies and parasitic infections
Reticulocytes	Elevated after acute hemorrhage, hemolysis
	Reticulocytes are immature red blood cells (RBC)
Thyroid Stimulating Hormone (TSH)	Elevated - Hypothyroidism (>5.5 mU/L)
	Very low - Hyperthyroidism (0.4 mU/L)
International Normalized Ratio (INR)	Atrial Fibrillation/Thrombosis
	PE: 2.0–3.0 times normal
	Bioprosthetic Valves: 2.0–3.0
	Prosthetic Valves 2.5–3.5

■ In alpha or beta thalassemia trait (or minor), the following results are found: normal to high ferritin/iron and normal to "below normal" TIBC/transferrin levels.

■ The gold standard test to diagnose thalassemia (or any anemia with abnormal hemoglobin such as sickle cell) is the hemoglobin electrophoresis.

DIAGRAMS

Discussion

Currently, examples of chest X-ray films and electrocardiogram strips have not been seen on the certification exams. The only diagram seen on the test at the moment is one of a chest with the four cardiac auscultory areas (aortic, pulmonic, tricuspid, and mitral) marked. The diagram is used for questions on either cardiac murmurs or heart sounds.

Example

Where is the best location to listen for the S3 heart sound?

a) aortic area
b) pulmonic area
c) tricuspid area
d) mitral area

The correct answer is option b: pulmonic area.

Question Dissection

Best Clue
■ There are no clues to this question.

Notes
■ The answer to this question is based on memory.
■ The best place to listen for the S3 heart sound is the pulmonic area.

GOLD STANDARD TESTS

Discussion

Do not confuse a screening test with a diagnostic test or the gold standard. Diagnostic tests are more specific and sensitive than screening tests. Some examples of diagnostic tests are tissue biopsies, cultures, and computed tomography or magnetic resonance imaging.

In contrast, screening tests are less specific and sensitive, but are more available and cost-effective. Some examples of screening tests are the hemoglobin and/or hematocrit (anemia), blood pressure (hypertension), Mantoux test or purified protein derivative (PPD) test (tuberculosis), and the fasting blood glucose (diabetes).

Although there are hundreds of laboratory and other diagnostic tests available, there are still many diseases for which there are no screening tests. This is because the ideal screening test is one that can detect disease at its earliest stages when it is potentially curable. A good example of a disease with no screening test is ovarian cancer. Although carcinoembryonic antigen (CEA) 125 testing and pelvic ultrasounds are currently available, they do not pick up the disease early enough. Therefore, screening all women for this cancer is currently not recommended.

Example

A middle-age nurse is having his PPD test result checked. A reddened area of 10.5 mm is present. It is smooth and soft and does not appear to be indurated. During the interview, the patient denies fever, cough, and weight loss. He is a nonsmoker. Which of the following is a true statement?

a) The PPD test result is negative.
b) The PPD test result is positive and a sputum culture and chest X-ray are necessary.
c) The PPD test should be repeated in 2 weeks.
d) Only a chest X-ray is indicated.

The correct answer is option a: The PPD result is negative.

Question Dissection

Best Clues
- The skin is not indurated.
- A red color alone does not mean a positive result. It can be due to a reaction to the preservative.
- When checking results within 48 to 72 hours, the induration is the important finding to look for.

Notes
- Test takers who read too fast or answer the question too rapidly are more likely to make errors with this type of question. When some test takers see the 10.5 mm size, they assume automatically that it is a positive result, especially with the erythema on the site. The induration and not the redness is what counts.
- When the question is read carefully, you realize that the PPD test result is negative because of the description of the smooth skin, which is not indurated.
- The skin must be indurated. Erythema is not an important criterion.
- For pulmonary TB, a sputum culture is the gold standard. Treatment is started with at least three anti-tubercular drugs because of the high rates of

resistance. When the sputum culture and sensitivity result is available, the treatment can be narrowed down based on the results of the culture and sensitivity test.

▪ Tuberculosis is a reportable disease. Others are Lyme disease, meningococcemia, Rocky Mountain spotted fever, measles, rubella, diphtheria, chlamydia, gonorrhea, HIV, and so forth.

▪ For someone who is younger than 35 years of age with a negative chest X-ray and who is asymptomatic, prophylaxis with isoniazid (INH) is recommended by the Centers for Disease Control and Prevention. After age 35 years, the risk of hepatitis from the drug is increased.

ARE TWO NAMES BETTER THAN ONE?

Discussion Only

Some diseases and conditions are known by two different names that are used interchangeably in the clinical area and in the literature. Sometimes, the alternate name is used in the exam questions. This can fool the test taker who is familiar with the disease but only recognizes it under its other name.

Examples

▪ degenerative joint disease (DJD) or osteoarthritis
▪ atopic dermatitis or eczema
▪ senile arcus or arcus senilis
▪ purulent otitis media or acute otitis media
▪ group A beta streptococcus or strep pyogenes
▪ tinea corporis or ringworm
▪ enterobiasis or pinworm
▪ vitamin B12 or cobalamin or cyanocobalamin (chemical name)
▪ scarlet fever or scarlatina
▪ otitis externa or swimmer's ear
▪ condyloma acuminata or genital warts
▪ tic douloureux or trigeminal neuralgia
▪ tinea cruris or jock itch
▪ tinea capitis or ringworm of the scalp
▪ thalassemia minor or thalassemia trait (either alpha or beta, it does not matter)
▪ giant cell arteritis or temporal arteritis
▪ asthma or reactive airway disease (infants and children)
▪ psoas sign or iliopsoas muscle sign
▪ light reflex or the Hirschsprung test
▪ sentinel nodes or Virchow's nodes
▪ the PPD test or the Mantoux test
▪ varicella or chickenpox

MAJOR DEPRESSION (UNIPOLAR DEPRESSION)

Discussion

On the test and in the clinical area, all depressed patients should be screened for suicidal and/or homicidal ideation. Avoid picking statements that do not address this issue directly. Avoid vague generalized statements. Incorrect answers are statements that are judgmental, that reassure the patient, that ignore cultural issues, that are disrespectful, or that do not address the issue of suicide (or homicide) in a direct manner.

Risk Factors for Suicide
- history of a suicide attempt
- family history of suicide
- plan to use a gun or other lethal methods
- being an elderly white male after the death of spouse
- history of bipolar or depressive disorder (during depressive cycle)

   Although females make more suicidal attempts, males have a higher rate of death because of the increased likelihood of using more lethal methods (i.e., guns, hanging).

Example

An NP working in a school health clinic is evaluating a new patient who has been referred to him by a teacher. The patient is a 15-year-old boy with a history of attention deficit hyperactivity disorder (ADHD). He complains that his parents are always fighting, and he thinks they are getting divorced. During the interview, he stares at the floor and avoids eye contact. He complains that he is having problems falling asleep at night. Which of the following questions is the best choice to ask this teen?

a) Do you want me to call your parents after we talk?
b) Do you have any plans to kill yourself or to hurt other people?
c) Do you have any close friends?
d) Do you want to wait to tell me about your plans until you feel better?

   The correct answer is option b: Do you have any plans to kill yourself or to hurt other people?

Question Dissection

Best Clues
- The patient makes poor eye contact, has insomnia, and conflict (parents are getting divorced).
- The patient is a teenage male.

Notes

■ When interviewing a teen, do it privately (without parents) as well as with the parent(s) present.

■ Although option c (Do you have any close friends?) is a question commonly asked of teenagers, it is incorrect because it does not produce information of suicidal/homicidal intent.

■ Always avoid picking answer choices in which an intervention is delayed. The question "Do you want to wait tell to me about your plans until you feel better?" is a good example of a choice to avoid.

■ There is always a question on depression. The diagnosis is based on a history of depressed mood and/or anhedonia (decreased interest in things that use to give the patient pleasure) accompanied by at least four of the following factors: agitation or slowing down (psychomotor retardation), sleep disturbances (either insomnia or hypersomnia), fatigue, poor concentration and memory, and suicidal ideation.

■ Depression is thought to be caused by a decrease in the neurotransmitters of the brain, especially serotonin and norephinephrine.

■ Teenagers are separating from their parents emotionally and place a high value on their privacy.

OTHER PSYCHIATRIC DISORDERS

Discussion

Other psychiatric disorders such as obsessive-compulsive disorder (OCD), anxiety, panic disorder, alcohol addiction, delirium, abuse, and attention deficit hyperactivity disorder (ADHD) may be included in the exams. The question may only be about a common drug for the disorder such as the fact that methylphenidate (Ritalin) and other stimulants show positive in a drug toxicology urine test. The most common psychiatric disorders are major depression, domestic violence, and alcohol abuse.

Example

Which of the following drug classes is indicated as first line treatment of both major depression and OCD?

a) selective serotonin reuptake inhibitors (SSRIs)
b) tricyclic antidepressants (TCAs)
c) mood stabilizers
d) benzodiazepines

The correct answer is option a: SSRIs.

Question Dissection

Best Clues

- Rule out benzodiazepines; they are used to treat anxiety or insomnia (process of elimination).
- Rule out mood stabilizers such as lithium salts, which is used to treat bipolar disorder (process of elimination).
- Use the process of elimination if you are not sure of the answer.

Notes

- The SSRIs are first line treatment for OCD, generalized anxiety disorder, panic disorder, social anxiety disorder (extreme shyness), and premenstrual mood disorder (fluoxetine or Prozac).
- Examples of SSRIs include fluoxetine (Prozac), sertraline (Zoloft), and paroxetine (Paxil).
- Do not discontinue the SSRI paroxetine (Paxil) abruptly. Wean the patient slowly.
- The TCAs are now considered second line treatment for depression. They are also used for post-herpetic neuralgia and migraine headache prophylaxis.
- Examples of TCAs are amitriptyline (Elavil) and desipramine (Norpramine).
- Avoid treating suicidal patients with TCAs because of the risk of hoarding the drug and then overdosing.
- TCA overdose can be fatal (due to development of fatal heart arrhythmias).
- Anticonvulsants such as carbamazepine (Tegretol) are also used for chronic pain.

ABUSIVE SITUATIONS

Discussion

Health care workers are required by law to report suspected and actual child abuse to the proper authorities. Abuse-related topics on the exam may include domestic violence, physical abuse, child abuse, elderly abuse, and sexual abuse.

Example

An 8-year-old boy with a history of ADHD is brought to the ER by his mother. She does not seem to want her son to be alone in the room with the NP. The NP notes several burns on the child's trunk. Some of the burns appear infected. The NP documents the burns as mostly round and approximately 0.5 cm in size. Which of the following questions is most appropriate to ask the child's mother?

a) Your son's back looks terrible. What happened to him?
b) Does your son have friends to play with outside of school?
c) Did you burn his back with a cigarette?
d) Can you please tell me what happened to your son?

The correct answer is option d: Can you please tell me what happened to your son?

Question Dissection

Best Clues
■ Option d is an open-ended question.

Notes
In general, an open-ended question is usually the best answer in abuse case scenarios when you are trying to interview the relative or the patient.

■ Both options a and c are judgmental questions and would likely make the boy's mother respond defensively and/or antagonistically.
■ The question posed in option b does not elicit specific information nor does it address the immediate issue of the burn marks on the boy's back.

Communication Tips
■ When a history is being taken, questions should be open ended.
■ Any question that is judgmental is wrong.
■ Do not pick answers that "reassure" the patient. Reassuring a patient is considered poor communication.
■ Do not ignore cultural beliefs. Integrate them into the treatment plan if they are not harmful to the health of the patient.

THE CAGE SCREEN

Discussion

The acronym CAGE is a mnemonic used to guide the screening of patients for alcoholism. Answering yes to two of four questions is highly suggestive of alcohol abuse. In the exams, you are expected to use higher level cognitive skills and apply the concepts of CAGE. One example is a question in which you are asked to pick the patient who is most likely (or least likely) to abuse alcoholic drinks.

The CAGE Screening Tool (a score ≥ 2 positive answers is suggestive of alcoholism) stands for:

C: Do you feel the need to *c*ut down?
A: Are you *a*nnoyed when your spouse/friend comments about your drinking?

G: Do you feel *g*uilty about your drinking?
E: Do you need to drink early in the morning? (*e*ye-opener)?

Example

Which of the following individuals is least likely to become an alcohol abuser?

a) A housewife who becomes annoyed when her best friend expresses concern about her drinking habit.
b) A carpenter who drinks one can of beer nightly when playing cards with friends.
c) A nurse who feels shaky when she wakes up and relieves this feeling by drinking wine.
d) The college student who tells his friend that he drinks only on weekends but feels that he should be drinking less.

The correct answer is option b: a carpenter who drinks one can of beer nightly when playing cards with friends.

Question Dissection

Best Clues
■ One bottle of beer at night is considered normal consumption (lack of risk factors).
■ There is no description of any negative effects on the carpenter's daily function, social environment, or mental state (lack of risk factor).

Notes
Any person who feels compelled to drink or use drugs regardless of the consequences to health, finances, career, friends, and family is addicted to the substance.

■ The housewife who becomes annoyed if her best friend talks to her about her drinking habit embodies the *A* (annoyed) in CAGE. This is a good example of an alcohol abuser becoming annoyed when someone close remarks about his or her drinking problem.
■ A nurse who feels shaky when she wakes up and gets relief after drinking is indicative of the *E* (eye-opener) in CAGE. An eye-opener is the compulsion to drink after waking up in order to get relief from the symptoms of alcohol withdrawal.
■ The college student who tells his friend that he drinks only on weekends but feels that he should be drinking less fits the *C* in CAGE (*c*ut down). This student is aware that he should cut down on his drinking. This student is a binge drinker.

ALL QUESTIONS ON THE EXAM HAVE ENOUGH INFORMATION

Discussion Only

Assume that all the questions on the exams contain enough information to answer them correctly. Do not read too much into a question or assume that it is missing some vital information. As far as the ANCC and AANP are concerned, all questions contain enough information to solve them correctly.

FACTOID QUESTIONS

Discussion

Questions that simply ask for facts are what I call "factoid" questions. Some of my review course students in the past have remarked that "you either know the answer or you don't" with these types of questions. This type of question depends on rote memory and an adequate review of the facts.

Example

Which of the following drugs is the latest recommendation as first line treatment for an uncomplicated case of hypertension by the Joint National Commission on the Evaluation, Management, and Treatment of High Blood Pressure (JNC 7)?

a) angiotensin-converting enzyme inhibitors
b) thiazide diuretics
c) calcium channel blockers
d) beta blockers

The correct answer is option b: thiazide diuretics.

Question Dissection

Best Clue
▓ There are no clues with this question.
▓ Memorization of the JNC 7 guidelines.

Notes
▓ Angiotensin-converting enzyme inhibitors are first line drugs except for patients with a comorbidity such as diabetes mellitus or microalbuminuria. These are the drugs of choice for people with diabetes because of their renal-protective properties.
▓ Beta blockers are indicated for patients with both hypertension and migraine.

▪ Beta blockers are contraindicated in patients with chronic lung diseases such as asthma, chronic obstructive pulmonary disease (COPD), emphysema, sarcoidosis, or chronic bronchitis.
▪ The beta blockers are contraindicated in lung disease because of the brochoconstriction resulting from blockade of the beta receptors of the lungs.

PHYSICAL ASSESSMENT FINDINGS

Discussion

Questions about physical exam findings are plentiful. The organ systems that seem to appear most often are HEENT, heart, lungs, eyes, musculoskeletal, and neurological systems. Questions include not only normal and abnormal physical exam findings, but also maneuvers such as cranial nerve testing, the Rinne and Weber, Phalen and Tinel, abdominal (i.e., Rovsings), and orthopedic maneuvers. Learn the classic presentation of disease and emergent conditions. A few questions on benign physical variants will also be included such as a torus palatinus and a fishtail or split uvula, which are discussed in chapter 3.

Example

A 6-year-old child complains of a new onset of severe pain over her left ear after taking swimming classes for 2 weeks. On physical exam, the right ear canal is red and swollen. Purulent green exudate is seen inside the ear canal. Which of the following is not a true statement?

a) Pulling on the tragus causes the child pain.
b) The tympanic membrane is not visible.
c) Most children have tinnitus associated with the condition.
d) The child does not have a higher risk of acute mastoiditis secondary to the infection.

The correct answer is option c: Most children have tinnitus associated with the condition.

Question Dissection

Best Clues
▪ A history of swimming is a risk factor for acute otitis externa (swimmer's ear).
▪ Classic clinical findings are a reddened and swollen ear canal with green exudate.

Notes
▪ Acute otitis externa is a superficial infection of the skin in the ear canal. It is more common during warm and humid conditions such as swimming and summertime.

- The most common bacterial pathogen is pseudomonas (gram negative).
- Otitis externa does not involve the middle ear or the tympanic membrane and does not cause tinnitus (as seen in Ménière's disease).

GRADING MURMURS

Discussion

Expect at least one question about grading heart murmurs. It is very helpful if you have a system to remember a large amount of this type of information. The grading system for murmurs is as follows:

- Grade I is a very soft murmur that is difficult to hear.
- Grade II is a murmur that is mild to moderately loud.
- Grade III is a loud murmur that is easy to hear.
- Grade IV is the first time a thrill is palpated.
- Grade V is when the murmur can be heard with the stethoscope partly off the chest.
- Grade VI when the murmur is so loud that it can be heard with the stethoscope off the chest.

Example

A loud heart murmur that is easily heard when the stethoscope is placed on the chest is which of the following?

a) Grade II
b) Grade III
c) Grade IV
d) Grade V

The correct answer is option b: Grade III.

Question Dissection

Best Clues
- No thrill is present (the murmur is less than a Grade IV).
- The only answer options left are Grade II and Grade III.
- The description of an "easily heard" murmur that is not accompanied by a thrill best describes a Grade III murmur.

Notes
- A good system of remembering heart murmurs is to remember that the first time a thrill is palpable is at Grade IV. Any murmur that is less than Grade IV does not have any thrill.

NEGATIVE POLARITY QUESTIONS

Discussion

Many test takers have problems solving negatively worded questions. These are questions with the following words in the stem: not, never, false, not true, least likely, and so forth. Some have two negative words together in one question (a double negative question).

One technique that helps in solving these questions is to simply drop the negative word in the sentence and make it into a positive one. If a question has two negative terms, one can be dropped, which makes it easier to comprehend.

Example

When you look at this question drop the second negative term, "except." This makes it easier to understand. Look for three false statements; the remainder should be the true one and the correct answer.

All of the following are false statements about colonic diverticula except:

a) Diverticulitis is more common in young adults.
b) Diverticulitis is associated with chronic low dietary intake of fiber.
c) All diverticula are infected with Gram-negative bacteria.
d) Supplementing with fiber such as psyllium (Metamucil) is not recommended.

The correct answer is option b: Diverticulitis is associated with chronic low dietary intake of fiber.

Question Dissection

Best Clues
■ Rule out answers that have "all inclusive" words (i.e., all, not, never) as seen in option c, "*All* diverticula are. . . ." This narrows your choices to three options.
■ Your knowledge of the pathophysiology and treatment of diverticulitis.

Notes
Careful reading is imperative in problems such as this one. Option d reveals that the word "not" (Supplementing with fiber such as psyllium (Metamucil) is *not* recommended), has reversed its meaning and changed it to a false statement. The answer can be ruled out because you are looking for the true statement.

Keep in mind in these types of questions what you are looking for: a true statement or a false one?

■ Diverticulitis is the result of inflamed and infected diverticula. It is more common in older or elderly adults.

- Diverticula are small pouch-like structures along the clonic wall. They are caused by chronic lack of fiber in the diet
- Diverticulitis maintenance treatment is fiber supplementation such as psyllium (Metamucil) or methylcellulose (Citrucel) that is taken two to three times a day with 8 ounces of water.
- Diverticulitis can be a life-threatening infection; if the diverticula rupture, the result will be an acute abdomen.

TWO QUESTIONS

Discussion

These questions are problematic because the two questions are interdependent on each other. To solve both correctly, the test taker must answer the first portion correctly (arrive at the diagnosis) in order to answer the second one correctly.

Fortunately, there are usually only one or two of this type of question on the entire test. These are two-part questions that are based on only one case scenario.

Example

Part One
A 14-year-old boy who had been camping is brought in by his mother. The teen returned home from a trip 2 weeks ago without any apparent health problems. Now, the patient complains of a bad headache for the past 6 hours along with high fever and chills. He denies a stiff neck. A rash that started on both his wrist and ankles is starting to spread toward his trunk. Which of the following conditions is most likely?

a) thrombocytopenia
b) Rocky Mountain spotted fever
c) idiopathic thrombocytopenic purpura (ITP)
d) Lyme disease

Part Two
Which of the following is the best treatment plan to follow?

a) Refer the patient to an infectious disease specialist immediately.
b) Refer the patient to a hematologist.
c) Order a CT (computed tomography) scan of the head.
d) Treat the patient with antiviral medication as soon as possible.

The correct answer to Part One is option b: Rocky Mountain spotted fever.
The correct answer to Part Two is option a: Refer the patient to an infectious disease specialist immediately.

Question Dissection

Best Clues

Part One

- A rash starts on the wrist and ankles; spreading centrally is a classic sign of Rocky Mountain spotted fever.
- Rule out ITP (hemorrhagic lesions) and thrombocytopenia (easy bruising). These are not considered rashes.

Part Two

- Picking the correct answer depends on selecting the correct diagnosis in the first question.

Notes

- Rocky Mountain spotted fever (5% of cases are fatal) results from a tick bite, the spirochete of which is *Rickettsia rickettsii*. Rocky Mountain spotted fever is treated with doxycycline or chloramphenicol.
- Thrombocytopenia and ITP, an autoimmune disorder, result from the breakdown of platelets in the spleen. ITP is self-limiting and is usually precipitated by a viral infection.
- Lyme disease is caused by the ixodes tick (deer tick) bite, the spirochete of which is *Borrelia burgdorferi*.
- Erythema migrans (a targetlike red rash) is seen during the early stage of the infection. Early Lyme Disease is treated with a 21-day course of doxycycline.
- The majority of the cases of Lyme disease occur in the northeast and mid-Atlantic states (i.e., CT, MA, NY, NJ, PA).

NORMAL PHYSICAL EXAM FINDINGS: PUBERTY TO ADOLESCENCE

Discussion

The pediatric section in chapter 3 combines the physical exam findings from the neonate to the late adolescent. Be aware that sometimes questions relating to normal growth and development are designed to look like pathology.

Example

A 9-year-old girl complains of an irregular menstrual cycle. She started menarche 6 months ago. Her last menstrual period was 2 months ago. She denies being sexually active. Her urine pregnancy test is negative. Which of the following would you advise the child's mother to do?

a) Consult with a pediatric endocrinologist to rule out problems with the hypothalamus-pituitary-adrenal axis (HPA).
b) Advise the mother that irregular menstrual cycles are common during the first year after menarche.
c) Advise the mother that her child is starting menarche early and has precocious puberty.
d) Ask the medical assistant to arrange for lab tests for a thyroid stimulating hormone, follicle stimulating hormone, and estradiol levels.

The correct answer is option b: Advise the mother that irregular menstrual cycles are common during the first year after menarche.

Question Dissection

Best Clues
■ The patient started menarche 6 months ago.
■ The pregnancy test is negative, ruling out pregnancy as the cause of the amenorrhea.

Notes
■ This question describes normal growth and development in puberty. Puberty starts when the child starts to develop secondary sexual characteristics. If it starts before the age of 8 years in girls and 9 years in boys, it is considered precocious puberty.
■ Irregular menstrual cycles are common during the first year after menarche.
■ Other pubertal changes to learn are the Tanner Staging system of secondary sexual development.

PREGNANT WOMEN

Discussion

The questions in this area concern normal physiologic changes as well as some emergent conditions seen only in pregnancy, such as preeclampsia, placenta abruptio, placenta previa, and ectopic pregnancy. Although most NPs do not manage pregnant women, the FNP is still expected to be familiar with both the normal physiological exam changes during pregnancy and some emergent conditions seen in this group of patients.

Example

A young primigravida who is at 32 weeks of gestation complains of a painful and "rock-hard" uterus 3 hours after slipping on an icy sidewalk. She complains of vaginal bleeding that started 1 hour after the incident. Which of the following is most likely?

a) placenta previa
b) placenta abruptio
c) bicornate uterus
d) premature labor

The correct answer is option b: placenta abruptio.

Question Dissection

Best Clues
▪ The classic presentation of placenta abruptio is a hard or hypertonic uterus that is painful and accompanied by vaginal bleeding.
▪ The history of a traumatic fall 3 hours before onset of symptoms.

Notes
▪ Placenta abruptio is the traumatic separation of the placental bed from the uterine wall, causing hemorrhage, which can be life threatening to both the mother and fetus. Women with mild cases are placed on strict bedrest.
▪ Placenta previa results when the placenta is implanted on the cervical neck or cervix itself. It is not usually seen until the third trimester. When the placenta is too large for the uterus to contain, the placenta starts to separate from the uterus, resulting in bleeding.
▪ Compared with placenta abruptio, the uterus is soft and painless in placenta previa. Both conditions are included in the differential diagnosis for vaginal bleeding.
▪ Bicornate uterus is a congenital condition where a woman's uterus contains two smaller lobes.
▪ Premature labor is treated with intravenously administered magnesium sulfate and strict bedrest. If the cervix becomes dilated (inevitable abortion), labor is imminent whether the fetus is viable or not.

PEDIATRIC GROWTH AND DEVELOPMENT

Discussion

Proportionally, more of the questions in the pediatric area, as compared to the area concerned with adults, deal with normal growth and development. The age categories range from birth, infancy, toddlerhood, early to late childhood, puberty and into adolescence.

The reflexes, maneuvers (i.e., the Ortolani), safety issues, foods, and immunizations are some of the topics that may be included.

Example

All of the following are considered normal physical findings in a newborn female except:

a) a small amount of blood from the vaginal canal
b) lanugo
c) roseola infantum
d) Babinski reflex

The correct answer is option c: roseola infantum.

Question Dissection

Best Clues
■ The child is a newborn female.
■ Knowledge of benign variants seen among infants.

Notes
■ High levels of maternal hormones in circulation stimulate the neonate's uterus to produce an endometrial lining. The lining is shed (just like in menstruation) when levels of maternal hormones drastically decrease after birth. This finding may be seen during the first or second week of life. If present afterward, it is abnormal.
■ Lanugo is the fine vellus hair over cheeks, shoulders, and the back. It is normal in neonates. Lanugo may be seen in women who have a history of anorexia nervosa.
■ Roseola infantum (or exanthema subitum) involves an abrupt onset of high fever, up to 105° Fahrenheit (F), lasting from 3 to 5 days. The infant feeds and behaves normally. After the fever diminishes, a rash appears on the trunk/abdomen and then resolves spontaneously after a few days. Roseola infantum is sometimes associated with febrile seizures. It is caused by herpes virus type 6 and type 7.
■ Babinski reflex is one in which the toes flare upward when the sole of the foot is stroked. It is normal in neonates (immature nervous system). This reflex disappears by age 2 years. Later the normal response is for the toes to curl down. If the Babinski reflex is present later, it is a sign of serious brain damage.

ADOLESCENCE

Questions of "catch up" on immunizations in an adolescent are usually present. The teen presented in the case ranges from the age of 14 to 16 years. The teen is usually due for a Td booster (the last series of the DTaP is given at around 3 to 4 years of age or at preschool). Therefore, teens are due for their first 10-year booster of tetanus.

Another possibility is the teen who received fewer than three shots of Hepatitis B during his initial series; he will need another booster of Hepatitis B.

Discussion

During this period of life, numerous changes are occurring, both physically and emotionally. Adolescents are thinking in more abstract ways and are psychologically separating from their parents. The opinions of their peers are more important than those of their parents. Privacy is a big issue in this age group and should be respected.

During an interview, the teen needs to be seen without the presence of a parent, and then together with the parent.

Example

Which of the following is the cause of the highest mortality among teenagers in this country?

a) suicide
b) smoking
c) motor vehicle or unintentional injuries
d) congenital heart disease

The correct answer is option c: motor vehicle and unintentional injuries.

Question Dissection

Best Clues

▓ Using the process of elimination, the two answers that most test takers choose are either suicide or motor vehicle accidents and unintentional injuries.
▓ Rule out smoking because the adverse health effects take decades to manifest (e.g., lung cancer, COPD).
▓ Rule out congenital heart disease because the question is about teens, not infants.

Notes

▓ The number one cause of mortality in this age group is motor vehicle accidents or unintentional/injuries.
▓ The second most common cause of mortality for this age group is death from suicide.
▓ Screening for depression is recommended in all adolescents during each wellness visit. Signs of a depressed teen include falling grades, acting out, avoiding friends, moodiness, crying jags, sleep disturbance, anhedonia, and so forth.
▓ Most deaths from congenital heart disease occur during early infancy.

LEGAL RIGHTS OF MINORS

Discussion

Certain legal issues exist in dealing with adolescents that are not usually seen in pediatric and adult patients. These are the issues of confidentiality and right to consent without parental involvement.

Example

All of the following can be considered as emancipated minors except:

a) A 15-year-old who is married
b) A 14-year-old single mother who has one child
c) A 17-year-old who is enlisted in the U.S. army
d) A 16-year-old who wants to be treated for dysmenorrhea

The correct answer is option d: A 16-year-old who wants to be treated for dysmenorrhea.

Question Dissection

Best Clues
■ Option d is the only one that doesn't fit the pattern. The other three options address nonclinical issues.

Notes
■ Emancipated minors are teens who are younger than 18 years of age who have the same legal rights as adults.
■ Emancipated minors can give full consent and sign contracts and other legal documents that are legally binding just as they would be if signed by an adult.
■ The criteria to be an emancipated minor in the United States are: any minor who is married, any minor who is a parent, and any minor who is enlisted in the U.S. military.

DIFFERENTIAL DIAGNOSIS

Discussion

Differential diagnosis is a systematic comparison of clinical findings to determine which of two or more diseases is the cause of symptoms.

The signs and/or symptoms can be so similar that it can be very challenging to distinguish one from another. On the exam, the process is easier than in "real life" because the patient presents with the disease's classic historical findings and/or its classic signs and symptoms.

Example

A 57-year-old male executive with a history of asthma walks into an urgent care center. The patient complains of an episode of chest pain in his upper sternum during physical activity, which is relieved after he stops the offending activity. He has had several episodes of the chest pain in the past. A fasting total lipid profile is ordered. The result reveals a total cholesterol of 245 mg/dL, an low-density lipoprotein (LDL) of 138 mg/dL and a high-density lipoprotein HDL of 32 mg/dL. Which of the following is most likely?

a) acute esophagitis
b) myocardial infarction (MI)
c) gastroesophageal reflux disease (GERD)
d) angina

The correct answer is option d: angina.

Question Dissection

Best Clues
▓ Chest pain that is precipitated by exertion and is relieved by rest is a classic presentation.
▓ Hyperlipidemia is a risk factor for heart disease.
▓ The patient's age and gender are classic demographic clues for a high-risk patient.

Notes
All four answer options present some of the differential diagnoses for chest pain. The differences and similarities are compared and the best fit is the correct answer (angina).

▓ The patient's condition is aggravated by meals (*angina*, acute esophagitis, MI, GERD).
▓ The pain is relieved fully by rest (*angina*).
▓ The risk factors for heart disease are present (*angina*, MI).
▓ The history does not fit accute esophagitis. Look for a recent intake of an offending substance.
▓ The patient is a male older than age 50 (*angina*, MI). Age is not a risk factor for acute esophagitis.
▓ Physical activity aggravates the patient's condition (*angina*, MI).

47

CLASSIC PRESENTATION

Discussion

It is commonly known that diseases exist in a spectrum from the subclinical phase into the resolution phase. Not all the classic signs or symptoms manifest in real life practice. As a matter of fact, a large number of diseases are asymptomatic and do not manifest until damage has been done to the body.

But on the exams, the classic presentation of disease is always the rule. The disease will be presented with the risk factors, demographics, and the signs and symptoms, as shown in the previous example. Certification exams are administered all over the country and this allows the test to be valid and statistically sound at a national level.

Example

While performing a routine physical exam on a 60-year-old man, the NP palpates a pulsatile mass in the patient's mid-abdominal area. A loud bruit is auscultated over the soft mass. Which of the following conditions is most likely?

a) This clinical finding is considered a normal variant.
b) This is a stool impaction in the lower segment of the colon.
c) This is an aortic abdominal aneurysm.
d) This finding is adenocarcinoma of the colon.

The correct answer is option c: This is an aortic abdominal aneurysm.

Question Dissection

Best Clues
- A pulsatile mass located in the middle of the abdomen is a classic sign.
- The presence of a bruit over a pulsatile mass.

Notes
- This question describes the classic case of an aortic abdominal aneurysm, which is more common in older patients. Mild cases are observed with serial abdominal ultrasounds performed by cardiologists. Severe cases are treated surgically.
- It is imperative that the blood pressure be tightly controlled in patients with aneurysms to decrease the chances of rupture.
- Stool impaction and colon cancer do not pulsate or have bruits.
- Colon cancer screening by colonoscopy is recommended for persons from the age of 50 years or older or in younger patients with risk factors such as positive family history, polyposis, or Crohn's disease.

UNCOMMON DISEASES

Discussion

Although these exams are on primary care disorders (including normal findings), it is possible to be questioned about unusual disorders that sometimes initially present in the primary care area.

In general, exotic or unusual diseases are used as distractors on the exam and are best avoided when guessing for the correct answer.

Example

An elderly Hispanic woman is complaining of a painful swollen area in her left lower leg on the shin area. The NP notes an indurated bright red skin lesion that has very distinct edges. The lesion has red streaks underneath the skin. It is warm to the touch and the patient is febrile. The patient's history includes a long drive of 6 hours the previous day. During the physical exam, the NP notes that the Homan's sign is negative. The skin does not have bullae or dark necrotic areas. The circumference of both calves is equal. Which of the following conditions is most likely?

a) deep venous thrombosis (DVT)
b) necrotizing fasciitis
c) erysipelas
d) inflamed psoriatic plaque

The correct answer is option c: erysipelas.

Question Dissection

Best Clues

- It is a classic presentation of erysipelas.
- Homan's sign is negative and both the legs are equal in circumference; therefore, it is not DVT.
- Although a plaque is described, there are no silvery scales present, therefore ruling out psoriasis.
- No necrotic areas or bullae are present and the patient has no systemic symptoms nor is she toxic; thus, necrotizing fasciitis can be ruled out.
- The only condition that has not been ruled out is erysipelas, the correct answer.

Notes

- Erysipelas is a subtype of cellulitis in which the infection goes deeper down and spreads to local lymphatic channels (looks like red streaks).
- Erysipelas is caused by Group A beta strep (Gram-positive).
- Erysipelas is usually found on the face or the lower leg.

- The typical treatment for erysipelas is a Penicillin G injection or Penicillin V PO for at least 10 days.
- On the exam, DVT is usually associated with a positive Homan's sign; if it is a negative exam, as in the previous example, then it is not DVT. The swelling in DVT usually involves the whole limb, not just a localized area.
- In real life, Homan's sign is not considered a reliable indicator for DVT.
- Necrotizing fasciitis (also known as flesh-eating bacteria) is an aggressive and serious infection and spreads very quickly. In the early phase it appears as a round red papule and with a small amount of central necrosis. An important clue is that the patient will complain of pain that is out of proportion to the size of the wound.
- During the height of a necrotizing faciitis infection, the patient is toxic and may have multiorgan failure. Large necrotic areas and bullae are seen with rapid spread of the infection on the limb.
- The treatment for necrotizing fasciitis is hospitalization, intravenous administration of high-dose antibiotics, and aggressive surgical debridement and/or amputation of the infected tissue to save the patient's life.

ETHNIC BACKGROUND

Discussion

Ethnic background is an important clue for certain genetic disorders. For example, people affected by thalassemia are often of Mediterranean ethnicity (i.e., Italians, Greeks, etc.) or of Asian descent (e.g., Chinese). A question on thalassemia minor/trait may include information on the patient's ethnic background. Sometimes, only labs are given with no information of the ethnicity.

A warning about ethnic background: it can also be a potent distractor. With the majority of disease, the ethnic background has no effect on the treatment plan or the patient's response to treatment. The next question is an example of this concept.

Example

Which of the following laboratory tests is a sensitive indicator of renal function in people of Asian descent?

a) serum blood urea nitrogen (BUN)
b) serum creatinine
c) serum albumin
d) serum BUN to creatinine ratio

The question in this example can also be phrased, "Which of the following laboratory tests is a sensitive indicator of renal function in people of Hispanic or African or Asian descent?"

The correct answer is option b: serum creatinine.

Question Dissection

Best Clues
- The question is asking for a "sensitive indicator" of renal function in the primary care area.
- Your memory of the role of creatinine in the body.

Notes
- A patient's ethnic background has no effect on the creatinine level, but gender, age, certain medications, and preexisting disease do.
- The other three renal tests are not as specific as the serum creatinine.
- If the results of a serum creatinine test are abnormal, the next step in the work-up is a 24-hour urine collection for protein and creatinine.

QUESTIONS ABOUT FOOD

Discussion

There are basically three kinds of food-related questions on the exam. You may be asked to pick the foods that have high levels of certain minerals such as sodium, potassium, calcium, or magnesium. Other questions about food address food and drug interactions or the types of foods that are contraindicated (or indicated) for a certain disease process.

Certain foods are recommended for certain diseases (i.e., hypertension, hyperlipidemia) because of their favorable effect. Conversely, certain foods are contraindicated for the condition because of adverse or dangerous effects.

Example

Which of the following foods are known to have high potassium content?

a) yogurt, banana, and red meat
b) aged cheese, red wine, and chocolate
c) most fruits and vegetables
d) low-fat ice cream, orange juice, and banana

The correct answer is option c: most fruits and vegetables.

Question Dissection

Best Clues
- Use the process of elimination.
- First, look at the answer option groups for inconsistencies in the list of foods.

51

- Rule out option d because of inconsistencies. Low-fat ice cream is not a good source of potassium.
- Rule out option a because of inconsistencies.
- If options a, b, and d are incorrect, the only one left is option c (most fruits and vegetables are rich in potassium).

Notes

- If one of the foods on the list in an answer option is incorrect, rule it out because the inconsistency makes it false.
- A common distractor in this type of question is to mix up foods that do not possess the same characteristics.
- The three conditions presented in which a food question might be found are migraine headache, diabetes, and hypertension.

Examples of Food Groups

- High sodium content: cold cuts, pickles, preserved foods, canned foods, hot dogs, and chips
- Calcium: low-fat dairy, yogurt, and cheeses
- Potassium: most fruits, most vegetables, orange juice, and bananas
- Magnesium: whole grains, whole wheat bread, and some nuts
- Folate: green leafy vegetables (e.g., spinach) and liver
- Unsaturated fats: olive oil, canola oil, and walnut oil
- Saturated fats: animal fats and coconut oil
- Iron: red meat, black beans, and liver
- Complex carbohydrates: whole grain bread, whole grains
- Simple carbohydrates: sugar, candy, cakes, white bread

Common Disorders Associated With Certain Foods

Hypertension

- Avoid high sodium foods such as cold cuts, pickles, preserved foods, canned foods, and hot dogs. Maintain an adequate intake of calcium (low-fat dairy, yogurt, and cheese), magnesium (whole grains, whole wheat bread, and some nuts), and potassium (most fruits, most vegetables, orange juice, and bananas).

Migraine headaches

- Avoid chocolate, aged cheese, red wine, and monosodium glutamate.

MAOI (monoamine oxidase inhibitor) such as Parnate or Nardil

- Avoid high tyramine foods such as red wine, beer, chocolate, and fermented foods.

MEDICATIONS

Discussion

On the exam, drugs are always listed in both their generic and brand name forms. It is not necessary to learn both names because both will appear together. Use the name that you can best remember (either brand or generic name). Drug class must be memorized along with the representative drug. When picking a drug to memorize, pick out the most commonly used drug in that class. These are usually the older versions of the drug. A good example is the macrolides. Erythromycin is still preferred and is seen more often on the answer options than azithromycin (Zithromax) or clarithromycin (Biaxin).

Safety issues are important to learn such as dangerous drug interactions and contraindications. Other areas to learn are the drug's FDA category, indication, and some well-known side effects. Drugs that are contraindicated in pregnancy and FDA Category X drugs are listed under the obstetrics section in chapter 3.

Example

Using the drug class as the answer option, which of the following class of drugs is the preferred treatment for community-acquired pneumonia in patients younger than the age of 60 with no comorbid condition?

a) macrolides
b) beta lactams
c) cephalosporins
d) new fluoroquinolones

Example

This is the same question as before, but the answer options have been given in the generic and brand name.

Using generic and brand names as the answer options, which of the following drugs is the preferred treatment for community-acquired pneumonia for patients younger than the age of 60 with no comorbid condition?

a) erythromycin (E-mycin)
b) amoxicillin (Amoxil)
c) cephalexin (Keflex)
d) levaquinolone (Levaquin)

Example

The following is an example of a more complicated question. Maria is a 16-year-old high school student who was diagnosed with ADD 1 year ago. She recently applied for a job and was rejected because of a positive result on her urine toxicology test. Which of the following medications is not associated with this finding?

a) amphetamine (Dexedrine)
b) dextroamphetamine salts (Adderall)
c) sertraline (Zoloft)
d) methylphenidate (Ritalin)

The correct answer in the first example is option a: macrolides.

The correct answer in the second example is option a: erythromycin (E-mycin).

The correct answer in the third example is option c: sertraline (Zoloft).

Question Dissection

Best Clues

■ The patient has ADD (diagnosis) and the treatment of choice is the amphetamines.

■ Rule out all three of the amphetamines on the list.

If you are not familiar with them, notice that two of the drugs have "amphetamine" in their names: amphetamine (Dexedrine) and dextroamphetamine salts (Adderall) so you can rule out these two options.

■ Ritalin is a well-known drug used in the treatment of ADD/ADHD; rule it out.

■ If you are guessing, look at the pattern. The only SSRI or antidepressant in the list is sertraline (Zoloft).

Notes

■ The correct answer in the third example is sertraline (Zoloft), an SSRI. It does not show up on a urine toxicology screen. The other three choices are all amphetamines (or stimulants).

■ Amphetamines are the first line drugs for treating ADHD and ADD.

■ Amphetamines should be taken in the morning and no later than lunchtime to minimize their adverse effect on sleep.

■ Amphetamines are contraindicated in patients with hypertension, stroke, acute MI, psychosis, or any conditions in which overstimulation may produce adverse effects.

DESCRIBING A FINDING VERSUS USING THE NAME

Discussion

A sign and/or symptom may be described instead of using its name. Be aware of this method when you see a description that you do not recognize.

In the following example, instead of the common name of "clue cell," it is being described as "squamous epithelial cells with numerous bacteria on the cells' surface."

Example

A 30-year-old woman who is sexually active complains of a large amount of light-colored vaginal discharge with milklike consistency after she finished a prescription of antibiotics. She denies itch or redness of the external vagina. A microscopy slide reveals squamous epithelial cells with numerous bacteria on the cells' surface. The vaginal pH is at 6.0. Which of the following is most likely?

a) trichomonas infection
b) bacterial vaginosis (BV)
c) candidal infection
d) normal finding

The correct answer is option b: BV.

Question Dissection

Best Clues
▨ Rule out candida. The sentence is describing a bacteria (candida is a yeast).
▨ Trichomonas is not a bacteria; it is a protozoan.
▨ The pH is alkaline, which is a classic sign of BV in addition to the clue cell and positive Whiff test.

Notes
▨ Instead of using the name "clue cell," the appearance of the clue cell is being described.
▨ Clue cells are "squamous epithelial cells with numerous bacteria on the cells' surface."
▨ Typically, BV produces an alkaline pH of 6.0; the vagina normally has an acidic pH of 4.0. Because the bacteria inside the vagina do not cause inflammation, BV is known as vaginosis (not vaginitis) and is not considered a sexually transmitted infection. The male sex partner needs no treatment. It is treated with metronidazole (Flagyl) or clindamycin (Cleocin) vaginal cream or oral Flagyl for 7 days.
▨ The vaginal discharge in candidal infection is white with a thick, curdlike consistency. It causes itching and redness of the vulvovaginal area (inflammation). Candida yeast is normal flora in the gastrointestinal tract.
▨ Trichomonas infection causes the vaginal discharge to be copious and bubbly. It also causes a lot of inflammation, resulting in itching and redness of the vulvovagina. It is considered a sexually transmitted infection. The sex partner also needs treatment.

ASKING THE SAME QUESTION TWICE

Discussion

A question can be used twice on the exam with some minor variations. It is unknown whether these questions are both valid or are sample questions that are being evaluated statistically. Unfortunately, there is no way to distinguish between the two. Therefore, it is best to assume that all questions in the exams are graded.

To avoid problems with these types of questions, it is best to treat both as valid. Do not automatically assume that both questions are the same. Slowly read each question so that you are able to pick out the differences between the two. The changes may seem minor, but they can completely change the meaning and answer to the question. In the following example, notice that the diagnosis is different for each question.

Example

The NP suspects that an older patient who is complaining of a headache in the right temple may have *giant cell arteritis*. A sedimentation rate is ordered. Which of the following is the expected result?

a) normal
b) borderline
c) markedly elevated
d) below normal

Example

The NP suspects that an older patient who is complaining of a headache in the right temple may have *trigeminal neuralgia*. A sedimentation rate is ordered. Which of the following is the expected result?

a) normal
b) borderline
c) markedly elevated
d) below normal

The correct answer in the first example is option c: markedly elevated. The correct answer in the second example is option a: normal.

Question Dissection

Best Clues
■ Notice that the diagnosis in each question is different (careful reading).
■ The given diagnosis is the best clue.
■ Picking the correct answer is dependent on factual memory.

Notes
■ When reading these two "similar" questions, the mind automatically assumes that it is the same question used twice. Therefore, the same answer is picked for both.
■ Get out of autopilot mode; read and compare both questions carefully.

■ Temporal arteritis is a systemic inflammatory process that affects the arteries.

■ The screening test is for the erythrocyte sedimentation rate, which is markedly elevated.

■ Trigeminal neuralgia is a headache due to local irritation, inflammation, or compression of cranial nerve V (CN 5 or the trigeminal nerve). It is not a systemic illness. Therefore, the sedimentation rate is normal.

BENIGN VARIANTS

Discussion

A benign variant is a physiologic abnormality that does not interfere with bodily process or function. There are few questions on benign variants. Some examples of the benign variants that have been seen on the exams include the geographic tongue, torus palatinus, and a split or fishtail uvula. Benign variants are listed under each organ system in chapter 3.

Example

A 32-year-old woman complains of a sore throat. On examination, the NP notices a midline bony growth on the hard palate of the mouth. The patient denies any changes or pain. It is not red, tender, or swollen. She reports a history of the growth since childhood. Which of the following conditions is most likely?

a) torus palatinus
b) geographic tongue
c) acute glossitis
d) hairy leukoplakia

The correct answer is option a: torus palatinus.

Question Dissection

Best Clues

■ A good clue is the description. A bony growth midline in the hard palate is the classic description of a torus palatinus.

■ The question describes "... a growth on the hard palate." Notice that the other clinical findings are all located on the tongue (glossitis, geographic tongue and hairy leukoplakia).

Notes

■ A torus palatinus is a benign growth (or tumor) of bone located midline on the hard palate. It is congenital and painless and does not interfere with function.

- A geographic tongue has multiple fissures on its surface and is benign. Patients may complain of a burning sensation when eating or drinking acidic foods.
- Hairy leukoplakia is pathognomic for HIV. It is not a benign variant. The name is derived from the appearance of elongated papillae that resemble dark hair on the lateral edges of the tongue.

Health Screening and Systems Review 3

HEALTH SCREENING RECOMMENDATIONS: U.S. PREVENTATIVE TASK FORCE

A. Primary Prevention (prevention of disease/injury)

Immunizations, seatbelts, airbags, and bicycle helmets
Habitat for Humanity (shelter)
Education for healthy population (i.e., exercise for students). If preexisting disease present, considered a tertiary prevention (i.e., diabetic diet).

B. Secondary Prevention (detection of disease early to minimize bodily damage)

All screening laboratory test are secondary prevention.

1. Mammography with Clinical Breast Exam

Baseline mammogram at age 35 years
- Age 40 or older: annual mammogram recommended

Higher Risk
- genetics (BRCA and BRCA 2), high breast tissue density, atypical hyperplasia (biopsy), high-dosed radiation
- personal history breast cancer, first degree relative breast cancer (mother, sister)
- Longer exposure to estrogen: early menarche, late menopause, nulliparity, age >30 years before having a child
- obesity (adipose tissue can synthesize small amounts of estrogen)

2. Pap Smear

All sexually active girls and women

- start at any age if sexually active
- virgins can start at 18 to 20 years of age

Higher Risk

- multiple sex partners (defined as > 4 lifetime partners)
- younger age onset of sex (immature cervix easier to infect)
- immunosuppressive patients and smokers

3. Prostate Specific Antigen (PSA) with Digital Rectal Exam (DRE)

Start screening all males at age 50 except those with high-risk factors

Higher Risk

- start screening earlier at age 40 years
- all Black males are at higher risk
- first degree relative (father or brother) with history of prostate cancer

4. Colon Cancer

Start screening with Hemoccult × 3 and a DRE by age 40 years

Colonoscopy: start at age 50 years if no risk factors (highest risk factor is older age)

Higher Risk (refer to gastroenterologist)

- start screening at younger ages if at higher risk
- history of familial polyposis (multiple polyps on colon)
- first degree relative with colon cancer, Crohn's disease

5. Sexually Transmitted Disease (STD) Testing

The Centers for Disease Control and Prevention (CDC) recommends screening all women between the ages of 20 to 24 years for STDs or sexually transmitted infections (STIs).

6. Tuberculosis (TB)

Purified protein derivative (PPD) or Mantoux test. Sputum cultures or chest X-rays are not used for screening. High-risk criteria discussed under TB section.

C. Tertiary Prevention (rehabilitation and avoidance of further bodily damage)

Tertiary prevention is any type of rehabilitation such as cardiac rehab, physical therapy, or speech therapy. It also consists of educational or support groups for people with pre-existing conditions such as Alcoholics Anonymous (or a group of people meeting to deal with a common problem), and education for patients with pre-existing disease (i.e., diabetes, hypertension) about how to avoid drug interactions, proper use of wheelchair or medical equipment, and so forth.

UNITED STATES HEALTH STATISTICS*

Mortality

Leading Cause of Death (all ages/gender)
■ Heart disease

Leading Cause of Death (adolescents)
■ Motor vehicle crashes

Leading Cause of Death (infants younger than 12 months)
■ Congenital anomalies

Leading Cause of Death (12 months to 9 years)
■ Unintentional injuries

Cancers

Leading Cause of Cancer Deaths
■ Lung cancer

Most Common Cancer Deaths by Gender

Males
■ Lung cancer

Females
■ Lung cancer

**Most Common Cancer and Cancer Death in Children
(ages 0–19 years)**
■ Leukemia

Most Common Cancer All Ages/Gender (prevalence only, not mortality)
■ Skin cancers (Squamous cell cancer is most common skin cancer.)

Exam Tips

■ Breast self-examination is commonly mistaken as primary prevention (it is secondary).
■ Chest X-ray is not a screening test for TB or lung cancer. Screening is not currently recommended for lung cancer because no test can detect it at an early stage.

---

* Adapted from the CDC (Centers for Disease Control) at http://www.cdc.gov/cancer/.

■ Read questions asking for mortality statistics carefully. Are they asking for the most common cause of death overall or are they asking for it by gender?

ORGAN SYSTEM REVIEW

DERMATOLOGY

Fast Facts | Danger Signals

Rocky Mountain Spotted Fever

It begins with acute onset of high fever and myalgia accompanied by a severe headache. By the 2nd to 3rd day, a petechial rash appears starting on the wrist and ankles (includes soles and palms) that spreads centrally toward the trunk and the face. Highest incidence is in the southeastern and south central areas of the United States.

Shingles Infection of the Trigeminal Nerve (ophthalmic branch)

The classic pattern and evolution of the rash is a good clue. Starts with a sudden onset of a crop of small papules that evolve into vesicles, which rupture easily and become crusted. Lesions are located over the trigeminal nerve ophthalmic branch distribution following the dermatomal pattern. The lesions are located over one side of the forehead/temple area and on the tip of the nose. Can cause corneal blindness.

Meningococcemia

Patient complains of the sudden onset of high fever, headache with a stiff neck, accompanied by nausea and/or vomiting. It is associated with petechial rashes to hemorrhagic lesions (purple color) over the entire body. Highest incidence is in college students residing in dormitories; vaccine is recommended for this population.

Erythema Migrans (early Lyme disease)

Presents as the classic round lesion (annular) that enlarges over time with central clearing (targetlike). Lesion appears from 3 to 30 days after the bite by the Ixodes tick infected with the spirochete Borrelia burgdorferi. Spontaneously resolves within a few weeks. If untreated, the infection becomes dessimated and affects many organ systems (e.g., musculoskeletal, nervous system, heart, etc.). Highest incidence is seen in the northeastern United States.

Stevens-Johnson Syndrome

Acute onset of severe vesicular to bullous lesions all over the body. They range from hives to blisters (bullae) and hemorrhagic lesions. Mucosal involvement with blisters on the conjunctiva, mouth, nares, genitals. History of current or recent antibiotic treatment with sulfas, penicillins, phenytoin, and other drugs can precede onset.

Erythema Multiforme

A milder form of Stevens-Johnson syndrome. Pink-to-red targetlike lesions, wheals, and blisters. No mucosal involvement. Look for history of antibiotic and other drug treatment such as sulfa drugs, penicillins, and other drugs.

Melanoma

Dark-colored moles with uneven texture, mixed colors, and irregular borders. May be pruritic. If melanoma is located in the nailbeds (ungual melanoma), it is usually more aggressive. Lesions can be located anywhere on the body including in the retina. Higher incidence in patients with a family history of melanoma.

Actinic Keratoses

Precursor lesion of squamous cell carcinoma appears as dry, red lesions with a rough texture. Lesions have been present for several years and slowly enlarge and do not heal. Located in sun-exposed areas of skin such as the cheeks, nose, face, neck, arms, and back. Diagnosed by skin biopsy and clinical appearance. More common in light-skinned individuals.

Fast Facts | Normal Findings

Anatomy of the Skin

Three layers: epidermis, dermis, and the subcutaneous layer
Epidermis: no blood vessels; gets nourishment from the dermis
Epidermis (two layers): topmost layer consists of keratinized cells (dead squamous epithelial cells); bottom layer is where melanocytes reside and vitamin D synthesis occurs
Dermis: blood vessels, sebaceous glands, and hair follicles
Subcutaneous layer: fat, sweat glands, and hair follicles

Vitamin D Synthesis

People with darker skin need longer periods of sun exposure to produce vitamin D. A deficiency of vitamin D in pregnancy results in infantile rickets (brittle bones, skeletal abnormalities).

Skin Lesion Review

- Bulla: elevated superficial blister filled with serous fluid and greater than 1 cm in size
- Example: second degree burns

- Vesicle: elevated superficial skin lesion less than 1 cm in diameter and filled with serous fluid
- Example: herpetic lesions

- Pustule: elevated superficial skin lesion smaller than 1 cm in diameter filled with purulent fluid
- Example: acne pustules

- Macule: flat nonpalpable lesion smaller than 1 cm in diameter
- Example: freckles, lentigines

- Papule: palpable solid lesion up to 0.5 cm
- Example: acne

- Plaque: flattened elevated lesions with variable shape that are more than 1 cm in diameter
- Example: psoriatic lesions

Fast Facts   Benign Variants

Lipoma

Benign fatty, cystic tumors located in the subcutaneous layer of the skin. Round-to-oval shape. Sizes vary and are located mostly on the neck, trunk, legs, and arms. Painless unless it becomes too large, irritated, or ruptured.

Melasma (mask of pregnancy)

Brown-to-tan stains located on the upper cheeks and forehead in some women who have been or are pregnant or are on oral contraceptive pills. More common in darker-skinned women. Stains are usually permanent and usually become lighter in color over time.

Nevi (moles)

Round macules to papules (junctional nevi) in colors ranging from light tan to dark brown. Borders may be distinct or slightly irregular. Atypical nevi at higher risk for melanoma.

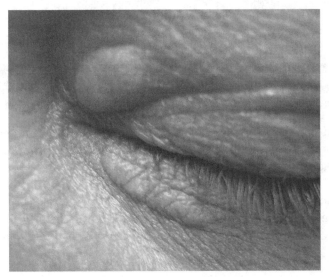

Figure 3.1. Xanthelasma

Seborrheic Keratoses

Soft and round wartlike fleshy growths on the trunk located mostly on the back. Lesions on the same person can range in color from light tan to black. Onset usually starts after the age of 50 years. Painless unless a lesion becomes irritated.

Vitiligo

Hypopigmented patches of skin with irregular shapes. Progressive and can involve large areas. Can be located anywhere on the body. More visible on darker skin.

Xanthelasma

Raised and yellow soft plaques that are located under the brow on the upper and/or lower lids of the eyes on the nasal side. May be a sign of hyperlipidemia if present in persons younger than 40 years of age.

Xerosis

Inherited skin disorder resulting in extremely dry skin. May involve mucosal surfaces such as the mouth (xerostomia) or the conjunctiva of the eye (xerophthalmia).

Fast Facts Topical Steroids

■ Avoid steroids if viral etiology is suspected because they will worsen the infection.

■ Do not use fluorinated topical steroids on infants, children, and facial skin (thin skin); use 0.5% to 1% hydrocortisone.

- Topical steroids: hypothalamus-pituitary-adrenal axis (HPA) suppression, striae, skin atrophy, telangiectasia, acne, and hypopigmentation.

Fast Facts | Disease Review

Psoriasis

An inherited skin disorder in which squamous epithelial cells undergo rapid mitotic division and maturation. The rapid turnover of skin produces the classic psoriatic plaque.

Special Findings
Koebner phenomenon: new psoriatic plaques form over areas of skin trauma
Auspitz sign: pinpoint areas of bleeding remain in the skin when a plaque is removed

Classic Case
Complaints of pruritic erythematous plaques covered with fine silvery white scales and pitted fingernails and toenails. The plaques are distributed in the scalp, elbows, knees, sacrum, and in the intergluteal folds. Patients with psoriatic arthritis complain of painful red, warm, and swollen joints (migratory arthritis).

Medications
Topical steroids and tar preparations (Psoralen drugs). Systemic drugs such as antimetabolites (i.e., methotrexate) are used for severe forms of the disease. Goeckerman regimen (UVB light and tar-derived topicals) may induce remission in severe cases.

Complications
Guttate psoriasis (drop-shaped lesions): rare form of psoriasis resulting from a beta-hemolytic streptococcus Group A infection (usually due to strep throat).

Actinic Keratosis

Precancerous lesions that are precursors to squamous cell carcinoma and caused by chronic sun exposure. Most commonly seen in older White patients with a history of long-term sun exposure, especially those with frequent episodes of sunburn during early childhood (before age 18 years).

Classic Case
Described under the "Danger Signals" section.

Medications
If only a small number of lesions, can be treated with cryotherapy. If larger numbers, fluorouracil cream 5% (5-FU cream), a topical antineoplastic agent, is used over several weeks.

Tinea Versicolor

A superficial skin infection caused by the yeasts *pityrosporum orbiculare* and *pityrosporum ovale.* Lesions appear as round macules that vary in color from flesh tones to hypo- or hyperpigmentation. The most common locations are on the face, shoulders, chest, and back.

Labs
Potassium hydroxide (KOH) slide: hyphae and spores ("spaghetti and meatballs")

Medications
Topical selenium sulfide or ketoconazole (Nizoral) shampoo or cream applied to affected areas twice daily (BID) × 2 weeks.

Eczema (atopic dermatitis)

A chronic inherited skin disorder marked by extremely pruritic rashes that are located on the hands, flexural folds, and the neck (older child to adults). The rashes are exacerbated by stress and environmental factors (e.g., allergens, cold and dry climate, etc.). This disorder is associated with other atopic disorders such as asthma or allergic rhinitis, and a positive family history (genetic factor).

Classic Case
Infants up to the age of 2 years have a larger area of rash distribution compared with teens and adults. The rashes are typically found on the cheeks, entire trunk, knees, and elbows.

Older children and adults have rashes on the hands, neck, and antecubital and popliteal spaces (flexural folds). The classic rash starts as multiple small vesicles that rupture, leaving painful bright red weepy lesions. The lesions become lichenified from chronic itching and can persist for months. Fissures form that can become secondarily infected with bacteria.

Medications
Topical steroids, systemic oral antihistamines, and skin lubricants (Eucerin, Keri Lotion, baby oil). Avoid drying skin (e.g., hot water baths, harsh detergents, chemicals, and wool clothing).

Contact Dermatitis

An inflammatory skin reaction that is due to contact from an irritating external substance. Lesions range from localized lesions to generalized rashes (e.g., seabather's itch). Common offenders are poison ivy (rhus dermatitis), nickle, latex, and others. Onset may occur within minutes to hours after contact.

Classic Case
New rashes are bright red and pruritic. The rashes rapidly evolve into bullous or vesicular lesions that easily rupture, leaving bright red moist and weepy areas that

are tender. Later, the rash becomes dried and crusty. Chronic scratching results in skin lichenification.

A classic finding to look for is the shape (linear or unusually shaped rash) and the asymmetric distribution (may only have one rash compared to eczema).

Medications

Topical steroids. Wet compresses to dry weeping lesions. Calamine lotion and oatmeal baths.

Generalized severe rash: oral prednisone for 12 to 14 days (wean). Avoid re-exposure.

Candidiasis

Superficial skin infection from the yeast *Candida albicans*. Environmental factors promoting overgrowth are increased warmth and humidity. Other factors associated with infections are decreased immunity states and diabetes mellitus.

Classic Case (infants)

Manifests either as diaper rash or oral thrush. Diaper rash is a bright red color with small, red, round lesions in the periphery (satellite lesions) that may burn.

Oral thrush: infant will have a sore throat and feed poorly with more frequent bouts of crying. Adherent white plaques with a red base (that are hard to remove) are seen on the pharynx. Treat diaper rash with Nystatin cream or use oral suspension for oral thrush.

Thrush in toddlers and adults may be seen with chronic steroid use (oral or inhaler form). Frequent episodes of candidiasis may signal human immunodeficiency virus (HIV) infection.

Acute Cellulitis

An acute skin infection caused by Gram-positive bacteria (rarely Gram-negative). Points of entry are skin breaks such as insect bites or abrasions, surgical wounds, and so forth. Infections range from local superficial infections to more serious deeper skin infections that may be life threatening. Usually caused by Gram-positive bacteria such as *Staphylococcus aureus* and *Streptococcus pyogenes*/beta strep group A.

Dog and Cat bites: *Pasteurella multocida* (Gram-negative)

Classic Case

Acute onset of diffused pink-to-red skin on the site of skin trauma that enlarges over the next several days. Infected skin will become indurated, swollen, and tender. Deeper infection of the skin is manifested by red streaks radiating from infected area under the skin secondary to infection of the lymphatic chains.

Labs

If discharge is present, order skin culture and sensitivity (C&S); if fever is present order complete blood count (CBC).

Medications

Dicloxacillin PO (orally) three times daily (TID) × 10 days (good choice if high rate of beta-lactam resistance). Cephalexin (Keflex) PO × 10 days (not active against beta-lactamase–resistant bacteria). Tetanus (Td) booster if last dose was more than 5 years ago. If penicillin-allergic, use a macrolide such as erythromycin, a cephalosporin, clindamycin, or quinolones that have gram-positive coverage such as levaquinolone (Levaquin) if patient is over the age of 18 years (contraindicated in children).

Complications

Osteomyelitis, tendon and fascial extension, and sepsis.

Erysipelas

A subtype of cellulitis involving deeper tissue involvement caused by beta strep.

Classic Case

Complaints of acne or insect bite that become infected. The lesion evolves into a raised and indurated bright pink plaque with a distinct raised edge. The plaque is usually located on the cheeks or lower legs.

Bites: Human and Animal

Human Bites

The "dirtiest" bite of all. Watch for closed-fist injuries of the hands (may involve tendon damage and joint capsule damage).

Dog and Cat Bites

Infected with *Pasteurella multocida*. Cat bites are more likely to be infected than dog bites.

Bat, Raccoon, or Skunk Bites

Do not forget to rule out rabies in addition to antibiotic treatment. Call local public health department and the CDC (1-800-CDC – INFO).

Treatment: Bites (human or animal)

- Amoxicillin/clavulanic (Augmentin) PO × 10 days (penicillin allergy, use clindamycin plus fluoroquinolone)
- Wound C&S testing if suspect infection
- Do not suture infected wounds or puncture wounds

- Tetanus prophylaxis (if last booster >5 years, needs booster)
- Certain animal bites (dog, cat, bat, raccoon, and skunk) may require rabies immunoglobulin plus rabies vaccine if animal suspected of being rabid
- Follow-up patient within 12 to 24 hours after treatment

Hidradenitis Suppurativa

A bacterial infection of the sebaceous glands of the axilla (or groin) by Gram-positive *Staphylococcus aureus*. Marked by flare-ups and resolution. The infection can involve one or both axillae. Chronic episodes of infection eventually leave sinus tracts and heavy scarring.

Classic Case
Complaints of an acute onset of painful red nodules and pustules under one or both axillae. The patient reports that some of the lumps start to drain pus. History of recurrent episodes.

Objective Findings
Affected axillae with large dark red nodules and pustules that are indurated. Some of the pustules fluctuate and rupture draining green purulent discharge (pus).

Labs
A C&S of purulent discharge.

Medications
Amoxicillin/clavulanate (Augmentin) PO BID or dicloxacillin TID × 10 days. No underarm deodorants. Muciprocin ointment to lower third of nares and under fingernails BID × 2 weeks to eliminate sources of infection (patient may be a carrier of the bacteria).

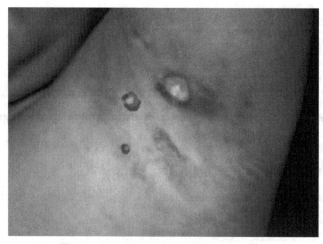

Figure 3.2. Hidradenitis Suppurativa

Impetigo

Acute bacterial superficial skin infection caused by Gram-positive bacteria such as *Streptococcus pyogenes* (beta strep) or *Staphylococcus aureus*. Very contagious and pruritic. More common in children and during warm and humid weather. Two types: bullous and nonbullous.

Classic Case

Complaints of an acute onset of pruritic pink-to-red maculopapular rashes and/or bullae that are covered with honey-colored crusts (dried serous fluid). History of traumatized areas of skin such as insect bites, acne, scratches, chicken pox, and so forth.

Labs

A C&S of the skin lesions.

Medications

Cephalexin (Keflex) QID, dicloxacillin QID × 10 days. If PCN allergic: Azithromycin 250 mg × 5 days (macrolides), clindamycin × 10 days. If few lesions with no bullae, topical 2% Muciprocin ointment (Bacitracin) × 10 days. Frequent handwashing, shower/bath daily to remove crusts.

Meningococcemia

A serious life-threatening infection caused by *Neisseria meningitidis* (Gram-negative diplococci) that is spread by respiratory droplets. College students living in dormitories are at higher risk. Associated with 20% mortality. If treated early, mortality is less than 5%. The bodily damage is due to endotoxin's effects on the endothelium of the blood vessels.

Classic Case

Described under the "Danger Signals" section.

Prophylaxis

Close contacts must be given oral antibiotic rifampin. Meningococcal vaccination recommended by the CDC for college students living in dormitories.

Labs

Lumbar punctures: culture cerebrospinal fluid (CSF).
Blood cultures, throat cultures, and computed tomography (CT) or magnetic resonance imaging (MRI) of the brain.

Medications

Systemic penicillin × 10 days; ceftriaxone (Rocephin) × 5 days if penicillin-allergic.
Hospital; high-dosed antibiotics, isolation precautions.

Complications
Tissue infarction and necrosis (e.g., gangrene of the toes, foot, fingers, etc.) causing amputation. Death.

Early Lyme Disease

Erythrema migrans is a skin lesion caused by the bite of an Ixodes tick infected with *Borrelia burgdorferi*. If untreated, infection becomes systemic and affects multiple organ systems.

Classic Case
Described under "Danger Signals" section.

Labs
Serum antibody titers immunoglobulin (Ig)M (early) and IgG (late).

Treatment
Early Lyme disease: doxycycline BID or tetracycline × 14 days (amoxicillin if pregnant).

Complications
Neurological system problems such as Guillain-Barré syndrome, migratory arthritis, chronic fatigue, and so forth.

Rocky Mountain Spotted Fever

Caused by the bite of a tick that is infected with the parasite *Rickettsia rickettsii*. The mortality rate ranges from 1 to 7% if untreated.

Classic Case
Described under "Danger Signals" section.

Labs
A CBC with white cell count, liver function test, CSF, antibody titers, skin biopsy of lesion.

Medications
Doxycycline BID or tetracycline four times daily (QID) × 21 days.

Complications
Death

Herpes Zoster (Shingles)

Reactivation of the varicella zoster virus (or herpes zoster virus). After an initial varicella/chicken pox infection, the virus becomes latent in a dermatome and is kept under control by an intact immune system. The elderly and immunocompromised are at higher risk for shingle breakouts and postherpetic neuralgia.

Classic Case

Complaints of sudden onset of groups of small vesicles on a red base, following linear pattern (dermatomal) on one side of the body. The vesicles rupture easily and are crusty when dry. If prodrome present, may complain of severe pain or itching or burning sensation on the site of the breakout.

Labs

Serum antibody titers IgM and IgG if not sure of diagnosis.

Medications

Acyclovir (Zovirax) five times a day or Valacyclovir (Valtrex) BID × 10 days for initial breakouts and 7 days for flare-ups.

Complications

Postherpetic neuralgia: more common in elderly and immunocompromised patients.

Treat with tricyclic antidepressants (low-dose amitriptyline) or anticonvulsants (Depakote) at bedtime. Infection on cranial nerve V (trigeminal nerve ophthalmic branch) can result in corneal blindness. Refer immediately to ophthalmologist or emergency room (described under the "Danger Signals" section).

Pityriasis Rosea

Cause unknown. Self-limiting illness (4–5 weeks) and asymptomatic.

Classic Case

Complaints of oval lesions with fine scales that follow skin lines (cleavage lines) of the trunk or a "Christmas tree" pattern of papulosquamous lesions.

"Herald patch": first lesion to appear and largest in size. Appears 2 weeks before full breakout.

Medications

No medications. Advise patient that lesions will take about 4 weeks to resolve. If high-risk sexually active adolescent or adult, check rapid plasma reagin (RPR) to rule out secondary syphilis.

Scabies

An infestation of the skin by the *Sarcoptes scabiei* mite. The female mite burrows under the skin to lay her eggs. Transmitted by close contact.

Table 3.1 Common Skin Rashes

Disease	Description
Impetigo	"Honey-colored" crusts. Fragile bulla.
Measles	Koplik's spots
Scabies	Very pruritic, especially at night. Interdigital webs, waist, axillae, etc.
Scarlet fever	"Sandpaper" rash with sore throat (strep throat)
Tinea versicolor	Hypopigmented round-to-oval shaped macular rashes located on the shoulders and the back—"Sunspots"
Pityriasis rosea	"Christmas tree" pattern rash; "Herald patch"
Molluscum contagiosum	Smooth papules 5 mm size that are dome-shaped with central umbilication with white plug
Erythema migrans	Red target lesions that expand and grow in size. Early stage of Lyme disease.
Meningococcemia	Purple-colored painful skin lesions all over body. Reportable disease. Rifampin prophylaxis. Close contacts.
Rocky Mountain Spotted Fever	From bite of tick infected with Rickettsia Rickettsii. Round red rashes with petechiae, maculopapular headache (HA) & fever. Reportable disease.

(*Note:* Rashes in italics are life-threatening)

Classic Case
Complaints of pruritic rashes located in the interdigital webs, axillae, buttock folds, waist, and the penis. The itching is worse at nighttime and interferes with sleep. Other family members may also have the same symptoms.

Objective Findings
The rash appears as serpiginous (snakelike) or linear burrows. Lesions can be papular, vesicular, or crusted. Higher incidence in crowded conditions (e.g., nursing homes) and in the homeless population.

Labs
Scrape burrow or scales with glass slide, use coverslip. Look for mites or eggs.

Medications
Permethrin 5% (Elimite): apply cream to entire body and head; wash off after 8 to 14 hours.

Must treat entire household. Wash linens and clothes in hot water.

Alternative: lindane (Kwell); remove in 8 to12 hours (contraindicated in pregnancy, infants, toddlers, seizure disorder). Out of favor as treatment due to neurotoxicity.

Tinea Infections (dermatophytoses)

An infection of superficial keratinized tissue (skin, hair, and nails) by tinea yeast organisms.

Labs
KOH slide of scales, hair, and nails (hyphae and spores); fungal cultures.

Medications
Topical azoles: over the counter (OTC) clotrimazole, miconazole. Terconazole (Terazole) is a prescription topical antifungal. Systemic oral antifungals: ketonazole, fluconazole (Diflucan) weekly for 6 months (pulse therapy). Antifungals have numerous drug interactions (warfarin, anticonvulsants, etc.). Hepatotoxic. Baseline liver function tests.

Tinea capitis (scalp)

More common in Black children. Patchy alopecia with "black dots" (broken hair shaft) and fragile hair shaft. Fine scales on scalp. Frequent itching of the scalp.

Medications
Treat only with oral systemic antifungals such as griseofulvin (Fulvicin) for several weeks.

Complications
Kerion: inflammatory lesions secondary to tinea capitis infection that permanently damage hair follicles, causing patchy alopecia.

Tinea pedis (athlete's foot)

Two types: scaly and dry form or moist type (strong odor). Moist lesions between toe webs that are white with strong unpleasant odor. Dry type with fine scales only.

Tinea corporis or Tinea circinata (ringworm of the body)

Ringlike pruritic rashes with a collarette of fine scales that slowly enlarges and some central clearing. Large numbers or severe cases can also be treated with oral antifungals.

Tinea cruris (jock itch)

Perineal and groin area with pruritic red rashes with fine scales. May be mistaken for candidal infection (bright red rashes with satellite lesions) or intertrigo (bright red diffused rash caused by a bacterial infection).

Tinea manuum (hands)

Pruritic round rashes with fine scales on the hands. Usually infected from chronic scratching of foot that is also infected with tinea (athlete's foot).

Tinea barbae (beard area)

Beard area affected. Scaling with pruritic red rashes.

Onychomycosis (nails)

Nail becomes yellowed, thickened, and opaque with debris. Nail may separate from nailbed (onycholysis). Great toe is the most common location.

Labs
Fungal cultures.

Medications
Oral itraconazole or terbinafine (Lamisil) for several weeks.
Mild cases: Ciclopirox 8% topical solution (Penlac) nail lacquer for several months. Works best in mild cases of the fingernails.

Acne Vulgaris (common acne)

Inflammation and infection of the sebaceous glands. Multifactorial causes such as high androgen levels, bacterial infection, and genetic influences. Found mostly on the face, shoulders, chest, and the back. Highest incidence in puberty and adolescence.

Mild Acne

Open comedones (blackheads) and closed comedones with small papules. Treat using topicals only. Benzoyl peroxide, erythromycin solution, or retinoic acid (Retin A) gel or cream.

Retin A photosensitivity reaction possible (use sunscreen).

Moderate Acne

Same as mild acne plus large numbers of papules and pustules. Treat with topicals plus oral tetracycline (category D) or minocycline (Minocin).

Tetracyclines: permanent discoloration of growing tooth enamel. Do not use if patient is younger than age 18. Tetracycline decreases effectiveness of oral contraceptives (use additional method).

Severe Cystic Acne

All of the moderate acne findings plus painful indurated nodules and cysts over face, shoulders, and chest.

Medications

Isotretinoin (Accutane) is a category X drug (extremely teratogenic). Curently, dispensed only by physicians. Patients need to sign special consent forms. Females must use two forms of reliable contraception and show two negative pregnancy tests before starting drug. Prescribe 1-month supply only. Monthly pregnancy testing results shown to pharmacist before refills. Pregnancy test 1 month after discontinued. Discontinue if the following are present: severe depression, visual disturbance, hearing loss, tinnitus, GI pain, rectal bleeding, uncontrolled hyper-triglyceremia, pancreatitis, or hepatitis.

Rosacea (Acne Rosacea)

Cause is unknown.

Classic Case

Complaints of chronic, small acnelike papules and pustules that erupt around the nose, mouth, and chin, which become exacerbated episodically. Seen mostly in adults to elderly with Celtic background (e.g., Irish, Scottish) with pale skin, blue eyes, and red-to-blond hair; more likely to blush with spicy foods and alcohol.

Medications

Metronidazole gel and/or oral tetracycline for several months.

Complications

Rhinophyma: hyperplasia of tissue at the tip of the nose from chronic severe disease.

Cheilosis

Skin fissures and maceration at each corner of the mouth. Multiple causes such as oversalivation, iron deficiency anemia, bacterial infection, vitamin deficiencies, and so forth.

Treat underlying cause. Apply triple antibiotic ointment BID to TID until healed.

Burns

First degree (superficial thickness)

Erythema only (no blisters). Painful. Cleanse with mild soap and water (or saline).

Cold packs for 24 to 48 hours. Topical OTC anesthetics such as benzocaine if desired.

Second Degree (partial thickness)

Red skin with superficial blisters (bullae). Painful. Use water with mild soap or normal saline to clean broken skin (not hydrogen peroxide or full strength Betadine). Do not rupture blisters. Treat with silver sulfadiazine cream (Silvadene) and apply dressings.

Third Degree (full thickness)

Painless. Entire skin layer, subcutaneous area, and soft tissue facia may be destroyed. Medicate for pain before debridement. Daily debridement to remove dead tissue. Treat with silver sulfadiazine cream (Silvadene) and apply dressings. Refer for facial burns, electrical burns, third degree burns, cartilaginous areas such as the nose and ears (cartilage will not regenerate). Burns over more than 10% of body.

Exam Tips

- Differentiate between contact dermatitis and atopic dermatitis. The best clue is the unilateral location and the shape of the lesions in contact dermatitis.
- A rash that is very pruritic at night and located on the interdigital webs and/or penis is scabies until proven otherwise.
- The dirtiest bite wound is the human bite.
- If allergic to penicillin, may also be allergic to cephalosporins (cross-reactivity of 10%). Instead, use macrolides such as azithromycin (Zithromax) or erythromycin.
- Do not confuse actinic keratosis (precursor to squamous cell cancer) with seborrheic keratoses (benign).
- Learn definition of bullae.
- Learn diagnoses for hidradenitis suppurativa, psoriasis, Rocky Mountain spotted fever, meningococcemia, Stevens-Johnson, contact dermatitis, rosacea.
- Instead of silvery scales, may see "covered with fine scales" with psoriasis.
- Psoralens (tar-derived topicals) used to treat psoriasis, antimetabolite (methotrexate).
- Working in oily environments (e.g., fast food cook) does not cause acne.
- Mild acne is treated only with topicals, not tetracycline. If the patient with moderate acne has been previously treated with topicals with no response, pick tetracycline as the next step.
- Accutane use in females: must use two forms of reliable birth control. Currently, it can only be prescribed by physicians with special training.
- "Herald patch" or a "Christmas tree pattern" is found in Pityriasis rosea.
- Postherpetic neuralgia prophylaxis: tricyclic antidepressants (TCA) amitriptyline (Elavil).
- A clue in a case scenario on cellulitis may be a patient walking barefoot, causing skin trauma.

- If beta strep group B infection in cellulitis, patient is also at risk for developing postglomerular nephritis as seen in strep throat. Treat for 10 days with a penicillin or macrolide.

Clinical Tips

- Use ophthalmic grade/sterile cream/ointments for rashes near the eyes.
- Pruritus may persist up to 2 weeks even after successful treatment of scabies.
- Human and cat bites are more likely to become infected compared with dog bites.
- On thin skin such as the facial and intertriginous areas (skin folds), use low potency topical steroids (e.g., hydrocortisone 1%). On thicker skin such as the scalp, back, or soles, may use higher potency steroids.
- Elavil is very sedating; give at bedtime.
- Antivirals (e.g., Zovirax) are most effective if given within 72 hours after onset of virus.

HEAD, EYES, EARS, NOSE, AND THROAT

Fast Facts | Danger Signals

Eyes

Herpes Keratitis
Damage to corneal epithelium caused by herpes virus infection usually from shingles. Complaints of eye pain, photophobia, and blurred vision in the affected eye. Diagnosed by using fluorescein dye strips with a black lamp in darkened room. Appears as fernlike lines. In contrast, corneal abrasions appear more linear.

Acute Closed-Angle Glaucoma
Elderly patient complains of acute onset of severe eye pain accompanied by headache, photophobia, nausea and/or vomiting, and blurred vision.

Periorbital Cellulitis
A child with a history of sinus infection has an acute onset of edema and redness in the periorbital area. Abnormal extraorbital muscles exam. Complains of double vision (diplopia). Accompanied by high fever, chills, and toxicity.

Ears, Nose, and Sinus

Battle's Sign
Fractures of the basilar area of the skull can present as bruising over the mastoid(s).

Look for clear golden fluid draining from the nose and/or ear. Testing the fluid with a urine dipstick will reveal if it is positive for glucose. A bruised area may be present over the mastoid area. Caused by trauma to the skull (from a motor vehicle crash, etc.).

Cholesteatoma
"Cauliflower-like" growth with foul-smelling discharge from an ear. On exam, there is no visibile tympanic membrane or ossicles (destroyed). If not removed, can erode into skull and the facial nerve (CN 7). A complication from chronic otitis media infections. Treated with antibiotics and surgical removal of the mass.

Cavernous Sinus Thrombosis
Classic finding are ophthalmoplegia, proptosis, chemosis, and Horner's syndrome. The cavernous sinus contains CN 3, 4, and 6 (EOMs), carotid artery and veins. Abnormal EOM exam. Caused by a blood clot in the cavernous sinus. Unusual life-threatening complication usually from a sinus or ear infection.

Pharynx

Peritonsillar Abscess
Complaints of severe sore throat and difficulty swallowing on one side of the throat. One tonsil is swollen and indurated and appears as a bulging red mass. The uvula is displaced away from the mass. Accompanied by systemic signs such as fever and chills.

Diphtheria
Complaints of severe sore throat and dysphagia. The posterior pharynx and respiratory tract are coated with a gray-to-yellow pseudomembrane that is hard to displace. Accompanied by systemic symptoms. Infection caused by corynebacterium diphtheriae (gram positive rod) that produces an exotoxin that affects heart, kidneys, and nerves. Rare in the United States.

Fast Facts Normal Findings

Eyes

Fundi: the veins are larger than arteries
Cones: for color perception
Rods: for detecting light, depth perception
Macula and fovea: central vision

Ears

Tympanic membranes: translucent off-white to gray with the "cone of light" landmark.

Tympanogram: most objective measure for presence of fluid inside middle ear.

Nose

Usually, only the inferior nasal turbinates are visible if not using a nasal speculum. Lower third of the nose is cartilage. Cartilage tissue does not regenerate. Injuries should be referred to a plastic surgeon.

Mouth

Tonsils may have "crypts" or small porelike openings that can have exudate with infections.

Posterior pharynx: Look for postnasal drip (acute sinusitis, allergic rhinitis).

Fast Facts Benign Variants

Torus palatinus

Painless bony protuberance located midline on the hard palate.

Fishtail or split uvula

Uvula is split into two sections ranging from partial to complete. Rule out occult cleft palate.

Nystagmus

A few beats of *horizontal nystagmus* on prolonged extreme-lateral gaze that resolve when the eye moves back toward midline is normal. Vertical nystagmus is always abnormal.

Fast Facts Abnormal Findings

Papilledema

Optic disc swollen with blurred edges caused by increased intracranial pressure (ICP) because of brain tumor, abscess, or pseudotumor cerebri.

Hypertensive retinopathy

Copper and silver wire arterioles.

Diabetic retinopathy

Microvascularization and microaneurysms.

Cataracts

- Opacity of the corneas.

Koplik spots

Measles: small, white papules on a red base with bluish-white centers inside the cheeks by the lower molars.

Hairy leukoplakia

Elongated dark-colored papillae on the lateral aspects of the tongue. Rule out HIV (human immunodeficiency virus) infection.

Leukoplakia of the tongue

A bright, white plaque usually located on the lateral edges of the tongue. Can be benign to cancerous.

Vocabulary

- Buccal mucosa: mucosal lining inside the mouth
- Palpebral conjunctiva: mucosal lining inside eyelids
- Bulbar conjunctiva: mucosal lining covering the eyes
- Hard palate: the "roof of the mouth"

Evaluation and Testing

Visual Tests

- Distance vision: use the Snellen chart to measure central distance vision.
- Near vision: use a newspaper to test.
- Peripheral vision: examine by using the "visual fields of confrontation" exam. Performed by using examiner's fingers to approach patient's peripheral line of vision. Slowly move the fingers forward until the patient can see them. Look for blind spots (scotoma).
- Color blindness: use the Ishihara chart.

Visual Test Results

Definition of a Snellen test result 20/60

- Top number (or numerator): the number of feet the patient stands away from the Snellen or picture eye chart (always at 20 ft and never changes)
- Bottom number (or denominator): the number of feet that the patient can see compared with a person with normal vision (20/20 or less). Number changes,

dependent on patient's vision. In this example, the patient can see at 20 ft what a person with normal vision can see at 60 ft.

Legal blindness: defined as a distance vision of 20/200.

Hearing Tests

Weber test

- Place the tuning fork midline on the forehead.
- Normal finding: no lateralization. If lateralization (hearing the sound in only one ear) occurs, the result is abnormal.

Rinne test

- Place tuning fork first on mastoid process; then front of the ear. Time each area.
- Normal finding: air conduction lasts longer than bone conduction.

Fast Facts | Disease Review

Herpes Keratitis

Damage to corneal epithelium caused by herpes virus infection, usually shingles.

Classic Case
Complaints of acute onset of eye pain, photophobia, and blurred vision in the affected eye. Look for a herpetic rash of the side of the temple and on the tip of the nose.

Labs
Use fluorescein dye strips with a black lamp in darkened room. Appears as fernlike lines. In contrast, corneal abrasions appear more linear.

Medications
Treated by ophthalmologist with high doses of Zovirax or Valtrex BID until resolved. No steroid ophthalmic drops (will worsen it).

Plan
- Refer to ophthalmologist immediately or to ER.

Hordeolum (stye)

A painful acute bacterial infection of a hair follicle on the eyelid.

Classic Case

Complaints of an itchy eyelid and an acute onset of a red papule or pustule on either upper or lower eyelid.

Medications

Antibiotic drops or ointment (e.g., sulfa drops, gentamicin gtts, etc.).

Plan

■ Warm packs BID to TID until abscess drains.

Chalazion

A chronic inflammation of the meibomian gland (specialized sweat gland on the eyelids).

Classic Case

Complaints of a gradual onset of a small nodule that moves under the skin of the eyelid and feels like a bead. Painless. May slowly enlarge over time.

Plan

■ If nodule enlarges or does not resolve in a few weeks, obtain a biopsy to rule out squamous cell cancer. If large sized and affects vision, surgical removal is an option.

Pinguecula

A yellow, triangular thickening of the bulbar conjunctiva (skin covering eyeball). Located on both the inner and outer margins of the cornea. Caused by chronic sun exposure.

Pterygium

A yellow, triangular thickening of the conjunctiva located either on the nasal or temporal cornea. Caused by chronic sun exposure resulting in UV-damage.

Plan (both pinguecula and pterygium)

■ Recommend use of good quality sunglasses. Growth can be removed surgically if it starts to encroach over iris and affect vision. If inflamed, short-term steroid eyedrops may be useful.

Subconjunctival Hemorrhage

Hemorrhage of blood that is trapped between the conjunctive and sclera of the eye due to broken arterioles from trauma or force.

Classic Case
Complaints of sudden onset of bright red blood on the eye that does not impede vision and is painless. Event preceded by severe coughing, sneezing, trauma. Higher risk if on aspiriin or warfarin (Coumadin). The trapped blood slowly changes color over a period of weeks from dark red, green, and then yellow until it resolves.

Plan
■ Watchful waiting and reassure patient. Follow up until resolution.

Primary Open-angle Glaucoma

Gradual onset of increased intraocular pressure (IOP) due to blockage of drainage of the aqueous humor. The optic nerve (CN 2) undergoes ischemic damage resulting in permanent visual loss. Most common type of glaucoma (60–70%).

Classic Case
Complaints of gradual loss of peripheral vision (lost first). Results in permanent blindness if not treated. Most commonly seen in elderly patients, especially those of African background or diabetics.

Labs
Tonometer: normal range IOP: 10 to 22 mmHg

Medications
Betimol (timolol): Beta-blocker eyedrops lower IOP. Side effects and contraindications same as oral form (bronchospasm, fatigue, depression, heart failure, and bradycardia). Contraindicated: asthma, emphysema, chronic obstructive pulmonary disease (COPD), 2nd to 3rd degree heart block, heart failure.

Plan
■ Refer patient to ophthalmologist.

Complication
Blindness

Primary Closed-angle Glaucoma

Sudden blockage of aqueous humor causes markedly increased IOP causing ischemia and permanent loss of vision.

Classic Case
Older patient complains of acute onset of severe frontal headache or eye pain accompanied by blurred vision and tearing. Reports seeing halos around lights. May be accompanied by severe nausea and vomiting.

Objective Findings
Pupils: fixed and mid-dilated and appears cloudy; pupil looks more oval than round. Conjunctival injection with an increase in lacrimation.

Plan
■ Refer to ER.

Macular Degeneration

Gradual changes in the pigment in the macula (area of central vision) results in blindness. Cause is unknown. Leading cause of blindness in the elderly in the United States. More common in elderly smokers. Two types: atrophic (dry form) and exudative (wet form).

Classic Case
Elderly smoker complains of a gradual or sudden painless loss of central vision. During the early phase, the patient will notice a distortion in central vision. Peripheral vision is preserved even with the profound loss of central vision.

Labs
Check central vision with Amsler Grid test the lines in the center of the grid are distorted. (See Figure 3.3).

Increase intake of antioxidants (vitamins C and E, beta-carotene, zinc) and the herbs lutein and bilberry. Refer to ophthalmologist.

Allergic Rhinitis

Chronic inflammatory reaction of the nasal mucosa secondary to exposure to allergens.

Seasonal or daily symptoms.

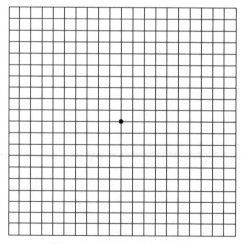

Figure 3.3. Amsler Grid*

---

* Adapted from an illustration by the National Eye Institute, National Institute of Health

Classic Case
Complaints of constant nasal congestion with clear mucus discharge accompanied by nasal itch and sneezing episodes. Coughing from postnasal drip worsens when supine.

Objective Findings
Nose: bluish and pale with boggy nasal turbinates. Postnasal drip with clear mucus.

Medications
Nasal steroid sprays daily (e.g., fluticasone or Flonase). Nedocromil sodium (Intal) nasal spray QID, works better for children. Zyrtec 10 mg daily or as needed (PRN) up to one time daily. May combine with decongestants (e.g., pseudoephedrine or Sudafed) PRN.

Complications
Acute sinusitis
Acute otitis media (AOM)

Epistaxis (nosebleeds)

Most nosebleeds in children and adults originate from the anterior lower one third of the nose that has a rich supply of small veins and arteries (Kiesselbach's plexus). Nosebleeds can be spontaneous or secondary to trauma. Posterior nasal bleeds can result in hemorrhage. Patients taking aspirin, using cocaine, having severe hypertension, or taking anticoagulants are at higher risk.

Classic Case
A school-age child complains of acute onset of nasal bleeding from "picking the nose" or frequent nasal blowing secondary to nasal congestion. Bright red blood is seen draining from one nare and sometimes on the posterior pharynx.

Plan
- Patient is sitting and leans forward. Apply pressure over nasal bridge for several minutes. Nasal decongestants (e.g., Afrin) to shrink tissue. Antibiotic prophylaxis for staph and strep PRN for severe cases.

Complication
Posterior nasal bleeds may hemorrhage (refer to ER).

Common Cold

A mild viral upper respiratory infection caused by up to 200 different types of viruses (e.g., rhinovirus and adenovirus). Colds occur throughout the year; most cases occur in the winter. A self-limiting infection (4–10 days). Most contagious from days 2 to 3.

More common in crowded areas and in children. Children average from three to eight colds per year. Transmission is by respiratory droplets, fomites.

Classic Case
School-age child presents with acute onset of sneezing and nasal itchiness that is followed by a sore throat. Nasal congestion, runny eyes, and rhinitis (or coryza) follow shortly, along with a low-grade fever and malaise. Usually resolves within 4 to 10 days.

Objective Findings
Nasal turbinates and pharynx: red and swollen. Lungs: clear. Cervical nodes: mobile, smooth, and small or "shotty" (0.5 cm size or less).

Plan
- Symptomatic treatment. Increase fluids and rest. Oral decongestants (e.g., pseudoephedrine/Sudafed) PRN. Antitussives (e.g., dextromorphan/Robitussin) PRN.
- Antihistamines (e.g., diphenhydramine/Benadryl) PRN. Frequent handwashing.

Complications
Acute sinusitis
Acute otitis media

Acute Otitis Media (AOM)

Also known as purulent otitis media. An acute infection of the middle ear cavity with bacterial pathogens secondary to temporary eustachian tube dysfunction. The infection is usually unilateral but may involve both ears. Highest incidence is from ages of 6 months to 3 years.

Organisms
Streptococcus pneumoniae (Gram-positive). High rates of beta-lactam–resistant strains. *Haemophilus influenza* (Gram-negative). *Moraxella catarrhalis* (Gram-negative).

Classic Case
Small child with the common cold of several days duration becomes febrile, irritable, and is noted to be frequently pulling at the painful ear.

Older children and adults with history of a recent cold or flare-up of allergic rhinitis complain of ear pain, a muffled sensation, and popping noises in the affected ear.

Objective Findings
Tympanic membrane: bulging or retraction with displaced light reflex (displaced landmarks). Erythema (may be due to coughing or crying in children).

Tympanogram: decreased mobility with flat line tracing (most objective finding).

Plan
- See the plan for acute sinusitis.

Acute Sinusitis (acute rhinosinusitis)

An infection of the sinuses by Gram-positive and Gram-negative bacteria. There are four paranasal sinuses (maxillary and frontal sinuses). The frontal sinuses are not present at birth and all the sinuses are developed in later childhood.

Organisms
Streptococcus pneumoniae (Gram-positive). High rates of beta-lactam–resistant strains. *H. influenzae* (Gram-negative). *M. catarrhalis* (Gram-negative).

Classic Case
Complaints of unilateral facial pressure that worsens when bending down, along with pain in the upper molar teeth (maxillary sinusitis) or frontal headache (frontal sinusitis). Coughing that is worse when supine (e.g., during sleep). Self-treatment with OTC cold and sinus remedies provides no relief of symptoms.

Objective Findings
Posterior pharynx: purulent mucoid postnasal drip. Infected sinus: tender to palpation.

Transillumination: positive ("glow" of light on infected sinus is duller compared with normal sinus).

Plan (both AOM and acute sinusitis)
- Duration of treatment 10 to 14 days.

First Line
- Amoxicillin is the "gold standard" for any age group.
- High beta-lactam–resistant strains: do not use amoxicillin.
- Close follow-up of infants and children. Evaluate again in 3 days. If not responding to amoxicillin, switch to second line antibiotic.

Second Line
Second line antibiotic treatment criteria: history of antibiotic use in the past 6 months or no response to amoxicillin.
- amoxicillin/clavulanate (Augmentin) PO BID
- cefuroxime (Ceftin) PO BID
- trimethoprim sulfamethoxazole (Bactrim DS) PO BID
- infants/young children: may use ceftriaxone, from one to three injections

- cephalosporins: second generation (cefprozil or Cefzil); third generation (ceftriaxone or Rocephin).

Penicillin-allergic Patients
- azithromycin (Z Pack) for 5 days
- trimethoprim sulfamethoxazole (Bactrim DS) BID
- infants/children: sulfamethoxazole/erythromycin (Pediazole) PO every 6 hours
- levofloxacin (Levaquin) if 18 years or older, take one tablet daily

Pain
Infants and children: topical benzocaine (Auralgan Otic drops), acetaminophen (Tylenol), ibuprofen (Advil).
Older child to adults: naproxen sodium (Anaprox DS), ibuprofen (Advil), acetaminophen (Tylenol).

Drainage
Infants: Do not give decongestants to this age group. They are not effective.
Older child to adults: Oral decongestants such as pseudoephedrine (Sudafed). Topical decongestants (e.g., Afrin), use only for 3 days maximum or will cause rebound congestion.

Complications (from both sinusitis and AOM)
Cholesteatoma (described under the "Danger Signals" section).
Mastoiditis: red and swollen mastoid that is tender to palpation. Treat with antibiotics.
Periorbital or orbital cellulitis (more common in children): look for edema and redness in the periorbital area. Complaints of diplopia and eye pain. Clinical exam reveals abnormal range of motion of the EOMs (extraocular muscles).
Bacterial meningitis: stiff neck, headache, photophobia, fever.
Cavernous sinus thrombosis (described under "Danger Signals" section).
Hearing loss or persistent fluid in the middle ear impedes language development. A child who does not speak by the age of 18 to 24 months needs to be evaluated for hearing loss.

Rhinitis Medicamentosa

Prolonged use of topical nasal decongestants (>3days) causes rebound effects that result in severe and chronic nasal congestion. If the patient stops using the nasal spray, severe nasal congestion results.

Otitis Externa (Swimmer's Ear)

Bacterial infection of the skin of the external ear canal (rarely fungal). More common during warm and humid weather.

Organisms
Pseudomonas aeruginosa (Gram-negative). *Staphylococcus aureus* (Gram-positive)

Classic Case
Complaints of external ear pain accompaned by green purulent discharge. History of recent activities that involve water such as swimming.

Objective Findings
Ear: pain with manipulation of the external ear or tragus. Purulent green discharge. Erythematous and swollen ear canal that is very tender.

Medications
Corticosporin ear drops QID × 7 days. Keep water out of ear during treatment period.

Complications
Malignant otitis media: aggressive spread of infection into surrounding soft tissue and bone. Hospitalize for high-dose antibiotics and surgical debridement. Seen in diabetics.

Acute Mononucleosis (infectious mononucleosis)

Infection by the Epstein-Barr virus that is transmitted through saliva by intimate oral contact. The classic triad to look for is pharyngitis, cervical lymphadenopathy, and fatigue.

Classic Case
Teenage patient presents with sore throat, enlarged cervical nodes, and fatigue. Fatigue can persist for several months. May complain of upper abdominal pain secondary to hepatomegaly and/or splenomegaly.

Objective Findings
Nodes: enlarged cervical nodes. Pharynx: erythematous. Tonsils red, sometimes with exudate (off-white). Hepatomegaly and splenomegaly. Avoid vigorous palpation of the abdomen.

Plan
▪ Order abdominal ultrasound (sonogram) especially if patient is an athlete. Avoid all contact sports until resolution (repeat abdominal ultrasound). Symptomatic treatment.

Complications
Ruptured spleen (may be fatal)
Airway obstruction from enlarged tonsils

Hepatitis.

Blood dyscrasias (atypical lymphocytes), repeat CBC until lymphocytes normalized.

Exam Tips

- Ruptured spleen is a catastrophic event. Avoid contact sports (several weeks) until ultrasound documents resolution.
- Betimol (timolol) has the same contraindications as oral beta blockers.
- Cholesteatoma description.
- Do not use amoxicillin if previous antibiotic used in the past 3 months. Pick second line choice such as Augmentin, Ceftin, Bactrim DS.
- Penicillin-allergic patients: use macrolides, sulfas (also avoid cephalosporins because 10% of patients are cross-reactive).
- Learn to recognize a description of eye findings such as the pinguecula, pterygium, and chalazion.
- Weber or Rinne are tests for the acoustic or the 8th cranial nerve.
- Lateralization on the Weber exam is an abnormal finding.
- Remember what 20/40 vision means: patient can see at 20 ft what a person with normal vision can see at 40 ft. The top number is always what the patient can see at 20 ft.

CARDIOVASCULAR SYSTEM

Fast Facts | Danger Signals

Acute MI (myocardial infarction)

Older adult male complains of mid-sternal chest pain that feels like heavy pressure on the chest. The pain is associated with numbness and/or tingling of the left jaw and the left arm. The patient is pale and diaphoretic with cool clammy skin.

Acute Abdominal Aneurysm

Elderly White male complains of severe back pain with acute onset. With impending rupture, the back pain becomes severe along with a "tearing" sensation inside the abdomen. When it ruptures, signs and symptoms of shock and collapse appear quickly. Sometimes the patient may have undiagnosed Marfan syndrome, a genetic disorder of the connective tissue marked by tall stature, aortic dilatation/aneurysm, hyperflexible joints, pectus chest deformity or "pigeon chest."

Congestive Heart Failure (CHF)

Elderly patient complains of a gradual or acute onset of dyspnea, dry cough, and swollen feet and ankles. Sudden or gradual increased weight. Bibasilar crackles on the lung base and the presence of the S3 heart sound are classic findings. History of preexisting heart disease. The patient is usually already taking medications to prevent CHF such as diuretics, Lanoxin, and antihypertensives. Precipitating factors include excessive fluid retention due to medications, acute illness, infections, and so forth.

Bacterial Endocarditis

Middle-age male presents with fever, chills, and malaise associated with skin findings occurring mostly on the fingers/hands and toes/feet. These include splinter hemorrhages on the nailbed (subungual hemorrhage), petechiae on the palate, violet-colored painful nodes on the fingers or feet (Osler nodes), and tender red spots on the palms/soles (Janeway lesions). A heart murmur may be present on cardiac exam.

Fast Facts | Normal Findings

Anatomy

Most of the left ventricular mass is located behind the right ventricle. The right ventricle sits anteriorly toward the chest. Most of the atria are located posteriorly facing the back. The lower border of the left ventricle is where the apical impulse is generated. The apical impulse is located at the fifth intercostal space (ICS) about 8 cm from the midsternal line.

Deoxygenated Blood

Enters the heart through the superior vena cava and inferior vena cava to the right atrium → tricuspid valve → right ventricle → pulmonic valve → pulmonary artery → lungs (pulmonary vein).

Oxygenated Blood

Exits from the lungs through the pulmonary veins to the
left atrium → mitral valve → left ventricle → aortic valve → aorta → general circulation.

Systole and Diastole

The mnemonic to use is "motivated apples." These two words give you several clues. It will remind you of the names of the valves that produce the sound and the type of valve.

Motivated

M (mitral valve)

T (tricuspid valve)

AV (atrioventricular valves)

Apples

A (aortic valve)

P (pulmonic valve)

S (semilunar valves)

Normal Heart Sounds

S1 (systole)
- closure of the mitral and tricuspid valves
- atrioventricular or AV valves (3 leaflets)

S2 (diastole)
- closure of the aortic and pulmonic valves
- semilunar valves (2 leaflets)

S3 heart sound
- pathognomic for CHF
- occurs during early diastole (ventricular gallop)
- always considered abnormal if it occurs after the age of 40
- May be a normal variant in some children or young adults if there are no signs or symptoms of heart or valvular disease.

S4 heart sound
Caused by the increased resistance from a stiff left ventricle. Usually indicates left ventricular hypertrophy. Considered as normal finding in some elderly with no heart disease.

- S4 occurs during late diastole (atrial gallop or "atrial kick")
- best heard at the apex (mitral area) by using the bell of the stethoscope

Summation gallop
- all heart sounds are present (from S1 to S4) and sound like a galloping horse
- a pathologic finding

Stethoscope Skills

Bell of stethoscope
- low tones such as the extra heart sounds (S3 or S4)
- mitral stenosis

Diaphragm of the stethoscope
- mid- to high-pitched tones such as lung sounds
- mitral regurgitation
- aortic stenosis

Benign Split S2

Best heard over the pulmonic area (or second ICS left side of sternum). Caused by splitting of the aortic and pulmonic components. A normal finding if it appears during inspiration and disappears at expiration.

Benign S4 in the Elderly

Some healthy elderly patients have an S4 (late diastole) heart sound. Also known as the "atrial kick" (the atria have to squeeze harder to overcome resistance of a stiff left ventricle). If there are no signs or symptoms of heart/valvular disease, it is considered a normal variant. Otherwise, it is associated with LVH (left ventricular hypertrophy).

Exam Tips

- S3 is a sign of CHF and S4 is a sign of LVH.
- A split S2 is best heard at the pulmonic area.
- Memorize the pneumonic "motivated apples" to help you remember the valves responsible for producing S1 and S2.
- Grading murmurs: first time thrill palpated is at Grade IV.

Clinical Tip

- S3 is pathognomic for CHF. Look for the sign if you suspect a patient has heart failure.

Ausculatory Areas

It is necessary to memorize the locations of the ausculatory areas. This will assist in solving questions about heart murmurs. There are only three sites to remember for the exam.

- Aortic area: second ICS to the right side of the sternum.
- Pulmonic area: second ICS to the left side of the sternum.
- Mitral area: fifth ICS to the left side of the sternum medial to the midclavicular line.

Grading System for Heart Murmurs

- Grade I: very soft murmur. Heard only at optimal conditions.
- Grade II: mild to moderately loud murmur.
- Grade III: loud murmur that is easily heard once the stethoscope is placed on the chest.

- Grade IV: first time a thrill is felt. A louder murmur.
- Grade V: very loud murmur heard with edge of stethoscope off chest.
- Grade VI: the murmur is so loud that it can be heard even with the stethoscope off the chest.

Fast Facts | Abnormal Findings

Pathologic Murmurs

- All diastolic murmurs are abnormal
- Late systolic murmurs
- Loud murmurs, pansystolic or holosystolic murmurs
- Murmurs associated with a thrill

Solving Questions: Heart Murmurs

To solve a murmur question correctly, there are two pieces of information needed. These two are the timing (systole or diastole) and location of the murmur.

Timing of Murmur

Systolic murmurs
- use the MR TRAS mnemonic

Diastolic murmurs
- use the MS. PRAR mnemonic

Location

A question about mitral stenosis will not have the word "mitral" included on the question because it is an obvious clue. Instead, the location will be described in other ways as shown in the following:

Mitral area

- fifth ICS on the left side of sternum medial to the midclavicular line
- apical murmur or the apex of the heart

Pulmonic area

- second ICS on the left side of the sternum
- left side of the upper sternum at the base of the heart

Aortic area

- second ICS to the right side of the sternum
- right side of the upper sternum at the base of the heart

Mnemonic Devices

"MR TRAS" (use for all systolic murmurs)
Systole or S1 murmurs are also described as holosystolic, pansystolic, early systolic, mid-systolic, or late systolic murmurs.

MR (Mitral Regurgitation)
A pansystolic (or holosystolic) murmur

- heard best at the apex or the apical area
- radiates to axilla
- loud-blowing and high-pitched murmur (use the diaphragm of the stethoscope)

Tricuspid Regurgitation
- not on the test at present

Aortic Stenosis
- a mid-systolic ejection murmur
- best heard at the second ICS at the right side of the sternum
- radiates to the neck
- a harsh and noisy murmur (use the diaphragm of the stethoscope)

Patients with aortic stenosis should avoid physical overexertion. These patients are at risk for sudden death. Monitored by serial cardiac sonograms with Doppler flow studies. Surgical valve replacement if moderately severe.

"MS. PRAR"
Diastole or S2 is also decribed as early diastole, late diastole, or mid-diastole. Diastolic murmurs are always indicative of heart disease.

MS (Mitral Stenosis)
A low-pitched diastolic rumbling murmur
- heard best at the apex of the heart or the apical area
- also called an "opening snap" (use bell of the stethoscope)

PR (Pulmonic Regurgitation)
- not on the test at present

AR (Aortic Regurgitation)
A high-pitched diastolic murmur
- best heard at the second ICS at the right side of the sternum
- high-pitched blowing murmur (use diaphragm of the stethoscope)

Exam Tips

- Memorize the ausculatory locations and mnemonics.
- Systolic murmurs use MR. TRAS.
- Diastolic murmurs use MS. PRAR.
- All murmurs with "mitral" in their names are described as located on the apex of the heart or the apical area or the fifth ICS on the left side of the sternum medial to the midclavicular line.
- There is only one ausculatory area on the right side of the sternum (aortic). Your job is to determine whether it is aortic regurgitation (MS. PR*AR*) or aortic stenosis (MR. TRA*S*).
- If you forget which side of the sternum the aortic or pulmonic area lies on (left? or right?): the "r" in aortic is for the "right side" and the "l" in pulmonic is for the "left" side.

Fast Facts | Disease Review

Pulsus Paradoxus

Also known as a paradoxical pulse. Measured by using the BP cuff and a stethoscope.

During inspiration: systolic pressure normally decreases slightly because of a slight increase of the pressure inside the chest cavity (positive pressure). Certain pulmonary and cardiac conditions cause an exaggerated decrease of the systolic pressure of >10 mmHg.

Pulmonary cause: asthma, emphysema (increased positive pressure).

Cardiac cause: tamponade, pericarditis, cardiac effusion (decreases movement of left ventricle).

Atrial Fibrillation

Any condition or substance that irritates or overstimulates the heart can cause atrial fibrillation. For example: hyperthyroidism, cocaine, caffeine or alcohol, heart failure, and so forth.

May be asymptomatic. Rate of stroke is 10 times higher in older patients.

Classic Case

Usually asymptomatic. If symptomatic, the patient complains of a sudden onset of heart palpitations and may suddenly feel weak or dizzy. Sometimes accompanied by chest pain or syncope.

Plan

- Diagnostic test is the 12-lead electrocardiogram (EKG).
- The internationalized normal ratio (INR) is used to monitor response to anticoagulation.

Medications

Anticoagulants decrease risk of thrombosis and emboli. For acute episodes of embolization, patient is hospitalized and started on intravenous (IV) heparin. Before discharge, the patient is switched to warfarin sodium (Coumadin) 2 to 10 mg/day. Duration of treatment depends on the patient's age, medical history, and if there are recurrent episodes.

Complications

Death from thromboembolic event (e.g., stroke, pulmonary embolism)

Anticoagulation Guidelines
Atrial Fibrillation
INR 2.0 to 3.0
Synthetic Valves
INR 2.5 to 3.5

Hypertension

Majority of patients have essential hypertension (90–95% of cases)—a multifactorial disorder that results from genetic, renal (renin/angiotensin), sympathetic nervous system, and environmental factors.

BP: peripheral vascular resistance (PVR) × CO (cardiac output).

Any changes in the PVR or CO result in a change in BP (increase/decrease).

Examples
- Sodium water retention increases vascular volume (increased CO).
- Angiotensin I to angiotensin II: increased vasoconstriction (increased PVR).
- Sympathetic system stimulation: epinephrine secretion causes tachycardia and vasoconstriction (increased cardiac output and PVR).
- Vasodilation (beta blockers): decreased resistance (decreased PVR).
- Severe hemorrhage: less blood volume (decreased CO).

Correct Blood Pressure Measurement
- Avoid smoking or caffeine intake 30 minutes before measurement.
- Patient should be seated on a chair with back and arm supported.
- Begin BP measurement after 5 minutes of rest (mercury sphygmomanometer preferred over digital machines).
- Two or more readings separated by 2 minutes should be averaged per visit.
- Higher number determines BP stage (BP 140/100 is Stage II instead of Stage I).

Secondary Hypertension

Most common causes are renal conditions (e.g., renal artery stenosis and renal failure). Rule out secondary cause in the following cases:

- patient is younger than 35 years at onset of hypertension
- severe hypertension or abrupt onset
- refractory to treatment

Physical Exam Findings

Eyes
- silver and/or copper wire arterioles
- arteriovenous (AV) junction nicking
- flame-shaped hemorrhages, papilledema

Heart
- S3 (heart failure)
- S4 (left ventricular hypertrophy)
- carotid bruits (narrowing due to plaque)
- peripheral edema (CHF or kidney disease)
- decreased or absent peripheral pulses (PVD)

Renal Artery Stenosis
- epigastric or upper abdominal quadrant bruit

Pheochromocytoma
- labile increased BP, sudden onset anxiety
- paroxysms of sweating
- severe headaches, palpitations

Hyperthyroidism
- weight loss, tachycardia, fine tremor, moist skin, anxiety
- atrial fibrillation

Kidneys
- bruit (renal artery stenosis)
- cystic renal masses (polycystic kidney)
- increased creatinine (renal insufficiency, renal failure)

Sleep Apnea
- increases blood pressure
- marked hypoxic episodes during sleep

Exam Tip

- Eye findings: learn to distinguish the findings in hypertension (copper and silver wire arterioles, AV nicking) versus diabetes (neovascularization, micro-aneurysms

Current Treatment Guidelines*

Stage I (BP systolic 140–139 mmHg or diastolic 90–99 mmHg)
- thiazide-type diuretics preferred for most patients

Stage II (systolic equal or >160 or diastolic equal or >100 mmHg)
- two drug therapy for most patients

---

* Adapted from Joint National Committee for the Assessment's *Evaluation and Treatment of High Blood Pressure in Adults*, 7th Report, 2003.

Table 3.2 — Hypertension Diagnosis and Management: JNC 7 Treatment Guidelines

Stage	Systole/Diastole	Treatment Recommendations
Normal	<120 mmHg <80 mmHg	Healthy lifestyle. Exercise.
Prehypertension	120 to 139 mmHg 80 to 89 mmHg	Lifestyle changes. Lose weight. Exercise.
Stage I	140 to 159 mmHg 90 to 99 mmHg	*Thiazide diuretics preferred for most cases.* Compelling condition: ACE inhibitors, ARBs, Beta-blockers, CCB or combination drug.
Stage II	>160 mmHg >100 mmHg	Two drug combination for most patients. Thiazide diuretic plus ACE inhibitor, ARB, Beta-blocker, calcium channel blocker or a combination drug.
Compelling Indications	Diabetes Kidney disease Heart failure Recurrent stroke Prevention	ACE inhibitors, ARBs, Thiazide diuretics. Beta-blockers and/or CCBs. ACE inhibitors, ARB. Thiazide diuretic, beta blocker, ACE inhibitors, ARB, Thiazide diuretic, ACE inhibitors.
Diet	Magnesium, potassium, calcium	Increase intake: magnesium (nuts, grains), potassium (most fruits, veggies), calcium (low fat dairy).

ARB: ACE Receptor Blocker, CCB: Calcium Channel Blocker
*Adapted from Joint National Committee on Prevention, Detection, Evaluation, and Treatment of High Blood Pressure (JNC 7), 2003.
Cardiac Risk Equivalents
1. Even if patient has no preexisting coronary heart disease (CHD), if > 20% risk of having a heart attack within next 10 years, treat as if patient has heart disease.
2. Examples are diabetics, chronic renal disease, microalbuminuria, etc.
3. Goal BP for these patients is 130/80.
4. Diabetics/kidney disease: ACE inhibitors or ARBs preferred (renal protective).

▓ thiazide-type diuretic and another drug class antihypertensive agent
▓ if other disease(s) present with compelling indications, consider other drug
Diabetics and CAD (coronary artery disease)
▓ goal is BP <130/80 mmHg

Compelling Indications
Diabetes mellitus (DM)
▓ Unless contraindicated, all diabetics should be on angiotensin converting enzyme (ACE) inhibitors or angiotensin II receptor blockers (ARB) because of their renal protective properties.
Angiotensin converting enzyme (ACE) inhibitors
▓ captopril (Capoten)

Angiotensin II receptor blockers (ARB)
- losartan (Cozaar)

Beta blockers
- propranolol (Inderal LA): noncardioselective
- atenolol (Tenormin)

Calcium channel blockers (CCBs)
- nifedipine (Norvasc)

Systolic Hypertension in the Elderly
- diuretics preferred or long-acting dihydropyridine CCBs (e.g., Norvasc)

Heart Failure
- ACE inhibitors or ARBs
- diuretics
- beta blockers

Post Myocardial Infarction (MI)
- beta blockers, ACE inhibitors, aldosterone antagonists

Target Organs

Rule out target organ damage.
- Brain: strokes
- Eyes: retinopathy, bleeding, blindness
- Heart: left ventricular hypertrophy, heart disease, acute MI, CHF
- Kidneys: proteinuria, renal failure

Lifestyle Recommendations

This is the "first line" therapy for both hypertension and diabetes.
- Lose weight
- Stop smoking
- Reduce stress level
- Reduce dietary sodium to less than 2.4 g/day
- Maintain adequate intake of potassium, calcium, and magnesium
- Limit ETOH intake to 1 oz (30 cc) or less per day for men and 0.5 oz or less per day for women
- Eat fatty, cold water fish (salmon, anchovy) three times a week
- Exercise moderately 30 to 45 minutes most days of the week

Obesity

BMI calculation (body mass index): weight (in kilograms) $\times$ (height in meters)^2

Exam Tips

- Remember BMI calculation factors (weight $\times$ height).
- Do not confuse BMI formula with the PEF (peak expiratory flow).
- PEF is height, age, and gender (mnemonic is "HAG"): weight is not a factor used for the PEF formula.

Dietary Sources of Recommended Minerals
- Calcium (low-fat dairy)
- Potassium (most fruits and vegetables)

Table 3.3	Basal Metabolic Index (BMI) Criteria

*Category	BMI
Underweight	<18.5
Normal weight	18.5 to 24.9
Overweight	25 to 29.9
Obese	30 to 39.9
Grossly obese	>40.0
Waist circumference	Males >40 inches
	Females >35 inches
	Higher risk of CAD

*Adapted from the National Heart Lung and Blood Institute, 2007.

- Magnesium (dried beans, whole grains, nuts)
- Avoid high sodium intake: cold cuts, ready-made foods, any pickled foods (cucumbers, eggs, pork parts)
- Omega 3 oils: salmon, anchovies (sardines), flaxseed oil

Labs
Kidneys: creatinine, urinalysis
Endocrine: thyroid profile, fasting blood glucose
Electrolyte: potassium (K+), sodium (Na+), calcium (Ca+)
Heart: cholesterol, HDL, LDL, triglycerides (complete lipid panel)
Anemia: complete blood count
Baseline EKG and chest X-ray (to rule out cardiomegaly)

Medications

Beta blockers
Block beta receptors on the heart and the peripheral vasculature. There are two types of beta blocker receptors: B1 (cardiac effects) and B2 (lungs and peripheral vasculature). Beta blockers decrease vasomotor activity, cardiac output by inhibiting renin and nonepinephrine release.

Note
- Avoid abrupt discontinuation after chronic use. May precipitate severe rebound hypertension. Wean slowly.

Contraindications
- second to third degree heart block (okay to use with first degree block)
- asthma, COPD, or chronic lung disease
- sinus bradycardia

Other Uses
- Migraine headache: for prophylaxis only (not for acute attacks)
- Glaucoma: to reduce intraocular pressure (i.e., Betimol Ophthalmic Drops)
- Resting tachycardia, angina, post-MI
- Hyperthyroidism and pheochromocytoma: to control symptoms until primary disease treated
- Beta blockers: ends in "OLOL": metoprolol (Lopressor) 100 mg
- QID to BID, propranolol (Inderal LA) 40 mg BID (only long-acting form used for hypertension [HTN]), propanolol (plain Inderal): shorter half-life (not for HTN treatment)

Calcium Channel Blockers (CCB)
Blocks calcium channels in the arterioles resulting in systemic vasodilation, which results in decreasing PVR. Depresses heart muscle and the AV node (decreases cardiac output).

Side Effects
- headaches (vasodilation)
- ankle edema (from vasodilation; considered benign)
- heart block or bradycardia (depresses cardiac muscle and AV node)

Contraindications
- second and third degree AV block
- bradycardia
- CHF

Examples
- Nifedipine (Procardia XL), amlodipine (Norvasc)
- Verapamil (Calan), diltiazem (Cardizem CD)

ACE Inhibitors and ARBs
- Block conversion of angiotensin I to II (more potent vasoconstrictor)
- Classified as FDA category C drug
- Causes fetal kidney malformations and hypotension of the fetus

Side Effects
- Hyperlakemia (increased risk if combined with potassium-spacing diuretics such as triamterene)
- Angioedema (rare but may be life-threatening)

Contraindications
- Precipitates acute renal failure if patient has renal artery stenosis
- Hyperkalemia (this is also a side effect for ACE and ARBs, will have additive effect)

Examples
- ACE inhibitors: Captopril (Capoten), enalapril (Vasotec), lisinopril (Zestril)
- ARBs: Losartan (Cozaar)

Alpha-1 Blockers

Also known as: Alpha-1 inhibitor or agonist (instead of blocker). Blocks alpha receptors in peripheral arteries resulting in profound vasodilation (large number of alpha-1 receptors in arterioles). Used to treat males with benign prostatic hyperplasia (BPH) and hypertension.

Side Effect
- dizziness, postural hypotension

Start at very low dose and titrate up slowly until good BP control. Given at bedtime because of common side effect of postural hypotension.

Example
- Terazosin (Hytrin)

Exam Tips

- ACE inhibitors: the drug of choice for diabetics; causes a dry cough (10%).
- Avoid combining ACE inhibitors with potassium sparing diuretics (e.g., triamterene, spironolactone) because of increased risk for hyperkalemia.
- Renal artery stenosis: ACE inhibitors precipitate acute renal failure.
- Alpha blockers are not first line drugs for hypertension except if patient has preexisting BPH.

Clinical Tips

- High cholesterol is not considered a risk factor for heart disease in patients over the age of 75.
- Over age 75: screening depends on life expectancy and functional status.
- Start niacin at low dose and gradually titrate up to avoid unpleasant side effects of flushing and headache. Advise to take with food and warn patient about side effects. Side effects usually fade by 2 weeks. Can take with ibuprofen 30 minutes before to minimize side effects.

Congestive Heart Failure

Left Ventricular Failure
- Crackles, cough, decreased breath sounds, dullness to percussion
- Paroxysmal nocturnal dyspnea, orthopnea

Right Ventricular Failure
- Jugular venous distention (JVD), enlarged liver, enlarged spleen
- Anorexia, nausea, abdominal pain, lower-extremity edema

Summary

An easy way to remember whether a sign or symptom is from the left or right side of the heart is: both Left and Lung start with the letter "L". Left is for "lung" and right is the "GI" tract (by default).

Deep Vein Thrombosis (DVT)

Thrombus/thrombi develop in the deep venous system of the legs or pelvis secondary to stasis, trauma to vessel walls, inflammation, or increased coagulation.

Causes of DVT
- Venous stasis: prolonged travel/inactivity, bedrest, CHF
- Inherited coagulation disorders: Factor C deficiency, Leiden, and so forth
- Increased coagulation due to external factors: oral contraceptive (OC) use; pregnancy; bone fractures, especially of the long bones; trauma; recent surgery; and malignancy

Classic Case (on exam)
An adult or elderly patient complains of gradual or acute onset of swelling of lower extremity after a history of travel (>3 hours). The extremity is painful, tender to palpation, and is red and warm. On physical exam, a positive Homan's sign is noted.

Plan
- Homan's sign: lower leg pain on dorsiflexion of the foot
- Complete blood count, platelets, clotting time (PT/PTT, INR)
- Contrast venography (gold standard)
- B-mode ultrasound with Doppler flow study, magnetic resonance imaging
- Hospital admission, heparin IV; then warfarin PO (Coumadin) for 3 to 6 months (1st episode) or longer. For recurrent DVT or in elderly, antithrombotic treatment may need to be ongoing for the rest of the patient's life.

Complications
Pulmonary emboli
Stroke and other embolic episodes

Exam Tips
- On the exam, a case of DVT will have a positive Homan's sign. In real life practice, most cases of DVT are asymptomatic.
- Choose low-tech procedures (e.g., ankle and brachial BP) over invasive or expensive tests unless the low-tech procedure has already been done.

Superficial Thrombophlebitis

Inflammation of a superficial vein due to local trauma. Higher risk in-dwelling catheters, certain IV drugs (i.e., potassium), secondary bacterial infection due to *Staphylococcus aureus*.

Classic Case
Complaints of a cordlike and indurated vein. The vein is warm and tender to touch with a surrounding area of erythema that does not involve the entire limb.

Plan
- Nonsteroidal anti-inflammatory drugs (NSAIDs) such as ibuprofen or naproxen sodium (Anaprox DS) BID.
- Warm compresses. Elevate limb.
- If septic, admit patient to hospital.

Complications
- Permanent damage to vein

Peripheral Vascular Disease (PVD)

Gradual narrowing and/or occlusion of medium to large arteries resulting in permanent ischemic damage to an extremity. Also known as occlusive arterial disease. Higher risk with hypertension, smoking, diabetes, and hyperlipidemia.

Classic Case
Older patient complains of pain on ambulation (intermittent claudication) that is relieved by rest. Symptoms become worse over time until walking distance is greatly limited.

Objective Findings
- Skin: cool skin, atrophic changes due to chronic poor circulation. Affected skin on the lower leg is hairless, shiny, and darker than unaffected skin (hyperpigmentation).
- Cardiovascular: decreased-to-absent pulses (popliteal, dorsal pedis, and posterior tibialis), increased capillary refill time, bruits over partially blocked arteries.

Plan
- Low-tech method: ankle and brachial BP before and after exercise
- Diagnostic method: Doppler ultrasound flow study, angiography
- Smoking cessation (smoking causes vasoconstriction), walk daily, pentoxifylline (Trental)
- Percutaneous angioplasty or surgery: severe cases

Complications
Gangrene of foot and/or lower limb
Amputation of limb

Raynaud's Phenomenon

Reversible vasospasm of the arterioles on the fingers and toes. Unknown cause. Associated with an increased risk of autoimmune disorders (e.g., thyroid disorder, pernicious anemia, rheumatoid arthritis). Affects mostly females (60–90%) with a gender ratio of females to males of 8:1. Personal or family history of autoimmune disease.

Classic Case

Adult female reports episodes of color changes in the fingertips ranging from white, blue, and red, which is accompanied by tingling and numbness of the fingertips. Attacks may last several hours. Reports a history of cold hands and feet (sensitivity to cold temperatures).

Plan

- Avoid touching cold objects, cold weather.
- Smoking cessation. Nifedipine (Norvasc), captopril (Capoten).
- Do not use any vasoconstricting drugs (e.g., Imitrex, ergots), B-blockers, etc.

Complication

- Ulceration in fingertips and toes

Exam Tip

- Think of the colors of the American flag as a reminder of this disorder.

Bacterial Endocarditis

Bacterial infection of the endocardial surface of the heart. Presentation ranges from full-blown disease to subacute endocarditis. Higher risk with poor dental hygiene, prosthetic valvular implants, mitral valve prolapse, and IV drug users. Bacterial pathogens are Gram-positive (e.g., viridans strep, staph aureus, etc.). Also known as infective endocarditis.

Diagnosed using the Duke criteria.

Classic Case

Described in the Danger Signals section.

Labs

Blood cultures × 3 (first 24 hours) with C&S, transesophageal ultrasound, echocardiogram, CBC with differential (leukocytosis), sedimentation rate (elevated), RF (rheumatoid factor) positive, etc.

Medications

IV antibiotic with penicillin, gentamicin, or vancomycin

Complications

Valvular destruction, abscess (myocardium)
Emboli

Infective Endocarditis (IE) Prophylaxis Guidelines

Highest Risk*
- Prosthetic Valve or Prosthetic Material used for Valve Repair
- Previous IE
- Congenital Heart Disease (CHD): unrepaired cyanotic CHD; completely re-paired CHD using prosthetic device or material; Repaired CHD with residual defects
- Cardic Transplant with Valvulopathy

High-Risk Procedures
Dental (e.g., cleaning, root canals), respiratory (e.g., tonsillectomy, bron-choscopy), GU (e.g., prostatectomy, vaginal hysterectomy), terminations.

Standard Regimen
- Adults: amoxicillin 2 g PO 1 hour before procedure
- Child: amoxicillin 50 mg/kg 1 hour before procedure

Penicillin-allergic Patients
- Clindamycin 600 mg, Biaxin 500 mg, or Keflex 2 g 1 hour before procedure

List of Cardiac Arrhythmias

- No EKG strips are included in the exam. A few arrhythmias are described in detail and the test taker is asked to "diagnose" them.

Paroxysmal Atrial Tachycardia (PAT)
Also known as Paroxysmal Supraventricular Tachycardia (PSVT or SVT). Tachy-cardia with peaked QRS complex and p waves present. May be terminated with carotid massage, calcium-channel blockers, or beta blockers. Heart rate ranges from 100 to 250 beats/min. Causes: digitalis toxicity, heart disease, ETOH intoxi-cation, hyperthyroid, stimulants such as theophylline, cocaine, and so forth.

Classic Case
Patient complains of a sudden onset of palpitations that may be accompanied by feelings of lightheadedness or dizziness, dyspnea, chest pain, and fatigue.

Atrial Fibrillation
An irregularly irregular rhythm with no p waves seen on the EKG. Heart rate ranges from 80 to 180 beats/min. Common arrhythmia. Causes are heart disease, hyperthyroid, excess alcohol or stimulants, and so forth.

Classic Case
Patient may be asymptomatic or may complain of palpitations, dyspnea, and angina.

---

* IE prophylaxis is no longer recommended for mitral valve prolapse.

Mitral Valve Prolapse (MVP)
Normal sinus rhythm associated with an S2 "click" followed by a systolic murmur. More common in tall and thin adult females. Higher risk of thromboemboli and infective endocarditis. Diagnosed by cardiac ultrasound. IE prophylaxis is no longer recommended by the AHA for MVP.

Classic Case
▓ Female adult patient may complain of fatigue, palpitations, lightheadedness.

Hyperlipidemia

Screening Guidelines*
　　　▓ Complete lipid profile (fasting) every 5 years starting at age 20 years)
　　　▓ Over age 40 years, screen every 2 to 3 years
　　　▓ Preexisting hyperlipidemia—screen annually or more frequently
Total Cholesterol
　　　▓ Normal <199 mg/dL
　　　▓ Borderline between 200 and 239 mg/dL
　　　▓ High: >240 mg/dL
HDL (high density lipoprotein)
　　　▓ HDL: >40 mg/dL. If <40 mg/dL, associated with increased risk of CAD even if normal LDL or cholesterol
LDL (low density lipoprotein)
　　　▓ LDL: <130 mg/dL for low risk patients with less than two risk factors
　　　▓ LDL: <100 mg/dL if high risk such as diabetics, hypertension, CAD
Triglycerides
　　　▓ Normal: <150 mg/dL
　　　▓ High risk of acute pancreatitis: >500 mg/dL
　　　▓ If a patient with high cholesterol also has high triglycerides, must treat hypertriglyceridemia first before LDL or total cholesterol

Coronory Risk Equivalent
High risk: defined as a coronary heart disease risk of >20% (chances of an MI over next 10 years is 20%). These patients are treated the same as diabetics and patients with existing heart disease. Therefore, their goal is an LDL <100 mg/dL. Preexisting heart disease, diabetics, and coronary risk equivalent >20%. Goal is LDL <100 mg/dL

Exam Tips

You must memorize some values. These are (not inclusive):
▓ Borderline cholesterol, high cholesterol, HDL, LDL goal for CHD or DM

---

* Adapted from *Third Report of the Expert Panel on Detection, Evaluation and Treatment of High Blood Cholesterol in Adults*, 2001.

■ Low HDL (<40 mg/dL) is a risk factor of CHD even though total cholesterol, triglycerides, and LDL are normal.

Risk Factors: Heart Disease*

■ Hypertension

■ Family history of premature heart disease (women with MI age <65 yr or men with MI age <55 yr)

■ DM (considered a CHD risk equivalent even if patient has no history of preexisting heart disease)

■ Dyslipidemia

■ Low HDL cholesterol: <40 mg/dL

■ Age (men older than 45 yr or women older than 55 yr)

■ Cigarette smoker

■ Obesity (BMI equal or >30 kg/m^2)

■ Microalbuminuria

Treatment Plan

■ Lifestyle changes such as weight loss, exercise most days of the week, better diet low in saturated fat, and smoking cessation

■ Encourage use of soluble fiber in diet (i.e., psyllium, fruit, vegetables) to enhance lowering of LDL (lowers LDL by blocking absorption in GI tract up to 10%)

■ If no changes in lipids after a trial of 6 months of lifestyle changes, consider antilipidemic drugs if more than two risk factors.

Treatment Goals

■ Decrease LDL first except if patient has very high triglyceride levels (high risk of acute pancreatitis)

■ High triglyceride levels >500 mg/dL must be treated first before treating high LDL level

American Heart Association: Therapeutic Lifestyle Changes Diet

■ Cholesterol: <200 mg per day

■ Total fat: 25 to 35%

■ Saturated fat: less than 7%

■ Monounsaturated fat: up to 20%

■ Polyunsaturated fat: up to 10%

■ Carbohydrates: 50 to 60% should be from complex carbohydrate foods (i.e., whole grains, fruits and vegetables).

■ Protein: 15% (soy can replace some animal products)

Medications and Patient Education

■ Do not drink ETOH while on these drugs because of increased hepatotoxicity. Avoid prescribing to alcoholics.

■ Advise patient to report symptoms of hepatitis or rhabdomyolysis. Stop taking drug if suspect reaction.

---

* Adapted from *JNC 7* (May 2003).

■ Rhabdomyolysis: muscle pain and aches that persist and are not associated with muscular exertion

■ Labs: order creatine phosphokinase (CPK) or creatine kinase (CK) and liver function tests (LFTs) (will be elevated)

■ Acute hepatitis: anorexia, nausea, dark colored urine, jaundice, and fatigue

■ Labs: order LFTs (elevated ALT [SGPT] and AST [SGOT])

■ ALT or serum glutamic phosphate transaminase (SGPT) and aspartate transaminase

HMG CoA Reductase Inhibitors (statins)

■ Pravastatin (Pravachol), Lovastatin (Mevacor), Simvastin (Zocor)

■ Best agent for decreasing LDL. Some statins also elevate HDL (i.e., Zocor).

■ Increased risk of hepatitis or rhabdomyolysis (rare) if on combination therapy with fibrates or nicotinic acid.

■ Side effects: hepatic toxicity, rhabdomyolysis (breakdown of skeletal muscle = acute renal failure).

Nicotinic Acid

■ Niacin (over the counter) daily to TID, Niaspan (slow-release niacin) daily

■ Very good agent for lowering triglycerides and elevating HDL level

■ Combining this drug with statins, fibrates or ETOH increases risk of hepatotoxicity

■ Side effects: flushing, itching, tingling, hepatotoxicity; GI effects such as abdominal pain

Fibrates

■ Gemfibrozil (Lopid), fenofibrate (TriCor)

■ Great for reducing triglycerides and elevating HDL

■ Combining this drug with statins, niacin or ETOH increases risk of hepatotoxicity

■ Side effects: hepatic and renal effects

Bile Acid Sequestrants

■ Cholestyramine (Questran Light), colestipol (Colestid), colesevelam (WelChol)

■ Works locally in the small intestines to interfere with the absorption of fats

■ May be used in combination with other Medications (statins, fibrates, niacin) without increasing risk for hepatoxicity. An alternative drug for patients who cannot tolerate statins, fibrates, and niacin. Not as effective as other agents. No hepatoxicity.

■ Interferes with absorption: fat-soluble vitamins (take MVI tabs daily), tetracycline, digoxin, and so forth

■ Side effects: bloating, flatulence, abdominal pain. Start at low doses and titrate up slowly.

PULMONARY SYSTEM

Fast Facts | Danger Signals

Pulmonary Emboli (PE)

Older adult complains of sudden onset of dyspnea and coughing. Cough may be productive of pink-tinged frothy sputum. Other symptoms are tachycardia, pallor, and feelings of impending doom. Any condition that increases risk of blood clots will increase risk of PE. These patients have a history of DVT, atrial fibrillation, estrogens, surgery, pregnancy, long bone fractures, and prolonged inactivity.

Impending Respiratory Failure (asthmatic patient)

Asthmatic patient presents with an acute asthmatic exacerbation that is not responding to treatment. Symptoms are worsening. Eventually, the patient becomes fatigued and diaphoretic and uses accessory muscles to help with breathing. Physical exam reveals tachycardia, tachypnea, and "quiet" lungs with no wheezing or breath sounds audible.

Treatment

Adrenaline injection STAT. Call 911. Oxygen by nasal cannula, albuterol nebulizer treatments, parenteral antihistamines (diphenhydramine [Benadryl], and cimetidine [Tagamet]), steroids.

After treatment, a good sign is if breath sounds and wheezing are present (a sign that bronchi are becoming more open). Usually discharge with steroids (e.g., Medrol Dose Pack).

Fast Facts | Normal Findings

Normal Findings
- Lower lobes: vesicular breath sounds (soft and low)
- Upper lobes: bronchial breath sounds (louder)

Egophony
- Normal: will hear "eee" clearly instead of "bah"
- Abnormal: will hear "bah" sound
- Normal: the "eee" sound is louder over the large bronchi because larger airways are better at transmitting sounds. The lower lobes have a softer sounding "eee."

Tactile Fremitus
- Instruct patient to say "99" or "1, 2, 3." Use finger pads to palpate lungs and feel for vibrations.

- Normal: stronger vibrations palpable on the upper lobes and softer vibrations on lower lobes.
- Abnormal: the findings are reversed. May palpate stronger vibrations on one lower lobe (i.e., consolidation). Asymmetrical findings are always abnormal.

Percussion

- Normal: resonance.
- Tympany or hyperresonance: COPD, emphysema (overinflation).
- Dull tone: bacteria pneumonia with lobar consolidation, pleural effusion (fluid or tumor).
- Use middle finger or index finger as the pleximeter finger on one hand. The finger on the other hand is the hammer. The liver sounds dull. The stomach area may be tympanic.

Whispered Pectoriloquy

- Normal: voice louder and easy to understand in the upper lobes. The voice is muffled and harder to understand in the lower lobes.
- Abnormal: clear voice sounds in the lower lobes or muffled sounds in the upper lobes.
- Instruct patient to whisper "1, 2, 3." Compare both lungs.

Fast Facts | Disease Review

Chronic Obstructive Pulmonary Disease (COPD)

COPD is a term that includes both emphysema and chronic bronchitis. Most patients have a mixture of both; one or the other may predominate. The disease is characterized by the loss of elastic recoil of the lungs and alveolar damage, which takes decades. The most common risk factors are smoking and older age. Currently, COPD affects 14 to 16 million Americans and is projected to increase as the baby boomer generation gets older.

Chronic Bronchitis

Defined as coughing with excessive mucus production for at least 3 or more months for a minimum of 2 or more consecutive years.

Emphysema

Permanent alveolar damage and loss of elastic recoil results in chronic hyperinflation of the lungs. Expiratory respiratory phase is markedly prolonged.

Risk Factors

- chronic smoking (etiology in up to 90% of cases of COPD), older age (>40)
- occupational exposure (coal dust, grain dust)
- alpha-1 trypsin deficiency: rare condition. Patients have severe lung damage at earlier ages. Alpha-1 trypsin protects lungs from oxidative and environmental damage.

Classic Case

Elderly male with a history of many years of cigarette smoking complains of gradually worsening dyspnea over several years that is starting to limit physical activity. The patient complains of getting easily short of breath on physical exertion. Accompanied by a chronic cough that is productive of large amounts of white-to-light-yellow sputum.

Objective Findings

Emphysema component: increased AP (anterior-posterior) diameter or barrel chest, decreased breath and heart sounds, hypoxia especially at night in sleep, and weight loss.

- Percussion: hyperresonance
- Tactile fremitus and egophony: decreased
- Chest X-ray: flattened diaphragms with hyperinflation
- Chronic bronchitis component: productive cough, wheezing and coarse crackles
- Acute exacerbations: fever, purulent sputum, increased symptoms of wheezing and dyspnea
- Treatment: Bactrim DS, Augmentin, Ceftin, Floxin BID × 10 days, Medrol Dose Pack PRN

Treatment: COPD

- Ipratropium (Atrovent) QID (anticholinergic)
- Add albuterol (short-acting B2 agonist) inhaler or Atrovent/albuterol mix (Combivent)
- Add long-acting theophylline (Theo-Dur; serum levels 8–12 UG/mL)
- Start oxygen therapy by nasal cannula at 2 to 3 L/min
- Consider prednisone (10–14 days) for exacerbations (up to 10% benefit)
- Start oxygen therapy earlier. Usually started at bedtime (oxygen desaturation worsens in the night). It is the only therapy for COPD shown in studies to prolong life.

Exam Tips

- Ipratropium (Atrovent) is an anticholinergic.
- The only treatment known to prolong life in COPD patients is supplemental oxygen therapy.

Bacterial Pneumonia

Bacterial lung infection results in inflammatory changes and damage to the lungs. The bacteria causing the most deaths in outpatients are the pneumococcus (Gram-positive).

Organisms

- *Streptococcus pneumoniae* or pneumococcus (Gram-positive)
- *Haemophilus influenzae*: more common in smokers (Gram-negative)
- *Mycoplasma pneumoniae* or *Chlamydia pneumoniae* (atypical bacteria)

Classic Case

Middle-age-to-elderly adult complains of a sudden onset of fever, chills, and productive cough. The phlegm is a green to rusty color. The patient complains of pleuritic chest pain with coughing and appears tired and ill.

Objective Findings

- Auscultation: crackles and decreased breath sounds (affected lobe)
- Tactile fremitus: increased
- Abnormal whispered pectoriloquy (whispered words louder)
- Percussion: Dullness over affected lobe

Labs

- Sputum for Gram-stain and culture, chest X-ray (gold standard), CBC
- CBC: leukocytosis (>10.5) with a possible "shift to the left" (increased band forms). Seen more in serious bacterial infections.
- Chest X-ray: lobar consolidation or diffuse patchy infiltrates. If smoker or high risk, repeat chest X-ray posttreatment (8–10 weeks) because it may be a presenting sign of lung cancer (due to mass blocking bronchioles).

American Thoracic Society (ATS) Guidelines

Outpatient Community-Acquired Pneumonia (CAP)*

Below age 60 with no comorbidity (e.g., asthma, diabetes, heart disease)

1) Macrolides are preferred
   - clarithromycin (Biaxin) BID × 10 days
   - azithromycin (Z-Pack) daily × 5 days
   - erythromycin QID × 10 days

Ages 60 years or older and younger patients with comorbidity

1) Second generation cephalosporin or IM Ceftriaxone preferred
   - cefuroxime axetil (Ceftin) BID × 10 to 14 days
   - amoxicillin clavulanate (Augmentin) BID × 10 to 14 days
2) Consider adding a macrolide or doxycycline if high suspicion of atypical bacterial infection
3) OR anti-pneumococcal quinolone as ONE drug therapy
   - Levaquin 500 mg QD × 7 to 14 days

Pneumonococcal Vaccine (Pneumovax)

Healthy patients

- single dose usually sufficient at age 65 years (lifetime)
- 60 to 70% effectiveness

---

* Adapted from the American Thoracic Society CAP Guidelines, 2001.

Underlying disease
- 50% effective

Severely immunocompromised
- only 10% effective

Recommended for:
- Persons age 65 years or older; nursing home residents
- Patients with preexisting heart and lung disease; asthma, CHD, and emphysema
- Impaired immunity: alcoholics/cirrhosis of the liver; splenectomy or asplenia; HIV infection; chronic renal failure
- Blood disorders: sickle cell anemia; Hodgkin's lymphoma, multiple myeloma

High-Risk Patients
Repeat vaccine in 5 to 7 years (boosts antibodies):
- HIV infection
- asplenia, chronic renal failure
- blood cancers: lymphoma, Hodgkin's disease, leukemia
- organ transplant patients (immunosuppressive therapy)

Atypical Pneumonia

An infection of the lungs by atypical bacteria. More common in children and young adults. Seasonal outbreaks. Also known as "walking pneumonia."

Organisms
- *Mycoplasma pneumoniae* (atypical bacteria)
- *Chlamydia pneumoniae* (atypical bacteria)
- *Legionella pneumoniae* (atypical bacteria): found in areas with moisture such as air conditioners (more severe with higher mortality)

Classic Case
A teenager complains of several weeks of fatigue and severe coughing that is mostly nonproductive. Gradual onset of symptoms. Illness started with a sore throat, clear rhinitis, and low-grade fever. Complains of malaise. Continues to go to work/school despite symptoms. May have coworkers with same symptoms.

Objective Findings
- Auscultation: wheezing and diffused crackles/rales
- Nose: clear mucus
- Throat: red with no pus
- Chest X-ray: diffuse interstitial infiltrates

Medications
- Macrolides: azithromycin (Z-Pack) × 5 days; clarithromycin (Biaxin) 500 mg BID × 10 days; erythromycin stearate 500 mg QID × 10 days

■ Antitussives (dextromorphan, Tessalon pearles) as needed (PRN)
■ Increase fluids and rest

Poor Prognosis: Pneumonia
■ Elderly: age 60 years or older
■ Multiple lobar involvements
■ Leukopenia
■ Alcoholics (aspiration pneumonia)

Acute Bronchitis

Acute viral or bacterial infection of the bronchi causes inflammatory changes that result in increased reactivity of the upper airways. Mainly manifested with dry cough that may last from 4 to 6 weeks.

Classic Case
Young adult complains of paroxysmal dry cough. May have mild wheezing and chest tightness. Cough keeps patient awake at night. Chest hurts from coughing.

Objective Findings
■ Lungs: clear to diffused wheezing. Normal or prolonged expiration.
■ Percussion: resonant
■ Chest X-ray: normal
■ Tactile Fremitus/Egophony: normal

Plan
■ Treatment is symptomatic. Increased fluids and rest. Stop smoking (if smoker).
■ Dextromorphan (Robitussin), Tessalon Perles (antitussives) PRN
■ Guaifenesin (expectorant/mucolytic) PRN
■ Albuterol inhaler (Ventolin) QID PRN

Classic Cases: Lung Infections
Bacterial Pneumonia
    ■ sudden onset, toxic, fever
    ■ cough productive of green-to-rusty-colored sputum
Atypical Pneumonia
    ■ gradual onset, low grade to no fever
    ■ always tired but continues working
    ■ cough
Acute Bronchitis
    ■ frequent paroxysms of dry cough
    ■ hard to catch breath when coughing spells occur

Exam Tips

■ Recognize classic case of bacterial pneumonia versus atypical pneumonia.
■ Preferred treatment for atypical pneumonia is macrolides.

Table 3.4 | Common Lung Infections

Disease	Signs & Symptoms
Bacterial Pneumonia (Community-acquired or CAP) Broad-spectrum beta lactams New quinolones (has gram positive coverage)	Acute onset. Fever & chills. Productive cough; green-to-rusty-colored sputum. Chest pain (pleurisy) with cough. Strep. pneumoniae (G. Pos.) Mycoplasma pneum. (G. Neg.)
Atypical Pneumonia Macrolide antibiotics	Gradual onset. Low grade fever. Sore throat. Cough. Wheeze. Chest pain w/ cough.
Viral Pneumonia Symptomatic treatment; antivirals Prophylactic antibiotics	Fever. Cough. Pleurisy. Myalgias. Breath sounds: rales, decreased breath sounds
Acute Bronchitis Symptomatic treatment only. NO antibiotics. Antitussives, mucolytics (guaifenesin)	Paroxysms of dry coughing. Wheezing. Can last up to 4 to 6 weeks.

American Thoracic Society Guidelines for Community-Acquired Pneumonia (CAP)
1) Age < 60 years (or no comorbidity):
Macrolides preferred: Erythromycin, Zithromax, Biaxin. All macrolides are category B except Biaxin (category C).
2) Age > 60 years or with comorbidity (i.e., COPD, asthma, CHD, etc.):
Broad-spectrum beta-lactams (Augmentin, Ceftin, Cefzil)
Plus doxycycline OR another macrolide (azithromycin, erythromycin)
Monotherapy: anti-pneumococcal quinolones (Levaquin, Avelox)
*Adapted from the ATS (American Thoracic Society) CAP Guidelines, 2001.

Clinical Tip

■ Pneumovax vaccine is underutilized. Offer to high-risk patients.

Tuberculosis (TB)

A lung infection caused by mycobacterium tuberculosis bacteria. Transmission is through respiratory droplets. Most common site of infection is the lungs (85%). Other sites are the kidneys, brain, lymph nodes, adrenals, bone, and so forth. A TB infection is controlled by an intact immune system. Macrophages sequester the bacteria in the lymph nodes (mediastinum) in the form of granulomas.

The majority of cases (90%) of active disease in the United States are reactivated infections. Reactivation occurs when the immune system is compromised or is less active (child younger than age 3 years and the elderly).

Miliary Tuberculosis
Also known as "disseminated TB disease." Infects multiple organ systems. More common in younger children (younger than the age of 5) and the elderly. Chest X-ray will show classic "milia seed" pattern.

Classic Case

Immunocompromised adult patient complains of fever, anorexia, fatigue, and night sweats along with a mild nonproductive cough (early phase). Aggressive infections (later sign) will have productive cough with blood-stained sputum (hemoptysis) along with weight loss (late sign).

Labs

Screening: PPD subdermally (Mantoux test).
Tine test is not acceptable test for screening.
Sputum culture and acid-fast bacilli stain (takes from 3 to 6 weeks).

Medications

- Active disease: use three drugs initially because of higher rates of resistant strains against INH (isoniazid) and rifampin. Narrow down number of medications only after C&S results.
- Treat a minimum of 6 months until culture is negative.
- HIV: treat for at least 12 months and until culture is negative.
- Ethambutol (causes optic neuritis). Avoid in patients with abnormal vision (e.g., blindness, retinal vein occlusion, etc.).

Direct Observed Treatment

- Highly recommended for pediatric and noncompliant patients.
- How: Patient is observed by a nurse when he or she takes the medications. Mouth, cheek, and area under the tongue checked to make sure the pill was swallowed adequately.

Recent PPD Converters

Recent Converters: defined as a person with history of negative PPD results, then converts to a positive (became infected).

At higher risk of active TB disease (up to 10%) in the first 1 to 2 years after seroconversion.

Prophylaxis

- Offer if younger than age 35 years with no history of liver disease or ETOH abuse.
- Prophylaxis not recommend if older than age 35; higher risk of drug hepatitis.
- INH 300 mg daily × 6 months (HIV positive, treat for at least 12 months). Also give pyridoxine (vitamin B6) if on INH. Order baseline LFTs.

Before Prophylaxis

Chest X-ray must be negative with no signs/symptoms of active TB disease.

History of Bacille Calmette-Guérin Vaccination

Affects PPD testing adversely with higher risk of false-positive results. Commonly given to patients from areas where TB is endemic (Asia, Africa, Latin America).

Anergy Testing

Used for patients suspected of being immunocompromised with a higher risk of false-negative test result.

Procedure

- The PPD is administered on the volar aspect of the left lower arm (as usual) and the "control" antigen is given on the right lower arm. "Control" agents used are tetanus, candida, or mumps antigens.
- Do not mix the two. Use tuberculin syringe to administer each agent.
- If control side is negative, unable to do PPD (invalid result).
- Consider other methods for detecting infection (e.g., bronchoscopy).

Booster Phenomenon

Two-step Testing

- recommended for elderly
- reduces incidence of false-negative PPDs

Elderly patient's immune system "forgets" how to react to the PPD antigens. When given a second dose of PPD in 7 to 10 days, helps decrease false negatives.

Explanation

- A person is negative after many years of no PPD testing.
- When redone again (first time), there is no reaction (false negative).
- If PPD repeated in 7 to 10 days, it will be positive (if TB infection present). Otherwise, if still a negative, more likely to be a true negative result.

PPD Testing Results (Mantoux)

Look for an induration (feels harder). The red color is not as important. If a PPD result is a bright red but is not indurated (skin feels soft), it is a negative result.

Equal or >5 mm:

- HIV (+)
- Positive chest X-ray findings or in close contact with a person with active TB.
- Any child with TB symptoms (especially before the age of 5).

Equal or >10 mm:

- Immunocompromised (e.g., chemo, bone morrow transplant, renal failure, diabetes, etc.).
- IV drug user, health care worker, prisoner, homeless.
- Comes from a high-prevalence country (i.e., in Asia, Latin America, or Africa).

Exam Tips

- A PPD result may be listed as 9.5 mm. It is a negative (by definition) unless the patient has the signs/symptoms and/or chest X-ray findings suggestive of TB.
- Memorize the criteria of the 10 mm results.
- Small children exposed to active TB have a high chance of coming down with the disease.

Asthma

Reactive Airway Disease (children)

Chronic inflammation of the bronchial tree results in an increase in airway responsiveness to stimuli (internal or external). By definition, airway obstruction must be reversible. High risks are a positive family history of allergies, eczema, and allergic rhinitis. Exacerbations may be severe and life threatening.

Classic Case

A school-age child with reactive airway disease with history of a recent bout of a viral URI complains of becoming more short of breath, wheezing, chest tightness, and having a dry cough at night. He or she starts using the albuterol inhaler more often to self-treat symptoms.

Trigger Factors for Asthma

- Viral URIs, airborne allergens
- Food allergies: sulfites, red and yellow dye, seafood, etc.
- Cold air or cold weather and fumes from chemicals or smoke
- Emotional stress and exercise (exercise-induced asthma)
- GERD (reflux of acidic gastric contents irritates airways)
- ASA or NSAIDs

Objective Findings

Wheezing with prolonged expiratory phase. As asthma worsens, the wheezing occurs during both inspiration and expiration.

Exacerbations

- Nebulizer treatments using albuterol/saline solution. May repeat in 15 minutes if poor relief of symptoms. If unable to reverse attack, call 911. Administer Epinephrine STAT.
- Discharge home with Medrol Dose Pack or prednisone tabs 40 mg/day × 4 days (no weaning necessary if 4 days or less).

Maintenance Medications

Inhaled corticosteroid BID

Depending on severity of asthma, can add leukotriene inhibitors (Singulair), mast cell stabilizers (great for kids), long-acting B2 agonist mixture (salmeterol combined with corticosteroid), and/or sustained-release theophylline.

Respiratory distress: tachypnea, using accessory muscles (intercostals, abdominal) to breathe, diaphoresis, and fatigue.

Exam Tips

- First line treatment for severe asthmatic exacerbation or respiratory distress is an adrenaline injection.

■ Severe respiratory distress: tachypnea, disappearance of or lack of wheezing, accessory muscle use, diaphoresis, and exhaustion.

Treatment Algorithm: Asthma*
Step 1: Mild Intermittent
■ albuterol (Ventolin) metered dose inhaler as needed

Step 2: Mild Persistent Asthma
■ albuterol (Ventolin) metered dose inhaler as needed
■ low-dose steroid metered dose inhaler
■ and/or cromolyn/ nedocromil (Intal inhaler)

Step 3: Moderate Persistent Asthma
■ albuterol metered dose inhaler
■ low- to medium-dose steroid metered-dose inhaler mixed with salmeterol (i.e., Advair)
■ leukotriene inhibitors (e.g., Singulair)
■ Consider sustained release theophylline (maintain levels at 10–20 mg/L)

Exercise-induced Asthma
Premedicate before activity with two puffs: albuterol (10–15 min.), or cromolyn (15–20 min.), or salmeteterol (30–60 min.).

Asthma Medications
"Rescue" Medicine
These drugs are used to relieve wheezing as needed (PRN).

■ Short-acting B2 agonists
■ albuterol (Ventolin) or pirbuterol (Alupent) 2 inhalations every 4 to 6 hours PRN
■ levalbuterol (Xopenex) nebulizer solution
■ quick onset (15 to 30 minutes) and lasts about 4 to 6 hours
■ used to relieve symptoms (wheezing) but does not treat underlying inflammation

Maintenance Medications
These drugs are anti-inflammatories. They must be taken daily to be effective
■ steroids: triamcinolone (Azmacort) BID
■ mast cell stabilizers: nedocromil sodium (Intal) QID
■ leukotriene inhibitors: zafirlukast (Singulair)
■ The only exception is the long-acting B2 agonist formoterol (Foradil) BID
■ Long-acting B2 agonists are *not* rescue drugs. Although taken daily, they are used to relieve bronchospasm. Slow onset of action (3 hours); use daily to maintain a blood level.

---

* From *Expert Panel Report II: Guidelines for the Diagnosis and Management of Asthma*, Feb. 1997.

Theophylline (Theo-24)

Drug class: methylxanthine or xanthine

Now used as third line drug for asthma because of risk of toxicity and multiple drug interactions such as the following:

- macrolides, quinolones
- cimetidine
- anticonvulsants such as phenytoin, carbamazepine (Tegretol)
- check blood levels: normal is 12 to 15 mg/dL

Asthma Treatment: In a Nutshell

- Every patient should be on a short-acting B2 agonist (albuterol) PRN.
- For children mast cell stabilizers (Intal, Tilade) work well (give 4-week trial).
- Inhaled corticosteroids. Dose depends on class of asthma.

Leukotriene inhibitors, long-acting B2 agonist mixture (salmeterol combined with corticosteroid) and sustained-release theophylline are added depending on severity of asthma and the response.

Exam Tip

- Do not confuse asthma "rescue" drugs from "maintenance" or "control" drugs.

Clinical Tips

- Chronic use of high-dose inhaled steroids can cause osteoporosis, mild growth retardation in children, glaucoma, cataracts, immune suppression, hypothalamic-pituitary-adrenal axis suppression, and so forth.
- Consider supplementing with calcium with vitamin D 1500 mg tabs QD for menopausal women and other high-risk patients (e.g., on long-term steroids).
- Bone density testing, annual eye exams if on long-term steroids (checking for cataracts and glaucoma).
- Monitor growth in children.

Smallpox (variola virus)

Eliminated in 1977. Infects respiratory or oropharyngeal mucosal surfaces. Incubation period: 2 weeks

Classic Case

Fever, headache, photophobia, myalgia, and fatigue. Characteristic rash has large nodules that appear mostly in the central area of the face, arms, and legs. Treatment is symptomatic. Mortality rate (variola major) is from 20 to 50%.

Plan

If vaccine given within 3 to 4 days postexposure, can lessen severity of illness. Vaccinia immune globulin available (pregnant, immunosuppressed, etc.).

Peak Expiratory Flow (PEF)
Pneumonic: HAG
PEF is based on height (H), age (A), and gender (G) (HAG).

Peak Expiratory Flow Rate: (PEFR or PEF)
Used by asthmatics to measure effectiveness of treatment, worsening symptoms, and exacerbations. Correlates well with the FEV_1 (forced expiratory volume at 1 second).

Spirometer Parameters
Green Zone: 80% to 100% of expected volume
■ maintain or reduce medications

Yellow Zone: 50 to 80% of expected volume
■ maintenance therapy needs to be increased or patient is having an acute exacerbation

Red Zone: below 50% of expected
■ if after treatment, patient's PER still below 50% expected, call 911. If in respiratory distress, give epinephrine injection and call 911.

Pulmonary Function Tests (PFTs)
Measures severity of obstructive or restrictive pulmonary dysfunction.
■ Obstructive dysfunction (reduction in airflow rates): asthma, COPD (chronic bronchitis and emphysema), bronchioectasis, etc.
■ Restrictive dysfunction (reduction of lung volume from decreased lung compliance): pulmonary fibrosis, pleural disease, diaphragm obstruction, etc.

Exam Tips

■ Do not confuse the formula for the PEF with the BMI.
■ PEF formula is based on: height, age, and gender.
■ BMI formula is based on: height and weight.

ENDOCRINE SYSTEM

Fast Facts Danger Signals

Severe Hypoglycemia

Blood glucose is <50 mg/dL. Complains of weakness, "feel like passing out," headache, clammy hands, and anxiety. Difficulty in concentration and thinking. If severe hypoglycemia is uncorrected, it will progress to coma.

Type 1 Diabetes Mellitus

School-age child with recent history of viral illness complains of excessive hunger and thirst. Urinating more than normal (polyuria). Starts losing weight despite eating a large amount of food. Breath has a "fruity" odor.

Thyroid Cancer

A single large nodule (>2.5 cm) on one lobe of the thyroid gland. Positive family history of thyroid cancer. History of facial, neck, or chest radiation therapy.

Pheochromocytoma

Random episodes of severe hypertension (systolic >200 mmHg or diastolic >110 mmHg) associated with abrupt onset of severe headache, tachycardia, and anxiety. Episodes resolve spontaneously, but occur at random. In between the attacks, patient's vital signs are normal.

Hyperprolactinemia

Can be a sign of a pituitary adenoma. Slow onset. When tumor is large enough to cause a mass effect, the patient will complain of headaches.

Fast Facts Normal Findings

- The endocrine system works in a "negative feedback" system. If low levels of "active" hormones occur, it stimulates production. Inversely, high levels of hormones stop production.
- The hypothalamus stimulates the anterior pituitary gland into producing the "stimulating hormones" (e.g., follicle-stimulating hormone [FSH]).
- These "stimulating hormones" tell the target organs (e.g., ovaries, thyroid, etc.) to produce "active" hormones (e.g., estrogen, thyroid hormone, etc.).
- High levels of these "active" hormones work in reverse. The hypothalamus directs the anterior pituitary into stopping production of the stimulating hormones (e.g., TSH, luteinizing hormone [LH], FSH, etc.).

Endocrine Glands

Hypothalamus (master gland)
Directs the anterior pituitary gland. Directly produces oxytocin, the hormone responsible for uterine stimulation in labor and milk production.

Pituitary Gland

Located at the sella turcica (base of the brain). Produces the "stimulating hormones" that turn on the "switch" of the target organs (e.g., ovaries, etc.). The target organ then synthesizes the active hormones (e.g., estrogen).

Anterior Pituitary Gland

Produces the following hormones that regulate the target organs (e.g., ovary, thyroid, etc.).

FSH (follicle stimulating hormone)
- stimulates the ovaries enabling growth of follicles (or eggs)
- production of estrogen

LH (luteinizing hormone)
- stimulates the ovaries to ovulate
- production of progesterone (by corpus lutea)

TSH (thyroid stimulating hormone)
- stimulates thyroid gland
- production of thyroid hormones T3 and T4

GH (growth hormone)
- stimulates somatic growth of body

ACTH (adrenocorticotropin hormone)
- stimulates the adrenal glands (two portions of gland: medulla and cortex)
- adrenal medulla (central portion of the gland) produces adrenaline (epinephrine) and noradrenaline (norepinephrine)
- adrenal cortex (outer portion) produces aldosterone (a mineral corticoid) that regulates sodium retention and excretion of potassium and cortisol (a glucocorticoid).

Posterior Pituitary Gland

Vasopressin (antidiuretic hormone [ADH]) and oxytocin are made by the hypothalamus but stored and secreted by the posterior pituitary.

Parathyroid Gland

Located behind the thyroid gland. Produces ADH.

Fast Facts | Disease Review

TSH
The best screening test for both hypothyroid and hyperthyroid disease:
- used to monitor response to thyroid replacement therapy
- used to monitor response to treatment for hyperthyroid disease

Hyperthyroid
Elevated free T4 and low TSH can detect up to 90% of hyperthyroid cases.

Table 3.5 | Diagnostic Labs: Endocrine System

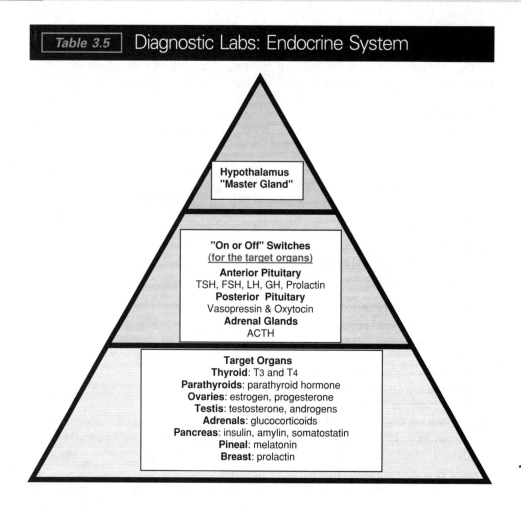

Hypothalamus "Master Gland"

"On or Off" Switches (for the target organs)
Anterior Pituitary
TSH, FSH, LH, GH, Prolactin
Posterior Pituitary
Vasopressin & Oxytocin
Adrenal Glands
ACTH

Target Organs
Thyroid: T3 and T4
Parathyroids: parathyroid hormone
Ovaries: estrogen, progesterone
Testis: testosterone, androgens
Adrenals: glucocorticoids
Pancreas: insulin, amylin, somatostatin
Pineal: melatonin
Breast: prolactin

Graves' Disease

An autoimmune disorder of the thyroid gland causing hyperfunction and pro-duction of excess thyroid hormones (T3 and T4). It is the most common cause of hyperthyroidism in this country. Higher incidence in women (8:1 ratio). These women are also at higher risk for other autoimmune diseases such as rheumatoid arthritis, pernicious anemia, and lupus.

Classic Case
Middle-aged female loses a large amount of weight rapidly, is irritable and anxious, experiences insomnia, frequent bowel movements (looser stools), amenorrhea, and heat intolerance.

Objective Findings
- Goiter: diffusely enlarged gland without nodules
- Hands/fingers: fine tremors, sweaty palms
- Cardiac: tachycardia
- Eyes: exophthalmos in later cases

Labs
Suppressed TSH, increased free T4 (free T4 better measure than total T4)

Medications
- Propylthiouracil (PTU): shrinks thyroid gland/decreases hormone production
- Methimazole (Tapazole): shrinks thyroid gland/decreases hormone production
- Adjunctive treatment: Given before thyroid under control to ameliorate symptoms such as hyperstimulation (e.g., anxiety, tachycardia, palpitations), which is treated with beta blocker propranolol (Inderal)
- Radioactive iodine: Permanent destruction of thyroid gland results in hypothyroidism. These patients need thyroid supplementation for the rest of their lives.
- For pregnant women: PTU is preferred; give lowest effective dose possible.

Exam Tips

- Radioactive iodine treatment results in hypothyroidism. Supplemented with thyroid hormone (e.g., Synthroid) for life.
- PTU preferred for pregnant women.
- Thyroid cancer risk factors (history of neck irradiation in childhood or a painless nodule > 2.5 cm).
- Chronic amenorrhea and hypermetabolism from hyperthyroidism may result in osteoporosis. Treat with calcium with vitamin D, Fosamax, weight-bearing exercises.

Clinical Tips

- TSH testing in neonates is a legal requirement in this country.
- Lack of thyroid hormone results in mental retardation and retarded somatic growth.

Thyroid Gland Tests
- Thyroid gland ultrasounds: used to detect goiter (generalized enlargement of the thyroid gland), multinodular goiter, single nodule, and solid versus cystic masses.
- Thyroid cancer: single painless nodule >2.5 cm, history of neck irradiation in childhood.
- Thyroid scan: shows metabolic activity of thyroid gland.
- Cold spot: not metabolically active (more worrisome; rule out thyroid cancer).
- Hot spot: metabolically active nodule and usually benign.

Diabetes Mellitus

A metabolic disorder affecting the body's metabolism of carbohydrates and fat.

Type 1 Diabetes

An autoimmune reaction stimulated by a viral infection. Massive destruction of beta cells in the Isles of Langerhans (pancreas) cause abrupt cessation of insulin production. Results in ketoacidosis from the breakdown of fatty stores that the body uses for fuel. If uncontrolled, ketosis will progress into coma or diabetic ketotic acidosis. Most patients are juveniles; occasionally adults (mature onset diabetes mellitus).

Type 2 Diabetes

Decreased secretion of insulin with peripheral insulin resistance resulting in a chronic state of hyperglycemia and hyperinsulinemia. Results in microvascular (retinopathy, nephropathy) as well as macrovascular (acute MI, strokes, atherosclerosis, or plaques on blood vessels) damage.

Target Organs

- the eyes, heart, vascular system, kidneys, and peripheral nerves, especially on the feet. Diabetes is the most common reason for chronic renal failure requiring dialysis and lower limb amputations in this country.

Type 2 Diabetes Mellitus (85 to 90% of cases in USA)

- Stronger genetic component compared with type 1 diabetes. Usually presents at age 40 or older (may appear at younger ages).
- Usually overweight or obese (BMI 30 or >).
- Hispanic, African-American, Asian, or American Indian, or positive family history.
- Metabolic syndrome (insulin resistance syndrome) present: defined as obese patient with hypertension, hyperglycemia, and dyslipidemia.

Diabetes Mellitus: Three Ways to Diagnose

- Symptoms of diabetes (polyuria, polydipsia, polyphagia) plus random blood glucose greater than 200 mg/dL.
- Fasting blood glucose equal or >126 mg/dL on two separate occasions.
- 2-hour blood glucose equal or >200 mg/dL during an OGTT (oral glucose tolerance test) with a 75 g glucose load.

Glycemic Parameters

- Fasting blood glucose: less than 126 mg/dL
- Post-prandial (2 hours after large meal): less than 200 mg/dL

Impaired Glucose Tolerance

A fasting blood glucose between 110 mg/dL and 126 mg/dL. These patients are considered at higher risk for type 2 diabetes. Another name for this condition is "prediabetes."

Labs
- Hemoglobin A1c (HbA1c): the average blood glucose levels over previous 3 months. No fasting required. Excess glucose attaches to the hemoglobin of the RBCs.
- Normal value for glycated Hb or Hb A1c: 4 to 6%.

Goal of Treatment
- HbA1c of 6% or less.
- Newly diagnosed diabetics: check HbA1c every 3 months until blood glucose controlled.
- Lipid profile at least once a year (or more if elevated).
- Urinalysis once a year. If urinalysis is normal, check urine for microalbuminuria, if positive, order 24-hour urine for protein and creatinine.
- Other: electrolytes (potassium, magnesium, sodium), liver function panel, TSH.

Diabetes Issues

Hypoglycemia
- High risk: 50 mg/dL or less
- Look for: dizziness, sweaty palms, nausea, rapid pulse, and weakness. Final result is syncope if not treated with glucose.
- Some patients may become confused ("hypoglycemic unawareness").
- Beta blockers block or blunt the symptoms of hypoglycemia.

Plan
- Every visit: check BP, weight, blood sugar diary.
- Check feet at every visit (5.07 U monofilament tool): look for vibration sense, light and deep touch, and numbness.

Recommendations for Preventative Care
- Flu shot every year
- Aspirin 81 mg per day
- Pneumovax vaccine age 60 (or earlier if at high-risk category)
- Ophthalmologist: annual dilated eye exam
- Podiatrist: once to twice a year especially with older diabetics
- BP: 130/80 mmHg

Skipping Meals and Illness in Diabetics
- Skipping a meal or exercising heavily will increase the risk of hypoglycemia in the evening and at bedtime.
- If patient is ill and unable to eat, consider withholding insulin/oral antidiabetic medications until patient can eat.

Exercise
- Increases glucose utilization and promotes weight loss. Some patients may have to reduce the usual dose or eat snacks before the activity and afterward.
- Snacking: simple carbohydrates (candy, juices) before or during exercise and complex carbohydrates (granola bars) after exercise (avoids postexercise hypoglycemia).
- Older diabetics: rule out preexisting CHD before starting exercise program by administering a stress test.

Diabetes Mellitus: Specific Eye Findings

Diabetes Mellitus
- microaneurysms
- neovascularization (fragile small arterioles in retina rupture easily causing bleeding and scarring on the retina)

Diabetic Foot Care
Patients with neuropathy should avoid excessive running or walking to minimize the risk of foot injury.
- Never go barefoot.
- Wear shoes that fit properly.
- Check feet daily, especially the soles of the feet (use mirror).
- Trim nails squarely (not rounded) to prevent ingrown toenails.
- Report redness, skin breakdown, or trauma to health care giver immediately (main cause of lower leg amputations in the United States).

Antidiabetic Agents

Thiazolidinediones
Rosiglitazone (Avandia), pioglitazone (Actos)
Reduces peripheral tissue resistance and reduces hepatic glucagon production (gluconeogenesis). Take daily at breakfast with a meal.

Contraindication
- History of moderate-to-severe CHF because of medication's effect of water retention (aggravates or will precipitate heart failure).

Labs
Monitor LFTs. Check baseline, then periodically thereafter.
Discontinue if LFTs elevated more than three times the upper limit of normal AST and ALT if there is muscle soreness or the patient is jaundiced.

Sulfonylureas
First generation: chlorpropamide (Diabinese) daily or BID
- Longer half-life with higher risk of hypoglycemia.
- Avoid in elderly or patients with history of hypoglycemic episodes.

Second generation: glyburide (DiaBeta) daily to BID, glipizide (Glucotrol XL) daily
■ Stimulates the pancreas to secrete more insulin. Take at least 30 minutes before meals.

Contraindication
■ ketoacidosis

Adverse reactions: hypoglycemia, photosensitivity, GI symptoms

Biguanides
Metformin (Glucophage)

Decreases gluconeogenesis and decreases peripheral insulin resistance. Very rarely may cause hypoglycemia. Preferred for obese patients (can cause weight loss).

Contraindications
■ Renal or liver disease, acidosis, alcoholics, renal insufficiency, hypoxia
■ Increased risk lactic acidosis (pH <7.25) during hypoxia, hypoperfusion, renal insufficiency

IV contrast dye testing: hold metformin on day of procedure and 48 hours after. Check baseline creatinine and recheck after procedure. Serum creatinine must be normalized before drug can be resumed.

Acarbose (Precose)
Inhibits the enzyme alpha-glucosidase in the small intestine, which reduces carbohydrate absorption. Does not cause hypoglycemia.

Side Effects
■ GI side effects such as bloating, flatulence, abdominal cramping, and pain. Common reason for noncompliance. Start patient on a low dose and titrate up slowly.

Repaglinide (Prandin)
A nonsulfonylurea drug. Rapid-acting with a very short half-life (<1 hr). Indicated for type 2 diabetics with postprandial hyperglycemia (defined as a blood sugar of >200 mg/dL 2 hours after a meal). Take before meals or up to 30 minutes after a meal. Because of its extremely short half-life, it is useful for treating the elderly and for patients with renal disease. Metabolized in liver.

Exam Tips
■ Do not use any oral antidiabetic drugs on type 1 diabetics.
■ Memorize the specific eye findings of diabetes versus hypertension.
■ Moderate-to-severe heart disease or heart failure is a contraindication because it causes water retention, which may precipitate CHF.

■ Mild type 2 diabetics do not need drug therapy if able to control blood glucose by diet and exercise alone.

Clinical Tip

■ In general, sulfonylureas are most effective in patients with type 2 diabetes of less than 5 years duration because their pancreas still produces small amounts of insulin (it gradually stops).

Diabetes Mellitus: Management

■ Lifestyle changes are first line treatment along with oral antidiabetics.
■ Weight loss improves metabolic control in type 2 diabetics.
■ Exercise increases cellular glucose uptake in the body.
■ Type 2 diabetics not well controlled on multiple oral agents, diet, and lifestyle changes are good candidates for basal insulin therapy.

Types of Insulin

This is not an inclusive list.

■ Short-acting insulin (Regular)
    Onset: 30 minutes
    Peak: 3 to 4 hours
    Duration: 6 to 8 hours
■ Intermediate-acting insulin (NPH or Lente)
    Onset: 1 to 2 hours
    Peak: 6 to12 hours
    Duration: 18 to 24 hours
■ Lantus (insulin glargine-recombinant)
    Considered a "basal insulin"
    Onset: 1 hour
    Duration: 24 hours with no pronounced peaks. Give once a day at the same time.
    Not indicated at present for children younger than 6 years of age.

Diabetes: Possible Complications

■ Eyes: cataracts, diabetic retinopathy, blindness
■ Cardiovascular: hyperlipidemia, CAD, MI, HTN
■ Kidneys: renal disease, renal failure
■ Feet: foot ulcers, skin infections, peripheral neuropathy, amputation
■ Gyne/GU: balanitis (candidal infection of the glans penis), candidal vaginitis

Diabetes: Other Findings

Dawn Phenomenon
It is a normal physiologic event for the plasma glucose to rise in the early morning because of the reduction of tissue sensitivity to insulin between 5 a.m and 8 a.m. (from physiologic spike of growth hormone).

Somogyi Effect (Rebound hyperglycemia)

Severe nocturnal hypoglycemia stimulates counter regulatory hormones such as glucagon to be released from the liver. The high levels of glucagon in the systemic circulation results in high fasting blood glucose by 7 a.m. The condition is caused by overtreatment with the evening and/or bedtime insulin (dose is too high). More common in type 1 diabetics.

- Diagnosis: check blood glucose very early in the morning (3 a.m.) for 1 or 2 weeks.
- Treatment: snack before bedtime or eliminate dinnertime NPH dose or lower bedtime dose.

GASTROINTESTINAL SYSTEM

Fast Facts | Danger Signals

Acute Appendicitis

School-age child complains of an acute onset of periumbilical pain that is steadily getting worse. Over a period of 12 to 24 hours, the pain starts to localize at McBurney's point. The patient has no appetite (anorexia). When the appendix ruptures, clinical signs of acute abdomen present such as involuntary guarding, rebound, and a boardlike abdomen. The Psoas and Obturator signs are positive.

Colon Cancer

Very gradual (years) with vague GI symptoms. Tumor may bleed intermittently and patient may have iron deficiency anemia. Changes in bowel habits, changes in stool or bloody stool. Heme positive stool, dark tarry stool, mass on abdominal palpation. More common in older patient (>50 years of age) especially if history of multiple polyps or Crohn's disease.

Zollinger-Ellison Syndrome

A gastrinoma located on the pancreas or the stomach; secretes gastrin, which stimulates high levels of acid production in the stomach. The end result is the development of multiple and severe ulcers in the stomach and duodenum. Complaints of epigastric to midabdominal pain. Stools may be a tarry color. Screening by serum fasting gastrin level.

Crohn's Disease

Right lower quadrant intermittent abdominal pain. Lower abdominal pain 1 hour after eating. Diarrhea with mucus. Fever, malaise, and mild weight loss. Abnormal liquid stools. Patients with Crohn's disease at higher risk for colon cancer.

Pyloric Stenosis

Projectile vomiting after meals in a young infant (2 weeks to 5.5 months). Painless olivelike smooth mass below the xiphoid process that is easier to palpate when feeding. Caused by hypertrophic pyloric sphincter.

Intussusception

Infant younger than 4 months appears in pain, crying all the time and pulls legs forward. Currant jelly stools (bright red color). Bowel sounds normal to hyperactive (affected areas). Caused by telescoping bowel causing ischemia and necrosis. May have signs of peritonitis and shock if discovered late.

Fast Facts | Normal Findings

Route of food or drink from the mouth:
Esophagus → stomach (hydrochloric acid, intrinsic factor) → duodenum (bile, amylase, lipase) → jejunum → ileum→ colon → cecum → rectum→ anus

Abdominal Contents

- Right upper quadrant: liver, gallbladder, ascending colon, kidney (right), and pancreas (small portion). Right kidney is lower than the left because of displacement by the liver.
- Left upper quadrant: stomach, pancreas, descending colon and kidney (left).
- Right lower quadrant: appendix, ileum, cecum, and ovary (right).
- Left lower quadrant: sigmoid colon and ovary (left).
- Suprapubic area: bladder, uterus, and rectum.

Fast Facts | Benign Variants

The appendix can be located in any quadrant of the abdomen.

Maneuvers: Acute Abdomen or Peritonitis
Psoas /Iliopsoas (supine position)
Used for acute appendicitis or any suspected retroperitoneal area acute process (e.g., ruptured ectopic pregnancy). Flex hip 90 degrees, ask patient to push against resistance (examiner's hand) and to straighten the leg.

Obturator Sign (supine position)
Used for acute appendicitis or any suspected retroperitoneal area acute process (e.g., ruptured ectopic pregnancy). Rotate right hip through full range of motion. Positive sign if pain with the movement or flexion of the hip.

Rovsing's Sign (supine position)
Deep palpation of the left lower quadrant of the abdomen results in referred pain to the right lower quadrant.

McBurney's Point

Localized area between the superior iliac crest and umbilicus in the right lower quadrant. Tenderness or pain is a sign of a possible acute appendicitis.

Markle Test (Heel Jar)

Instruct patient to raise heels then drop them suddenly. An alternative is to ask the patient to jump in place. Positive if pain elicited or if patient refuses to perform because of pain.

Involuntary Guarding

With abdominal palpation, the abdominal muscles reflexively become tense or "boardlike."

Rebound Tenderness

Patient complains that the abdominal pain is worse when the palpating hand is released versus the pain felt during deep palpation.

Fast Facts Disease Review

Irritable Bowel Syndrome (IBS)

A chronic functional disorder of the colon (normal colonic tissue) marked by exacerbations and spontaneous remissions. Commonly exacerbated by excess stress.

Classic Case

A young adult to middle-aged female complains of intermittent episodes of moderate-to-severe cramping pain in the lower abdomen, especially on the left lower quadrant. Bloating with flatulence. Relief obtained after defecation. Stools range from diarrhea to constipation, or both types with increased frequency of bowel movements.

Objective Findings

- Abdominal exam: tenderness in lower quadrants during an exacerbation. Otherwise the exam is normal.
- Rectal exam: normal with no blood or pus.
- Heme negative stools.

Plan

- Increase dietary fiber. Supplement fiber with Metamucil (psyllium).
- Antispasmodics (e.g., Bentyl) as needed. Decrease life stress.
- Rule out: amoebic, parasitic, or bacterial infections, and inflammatory disease of the GI tract. Check stool for ova and parasites (especially diarrheal stools) with culture.

Gastric Ulcer and Duodenal Ulcer Disease

Gastric ulcers have higher risk for malignancy (up to 10%) compared with duodenal ulcers, which are mostly benign. Duodenal ulcers are five times more prevalent than gastric ulcers (seen more in elderly).

Etiology
- *Helicobacter pylori* (Gram-negative bacteria)
- Chronic NSAIDs that disrupt prostaglandin production. Results in reduction of GI blood flow with reduction of protective mucus layer.

Classic Case
Middle-aged to older adult complains of epigastric pain, burning/gnawing pain, or ache (80%). Pain relieved by food and/or antacids (50%) with reoccurrence from 2 to 4 hours after a meal. Self-medicating with OTC antacids. May be taking NSAIDs or aspirin.

Objective Findings
- Abdominal exam: normal or mildly tender epigastric area during flare-ups.
- Hemoccult can be positive if active bleeding.

Plan
- Gold standard: biopsy of gastric and/or duodenal tissue (by upper endoscopy).
- Urea Breath Test: not as sensitive as a biopsy; positive with active infection.
- Titers: *H. pylori* IgM and IgG levels.
- Fasting gastrin levels to rule out Zollinger-Ellison syndrome as needed.

H. Pylori-Negative Ulcers

Do not prescribe antibiotics because there is no infection. Treat symptoms. Encourage lifestyle changes.
- First line: H2 blockers: ranitidine (Zantac) × 4 to 6 weeks
- If no relief or poor result, switch to a proton pump inhibitor (PPI): omeprazole (Prilosec) daily × 4 to 6 weeks

H. Pylori-Positive Ulcers

Two types of regimens:
1. Therapy 1
- Omeprazole (Prilosec) QD plus
- Clarithromycin (Biaxin) BID plus
- Amoxicillin 1 g BID
- Add an H2 antagonist or PPI × 4 to 6 weeks after

2. Therapy 2
- Bismuth subsalicylate tab 600 mg QID plus
- Metronidazole tab 250 mg QID plus

- Tetracycline 500 mg caps QID × 2 weeks
- Plus: Ranitidine 150 mg daily × 4 to 6 weeks after

Exam Tips

- Distinguish if question concerns *H. pylori*-negative ulcers or *H. pylori*-positive ulcers.
- Both treatment regimens have appeared on the exams before.

Clinical Tips

- Today, most clinicians start with PPIs versus H2 antagonists. But on the test, follow the stated regimens.

Gastroesophageal Reflux (GERD)

Acidic gastric contents regurgitate from the stomach into the esophagus. Chronic GERD causes damage to squamous epithelium of the esophagus and may result in Barrett's esophagus (a precancer), which increases risk of squamous cell cancer.

Classic Case

Middle-aged or older adult complains of chronic heartburn of many years duration. Symptoms associated with large and/or fatty meals and is worsened when supine. Long-term history of self-medication with OTC antacids. May be on chronic NSAIDs, aspirin, or alcohol.

Objective Findings

- Acidic or sour odor to breath
- Reflux of sour acidic stomach contents especially with overeating
- Thinning tooth enamel caused by increased hydrochloric acid in mouth
- Sore red throat (not associated with a cold)
- Chronic coughing

Labs

Gold standard: esophageal motility studies

Plan

- Lifestyle changes include: avoid large or high-fat meals especially 3 to 4 hours before bedtime, lose weight, avoid mints (relaxes gastric sphincter), avoid caffeine, alcohol, aspirin, and NSAIDs.

Medications

H2 blockers (ranitidine) × 4 to 6 weeks.
If no relief, start on PPI such as omeprazole (Prilosec) × 4 to 6 weeks.

Complication

Barrett's esophagus (a precancer for esophageal cancer).

Exam Tip

■ Barrett's esophagus is a precancer.

Clinical Tip

■ Any patient with at least a decade or more history of chronic heartburn should be referred to a gastroenterologist for an endoscopy to rule out Barrett's esophagus.

Diverticulitis

Diverticula are small pouchlike herniations on the external surface of the colon secondary to a chronic lack of dietary fiber. Diverticulitis is infected diverticula. Higher incidence in Western societies.

Classic Case
Elderly patient presents with acute onset of fever with left lower quadrant abdominal pain with anorexia, nausea, and/or vomiting, constipation, or diarrhea. Hematochezia (bloody stool) if hemorrhaging.

Objective Findings
If signs of an acute abdomen are present (e.g., rebound, boardlike), refer to ER. If diverticula not inflamed, normal abdominal exam.

Labs
Sigmoidoscopy after barium enema (can see diverticula the best) but not during acute exacerbation.

Plan
■ Chronic therapy: high-fiber diet with fiber supplementation such as psyllium (Metamucil) or methylcellulose (Citrucel).
■ Outpatient treatment for very mild cases only. If no response in 72 hours or if condition worsens, refer to ER.

Medications
Trimethoprim/sulfamethoxazole BID or Cipro BID.
metronidazole 500 mg × 6 hours × 7 to 10 days.
Close follow-up. For moderate-to-severe cases: hospitalize.

Acute Pancreatitis

Acute inflammation of the pancreas secondary to many factors such as elevated triglyceride levels, cholecystitis, cholelithiasis, alcohol abuse, and infections. Elevated triglycerides (>800 mg/dL) create a very high risk of acute pancreatitis.

Classic Case

Adult-to-older patient complains of an acute onset of guarding and tenderness over the epigastric area or the upper abdomen. The classic finding is of epigastric abdominal pain that radiates to the mid-back and anorexia. May be accompanied by fever, tachycardia, and signs and symptoms of shock. Refer patient to ER.

Objective Findings

■ Cullen's sign: bluish discoloration around umbilicus (hemorrhagic pancreatitis).
■ Gray Turner's sign: bluish discoloration on the flank area (hemorrhagic pancreatitis).
■ Hypoactive bowel sounds (ileus), jaundice, guarding, and boardlike upper abdomen if peritonitis.

Labs

Elevated pancreatic enzymes such as serum amylase, lipase, and trypsin.
Elevated AST, ALT, gamma glutamyl transferase (GGT), bilirubin, and leukocytosis.

Complications

Death
Acute hepatic injury
Diabetes

Viral Hepatitis

Laboratory Tests
Hepatitis A, B, and C

Hepatitis A

■ No chronic or carrier state exists.
■ Transmission: fecal and oral route from contaminated food.
■ Self-limiting infection. Treatment is symptomatic.
■ Vaccine available (Havrix) and recommended for travelers to areas where Hepatitis A is endemic.

IgG anti-HAV (Hepatitis A virus antibody IgG type) positive

■ Antibodies present (immunity from previous Hepatitis A infection or from vaccine [Havrix]).
■ No virus present and not infectious.

IgM anti-HAV (Hepatitis A virus antibody IgM type) positive means

■ Acute infection
■ Virus is present (infectious). No immunity.

Hepatitis B

■ Transmission: sexual secretions (semen, vaginal secretions, and saliva), blood, blood products, organs.

- HBsAg (Hepatitis B surface antigen).
- Screening test for Hepatitis B: if positive, patient has a current infection and is infectious.
- May be from either an acute infection or chronic Hepatitis B infection.

Anti-HBs (Hepatitis B surface antibody) positive means
- Antibodies present and immune against Hepatitis B virus.
- Not infectious.
- May be from either a past infection or from Hepatitis B vaccine.

HBeAg (Hepatitis B "e" antigen")
- Indicates active viral replication. Infectious.
- Persistence indicates chronic Hepatitis B.

Chronic Hepatitis Infection: Two Types
- Chronic infection with mildly elevated LFTs.
- Chronic and active infection with elevated LFTs (active viral replication). Patient is at higher risk for cirrhosis, liver failure, and liver cancer.

Anti-HCV (antibody Hepatitis C virus)
- Screening test for Hepatitis C.
- Up to 85% of cases become carriers.

Unlike Hepatitis A and B, a positive anti-HCV (antibody) does not always mean that the patient has recovered from the infection and has developed immunity. It may instead indicate current infection.

If this test is positive, order HCV RNA or HCV polymerase chain reaction (PCR). If this test is positive, indicates current infection.

Hepatitis C
- Transmission: IV drug use (50%), blood or blood products, and sexual intercourse. In 40% of cases, the mode is unknown.
- High risk groups: IV drug users, hemophiliacs, or anyone with history of frequent transfusions.
- Highest risk for chronic hepatitis infection and cirrhosis (30%). Cirrhosis markedly increases the risk for liver cancer or liver failure. Refer to GI for management.
- Treatment: alpha interferon injections and ribavirin. Liver biopsy to stage disease.

Fast Facts | Disease Review

Acute Hepatitis

An acute liver inflammation with multiple causes. Examples include viral infection, hepatotoxic drugs (e.g., statins), excessive alcohol intake, toxins, and so forth.

Classic Case

Sexually active adult complains of a new onset of fatigue, nausea, and dark-colored urine for several days. New sexual partner (<3 months).

Objective Findings

Skin and sclera have a yellow tinge (jaundiced or icteric).
Liver: tenderness over the liver from percussion and deep palpation.

Labs

ALT and AST: elevated up to 10 times normal during the acute phase of the illness.
Other LFTs may be elevated such as the serum bilirubin and GGT.

Plan

- Treat the cause (if possible).
- Avoid hepatotoxic agents such as alcoholic drinks, acetaminophen, and statins (e.g., pravastatin or Pravachol).
- Treatment is supportive.

Liver Function Tests (LFTs)

The following results are normal laboratory reference ranges for adults to elderly.

Serum AST (aspartate aminotransferase)

Also known as serum glutamic oxaloacetic transaminase (SGOT).
- Normal: 5 to 50 u/L.
- Present in the liver, heart muscle, skeletal muscle, kidney, and lung.
- Not specific for liver injury because it is also elevated in other conditions (e.g., acute MI).

Serum ALT (alanine aminotransferase)

Also known as serum glutamic pyruvic transaminase (SGPT).
- Normal: 5 to 40 u/L.
- This enzyme is found mainly in the liver. A positive finding indicates liver inflammation.
- More specific for hepatic inflammation than AST.

AST/ALT Ratio (or SGOT/SGPT ratio)

- A ratio of 2.0 or higher may be indicative of alcohol abuse.

Serum GGT (gamma glutamyl transpeptidase)

- Sensitive indicator of alcohol abuse. May be a "lone" elevation.
- Elevated in liver disease and acute pancreatitis.

Alkaline Phosphatase (ALP)

- An enzyme produced primarily by the bone and liver. Smaller amounts are produce by the placenta, the intestines, and the kidneys.
- Higher levels seen during growth spurts in children and teens.
- May also be elevated with healing fractures, osteomalacia, and malignancy.

Exam Tips

- PCR tests are not antibody tests. They are testing for presence of viral RNA. A positive result means that the virus is present.
- Hepatitis C has highest risk of cirrhosis and liver cancer.
- A lone elevation in the GGT is a sensitive indicator of possible alcoholism.
- Alkaline phosphatase is normally elevated during the teen years.
- Be prepared for a case scenario of a patient's titer results and to identify type of hepatitis patient is infected with (see the following).

Viral Hepatitis: Case Studies

Patient A
- HBsAg: negative
- Anti-HBs: positive
- HBeAg: negative

Results are indicative of either
- History of old Hepatitis B infection that has resolved.
- History of vaccination against Hepatitis B.

Patient B
- HBsAg: positive
- HBeAg: positive
- Anti-HBs: negative
- anti-HAV: positive
- anti-HCV: negative

Results are indicative of
- Hepatitis B infection.
- History of previous Hepatitis A infection and immunity.

Patient has Hepatitis B infection and is infectious. A positive HBeAg test indicates that patient is a carrier and has the virus.

Exam Tip

- There will be a serology question. You will have to figure out what type of viral hepatitis the patient has (A, B, or C).

RENAL SYSTEM

Fast Facts | Danger Signals

Acute Pyelonephritis

Patient presents with acute onset of high fever, chills, dysuria, frequency, and flank pain. The flank pain is described as a deep ache. May have history of recent bladder infection.

Acute Pyelonephritis (child)

Acute onset of high fever, chills, dysuria, and frequency. Complains of unilateral flank pain associated with nausea and/or vomiting. Acute pyelonephritis in a child signals a urinary or renal abnormality. Refer to pediatric urologist.

Wilm's Tumor (nephroblastoma)

Smooth abdominal tumor that does not cross the midline and is usually asymptomatic. If symptomatic, child complains of abdominal pain and has a poor appetite, hematuria, and hypertension. Higher incidence in Black female children (ages 2–3 years).

Recurrent Urinary Tract Infections (child)

Child complains of painful urination, frequency, and is taking longer than normal to void (if toilet trained). May have hematuria. A sign of renal or urologic abnormality. Refer to pediatric urologist.

Acute Renal Failure

Peripheral edema, weight gain (water retention), and oliguria. May be anorexic and lethargic. Rapid decrease in renal function. Elevated urinary and serum creatinine.

Fast Facts Normal Findings

Kidneys

The kidneys are located in the retroperitoneal area. The lower half of the right kidney falls below the rib cage. It is lower than the left kidney because of displacement by the liver.

The basic functional units of the kidneys are the nephrons, which contain the glomeruli.

Function
Kidneys are the body's regulators of electrolytes, fluids, and bicarbonate (affects blood pH). They also produce the hormone erythropoietin, which stimulates bone marrow into producing more RBCs. Water is reabsorbed back to the body by the action of antidiuretic hormone and aldosterone. Kidneys excrete water soluble waste as urine. The average daily urine output is 1,500 mL.

Fast Facts Laboratory Testing

Serum Creatinine
Male 0.7 to 1.3 mg/dL
Female 0.6 to 1.1 mg/dL

Serum creatinine is an indirect measure of renal function. Creatinine is the end product of creatine metabolism, which comes mostly from muscle. Creatinine clearance is fairly constant and is not affected by fluid status or dietary intake of meat.

Creatinine clearance is doubled for every 50% reduction of the glomerular filtration rate. Elevated values are seen during acute or chronic renal failure, from nephrotoxic drugs, and so forth.

Urinalysis

Epithelial cells
- Large amounts in a urine sample indicate contamination.

Leukocytes
Normal white blood cells (WBCs) in urine: ≤ 10 WBCs/μL.
- Presence of leukocytes in urine (pyuria) is abnormal in males and indicates infection. The urinalysis is a more sensitive test for infection in males as compared with females.

Urine for C&S
- $\geq 10^5$ CFU/mL of bacteria (CFU or colony forming units) indicates infection.
- Lower values indicative of bacteriuria.

Red Blood Cells
- Seen in kidney stones and some lower urinary tract infections (UTIs).

Protein
- Indicates kidney damage.
- May be present in acute pyelonephritis. May also see casts.
- Urine dipsticks only pick up albumin, not microalbumin (Bence Jones proteins).

Nitrites
- Indicative of infection.
- Is due to breakdown of nitrates by certain bacteria.

Fast Facts Disease Review

Urinary Tract Infections (UTIs)
Infection of the lower urinary tract predominantly from Gram-negative bacteria such as *Escherichia Coli* (85%). Others are *Staphylococcus saprophyticus* (4%), and *Klebsiella* (3%). UTIs in children younger than age 3 are more likely to progress to pyelonephritis.

Risk Factors
- Failure to void after sex or increased sexual intercourse (honeymoon bladder).
- Diaphragm and spermicide use.
- Diabetes mellitus.
- Pregnancy.
- History of a recent UTI.
- Renal calculi, ureteral strictures, tumors.

Classic Case
A sexually active female complains of new onset of dysuria, frequent urge to urinate, and nocturia. May also complain of suprapubic discomfort.

Plan
- Urinalysis: leukocyte positive (WBCs $\geq 10/\mu L$), positive nitrites, RBCs.
- Urine for C&S.

Medications
Treat $\times$ 3 days if uncomplicated UTI. Treat $\times$ 7 days for complicated UTIs.
Trimethoprim/sulfamethoxazole (Bactrim, Septra) BID, amoxicillin (Amoxil) TID.
Nitrofurantoin (Macrodantin) BID.
Ciprofloxacin (Cipro) or ofloxacin (Floxin) BID (age 18 years or older).

Complications
Acute pyelonephritis.

Urinary Tract Infections: Uncomplicated Versus Complicated

Uncomplicated UTIs
Healthy females age 18 years or older can have the "3-day" treatment regiment. These patients do not need urine C&S before or after treatment. Studies show that women reporting UTI symptoms have 90% sensitivity in identifying their infection.

Complicated UTIs
Must treat these patients for a minimum of 7 days.
- Diabetics
- Pregnant women
- Children
- Elderly

■ HIV patients or anyone who is immunocompromised.

■ History of one kidney only (or only one functioning kidney).

Labs
Urinalysis and urine C&S before and after treatment to document resolution.

UTIs: Special Categories

Pregnant women
Hormones cause dilation of the ureters and urinary stasis (kidneys and bladder). Treat even asymptomatic bacteriuria in this group. They are at higher risk (30%) for acute pyelonephritis and obstetric complications such as premature labor and low birth weight.

Use Category B antibiotics for lactating and pregnant women. Penicillins, cephalosporins, macrolides (except Biaxin, which is Category C) are considered safe.

Sulfa drugs (Bactrim)
Avoid during the third trimester because of the increased risk of hemolysis and hyperbilirubinia.

Elderly
UTIs can quickly progress to pyelonephritis and sepsis. It is one of the leading causes of death in this population.

Children
UTIs in this population are indicative of possible urologic or renal abnormality especially in infants and young children. In children younger than 3 years of age, there is a higher risk of progression to pyelonephritis. Refer patient to urologist.

Males
UTIs are not normal in males. Rule out ureteral stricture, infected kidney stones, anatomic abnormality, acute prostatitis, STDs, and so forth. Must be evaluated further. Refer patient to urologist.

Exam Tip

■ The serum creatinine is preferred to BUN when checking renal function.

Clinical Tip

■ Do not use fluoroquinolones or quinolones on pregnant women, children, or any patient below the age of 18 years (interferes with cartilage development).

Recurrent Cystitis (three or more per year for females)

Rule out urologic abnormality: infected stones, reflux, fistulas, and ureteral stenosis.

Consider prophylactic antibiotics for 6 to 12 months after ruling out pathology.

Medications
- Trimethoprim sulfa (40 mg/200 mg) 0.5 tab at bedtime
- Nitrofurantoin (Furadantin) 100 mg tablet at bedtime
- Postcoital UTIs: one tab (Bactrim DS) after sex

Acute Pyelonephritis

Acute bacterial infection of the kidney(s) most commonly caused by Gram-negative bacteria. Bacteria gain entry through the urethra and ascend up the urinary tract into the kidney.

Most common pathogens are Gram-negative bacteria such as *Escherichia Coli*, *Proteus*, and *Klebsiella* (Gram-negative anaerobe).

Classic Case
Patient presents with acute onset of high fever, chills, and one-sided flank pain. Complains of dysuria, frequency, and urgency. Anorexia with nausea and/or vomiting. May appear toxic.

Physical Exam
- CVA tenderness on one kidney (sometimes both).
- Urine dipstick: leukocytes, blood, casts, protein.
- Urine C&S: presence of 10^5 CFU (colony-forming units)/mL.
- CBC: leukocytosis, neutrophilia (>75%).
- Bands or stags (immature neutrophils) may be seen on the CBC (shift to the left).

Plan
- Treat adults as outpatient if not toxic with close follow-up.
- Ciprofloxacin (Cipro) or ofloxacin (Floxin) BID × 14 days (do not use if <18 years).
- Trimethoprim/sulfamethoxazole (Bactrim, Septra) BID × 14 days.
- Close follow-up: 12 to 24 hours.
- If toxic or has a coexisting condition that compromises the immune system, refer or hospitalize.
- Must hospitalize children and pregnant women for IV antibiotics.

Exam Tips

- Right kidney sits lower than the left kidney because of displacement by the liver.

- Large numbers of epithelial cells in the urine means contamination.
- Memorize the normal WBC count (10.5) and the neutrophil (or segs).
- Neutrophils make up from 50% to 75% of all the WBCs in a sample.
- If band forms (immature WBCs) are seen, it is indicative of a serious bacterial infection.

HEMATOLOGY/BLOOD DISORDERS

Fast Facts | Danger Signals

Hodgkin's Lymphoma

Night sweats, fevers, and pain with ingestion of alcoholic drinks. Generalized itching not associated with hives. Painless and enlarged lymph nodes. Anorexia and weight loss. Higher incidence from teens to adults and older adults (>50 years), males, and Whites. A cancer of the beta lymphocytes.

Non-Hodgkin's Lymphoma

Fever, night sweats, and weight loss. Painless enlarged lymph nodes. Bone pain. A cancer of the lymphocytes.

Acute Leukemia

Fever, fatigue, and weight loss. Bleeding gums, nose bleeds (epistaxis), pallor, easy bruising, petechiae, and bone pain. A cancer of the hemapoietic progenitor cells.

Acute Lymphocytic Leukemia (ALL)

Signs and symptoms the same as in acute leukemia. Makes up 80% of childhood leukemias. Peaks from ages of 3 to 7 years (up to 20% are adults).

Hemolytic Disease of the Newborn

May be jaundiced (icteric) on delivery or within first 24 hours of life. Sometimes born with splenomegaly. Generalized edema with severe anemia (hydrops fetalis).

- Mild cases: these infants are born with mild anemia and usually do not require treatment.
- Markedly elevated bilirubin (>5 mg/dL) in severe cases due to Rh or ABO incompatibility.

Vitamin B12 Deficiency

Gradual onset of paresthesias starting in the hands and/or feet (or both) that slowly progresses. CBC reveals a macrocytic anemia. Peripheral smear shows multisegmented neutrophils.

Acute Hemorrhage

Sudden and rapid drop in the hemoglobin (< 6 g/dL) and hematocrit values. Signs and symptoms of shock such as pallor, clammy skin, tachycardia, and hypotension.

Neutropenia

Frequent infections (especially bacterial). Fever, sore throat, and oral thrush. Defined as an absolute neutrophil count of less than $1,500/mm^3$.

Thrombocytopenia

Easy bruising, bleeding gums, spontaneous nosebleeds, hematuria, and so forth. Platelet count $100,000/mm^3$. Platelet count $<20,000/mm^3$ increases risk of spontaneous bleeding.

Fast Facts | Laboratory Testing

Laboratory Norms

Hemoglobin
- Males: 13.0 to 18.0 g/dL
- Females: 12.0 to 16.0 g/dL

Hematocrit
The proportion of RBCs in 1 mL of plasma.
- Males: 37% to 49%
- Females: 36% to 46%

MCV
A measure of the average size of the RBCs in a sample of blood. Decreased in microcytic anemias. Elevated in the macrocytic anemias.
- Normal: MCV 80 to 100 fL

Mean Corpuscular Hemoglobin Concentration (MCHC)
A measure of the average color of the RBCs in a sample of blood. Decreased in iron deficiency anemia and thalassemia. Normal in the macrocytic anemias.
- Normal: 31.0 to 37.0 g/dL

Mean Corpuscular Hemoglobin

Indirect measure of the color of RBCs. Decreased values means pale or hypochromic RBCs. Decreased in iron deficiency anemia and thalassemia. Normal with the macrocytic anemias.

■ Normal: 25.0 to 35.0 pg/cell

TIBC

A measure of available transferrin that is left unbound (to iron). Transferrin is used to transport iron in the body. Elevated in iron deficiency anemia. Normal in thalassemia, B12, and folate deficiency anemia.

■ Normal: 250 to 410 μg/dL

Serum Ferritin

The storage form of iron. Produced in the intestines. Stored in body tissue such as the spleen, liver, and bone marrow. Correlates with iron storage status in a healthy adult.

Markedly decreased in iron deficiency anemia but normal to high in thalassemia trait.

■ Normal: 20 to 400 ng/mL

Serum Iron

Decreased in iron deficiency anemia. Normal to high in thalassemia and the macrocytic anemias. Not as sensitive as ferritin. Affected by recent blood transfusions. Avoid iron supplements 24 hours before testing.

■ Normal: 50 to 175 μg/dL

Red Cell Distribution Width

A measure of the variability of the size of RBCs in a given sample. Elevated in iron deficiency anemia.

Reticulocytes (also called stabs)

Immature RBCs that still have their nuclei. After 24 hours in circulation, reticulocytes lose their nuclei and mature in an RBC (no nuclei). The bone marrow normally will release small amounts to replace damaged RBCs. RBCs survive 120 days before being broken down by the spleen into iron and globulin (recycled) and bilirubin (excreted).

■ Normal: 0.5% to 2.5% (of total red cell count)

Reticulocytosis (>2.5%)

An elevation is seen in 2 to 3 days when the bone marrow is stimulated by supplementation of iron, folate, or B12 (after deficiency) and after acute bleeding episodes. Chronic bleeding does not cause elevation of the reticulocytes.

If there is no reticulocytosis after an acute bleeding episode or after appropriate supplementation, considered abnormal. Rule out bone marrow failure.

Serum Folate and B12
Low values if deficiency exists. Deficiency will cause a macrocytic anemia.
▤ Normal folate level: 3.1 to 17.5 ng/mL
▤ Normal B12 level: >250 pg/mL

White Blood Cells and Platelets

White cell differential: percentage of each type of leukocyte in a sample. The differentials of each type should add up to 100%.
▤ normal white cell count: 4.5 to 10.5 × 10^3/uL (4,500 to 10,5000/10 mm^3)
▤ neutrophils or segs (segmented neut.): 45% to 75%
▤ band forms or stabs (immature neutrophils): 0 to 5%
▤ lymphocytes: 16 to 46%
▤ monocytes: 4 to 11%
▤ eosinophils: 0 to 8%
▤ basophils: 0 to 3%

Fast Facts   Benign Variants

Mildly elevated total RBC counts, hemoglobin, and hematocrit seen in people living in high altitudes.

Fast Facts   Disease Review

Microcytic Anemias

Anemia is simply defined as a decrease in the hemoglobin/hematocrit value below the norm for the patient's age and gender.

Iron Deficiency Anemia

Microcytic and hypochromic anemia (small and pale RBCs) caused by deficiency in iron. It is the most common type of anemia in the world for all races, ages, and genders.

Classic Case
Pallor of the conjunctiva and nailbeds. Complaints of daily fatigue and a sore red tongue (glossitis). Cravings for nonfood items such as ice or dirt (pica). Severe anemia will have spoon-shaped nails (koilonychia), dyspnea, and tachycardia.

Etiology
Most common cause is chronic bleeding. In reproductive-age females from heavy periods and in males/menopausal females from gastrointestinal blood loss; rule out cancer. Chronic gastritis (NSAIDs), postgastrectomy, increased physiologic

requirements such as in pregnancy. In infants, rule out feeding on cow's milk before age 12 months.

Labs
Decreased
- hemoglobin and hematocrit
- MCV <80 fL
- MCHC (pale color)
- ferritin and iron

Increased
- TIBC
- ferritin level

Abnormal peripheral smear: anisocytosis (variations in size) and poikilocytosis (variations in shape).

Plan
- Identify cause of anemia and correct if possible.
- Ferrous sulfate 325 mg PO BID to TID × 3 to 6 months.
- Treat iron deficiency anemia for 3 to 6 months to restore ferritin.
- Common side effects to taking iron supplements: constipation, dark stools, stomach upset.

Thalassemia Minor or Trait

A genetic disorder of the bone marrow where it manufactures small and pale RBCs that result in a mild hypochromic microcytic anemia. The bone marrow produces abnormal hemoglobin (defective alpha or beta globin chains). In addition, there is a reduction in hemoglobin synthesis. Affects ethnic groups such as Mediterraneans (Italians, Greeks) or Asians.

Classic Case
Discovered incidentally because of abnormal CBC results that revealed microcytic and hypochromic RBCs. Total RBC count may be mildly elevated. Ethnic background is either Mediterranean or Asian. Patient asymptomatic.

Plan
Gold standard diagnostic test: hemoglobin electrophoresis
- Hemoglobin electrophoresis: in beta thalassemia abnormal (elevated Hgb. A2, Hgb F) and in iron deficiency anemia, it is normal.
- Blood smear: microcytosis, anisocytosis, poikilocytosis.
- Serum ferritin and iron level normal (not a "deficiency" anemia).
- Educate patient about possibility of having child with disease if partner also has the trait. There is a one in four chance (25%) of having a child with the actual disease.

Table 3.6	Diagnostic Labs: Anemia

Anemia	Laboratory Tests
Iron deficiency Microcytic Hypochromic	TIBC ↑ Ferritin level ↓ MCV < 80
Thalassemia Microcytic Hypochromic	Hgb. electrophoresis
Pernicious anemia Macrocytic	MCV >100 Anti-parietal antibodies ↑ B12 level ↓ Neuro signs/symptoms
Folate deficiency Macrocytic	Folate level ↓ MCV >100
B12 deficiency Macrocytic	B12 level ↓ MCV > 100. Pernicious anemia is the most common cause
Sickle cell Hemolytic anemia	Hgb. electrophoresis Hemoglobin S present
Normocytic	MCV between 80–100 fL. Common in autoimmune disease, rheumatoid arthritis, lupus

Exam Tip

■ Learn to differentiate thalassemia from iron deficiency anemia.

Macrocytic/Megaloblastic Anemias

Vitamin B12 Deficiency Anemia

Deficiency in vitamin B12, which is necessary for the health of the neurons and the brain. Total body supply of B12 lasts 3 to 4 years. Chronic deficiency results in peripheral neuropathy that is progressive and can result in dementia if not corrected. Neurologic damage may not be reversible. Highest incidence in older women.

Pernicious Anemia

An autoimmune disorder caused by the destruction of parietal cells (by antiparietal antibodies) resulting in cessation of intrinsic factor production. Must have intrinsic factor to absorb Vitamin B12 in the small intestine. Most common cause of B12 deficiency anemia.

Other causes: gastrectomy, strict vegan diet, and small bowel disease.

Vitamin B12 sources: all foods of animal origin (meat, poultry, eggs, milk, cheese)

Classic Case
Older to elderly female complains of gradual onset of paresthesias of her feet and/or hands that is slowly getting more severe. Neuropathic symptoms may include any of the following:
- tingling/numbness of hands and feet
- neuropathy starts in peripheral nerves and migrates centrally
- difficulty walking (gross motor)
- difficulty in performing fine motor skills (hands)

Plan
Clinical findings may include
- Decreased reflexes in affected extremity, weak hand grip, decreased sensation
- Glossitis (not a specific finding as it is found in other disorders)
- Differential diagnosis: folate deficiency anemia

Labs
- Check for both B12 level and folate level (both levels must always be checked together)
- Positive: antiparietal antibody (to rule out pernicious anemia), 24-hour urine for methylmalonic acid (MMA), Schilling test
- Peripheral blood smear: macro-ovalocytes, hypersegmented neutrophils
- Decreased B12 level (less than 100 pg/L)

Medications
Lifetime supplementation of B12 (100 μg injections, oral, or nasal B12 spray)

Exam Tips
Pernicious Anemia (PA) results in
- B12 deficiency anemia
- Macrocytic/megaloblastic anemia
- Neurologic symptoms

Clinical Notes
- Missing a diagnosis of B12 deficiency can result in the patient developing irreversible neurological damage.
- Any patient complaining of neuropathy should have B12 levels checked.

Folic Acid Deficiency Anemia
Deficiency in folate results in RBC changes (macrocytosis) that manifest as macrocytic anemia. Total body supply of folate lasts 2 to 3 months.

- Most common cause is inadequate dietary intake (overcooking vegetables)
- Higher risk: alcoholics, elderly
- Increased physiologic need in pregnancy, chronic illness
- Drugs interfering with folate absorption: phenytoin, trimethoprim-sulfa, methotrexate

Classic Case

An alcoholic older male complains of tiredness, fatigue, and a reddened and sore tongue (glossitis). Pallor. No neurological complaints.

Plan

- CBC: decreased hemoglobin and hematocrit, increased MCV
- Peripheral smear: macroovalocytes, hypersegmented neutrophils
- Folate level below normal

Medications

- Correct primary cause. Improve diet (add leafy green vegetables, grains, beans, liver). Stop overcooking vegetables.
- Folic acid 1 to 5 mg per day.

Summary

- Pernicious anemia results in B12 deficiency.
- Pernicious anemia is a macrocytic anemia.
- Learn foods that are rich in both folate and B12.
- Red blood cell size is described in many ways such as: MCV <80: microcytic and hypochromic RBCs, small and pale RBCs and MCV >100: macrocytes or macroovalocytes, larger than normal RBCs or RBCs with enlarged cytoplasms.
- Iron deficiency anemia versus Thalassemia Trait: Ferritin level, low in iron deficiency and normal to high in thalassemia.
- Serum iron: decreased in iron deficiency and normal to high in thalassemia.
- TIBC: elevated in iron deficiency and normal or borderline in thalassemia.
- MCHC or color: decreased in iron deficiency and normal in thalassemia.
- Hb Electrophoresis: normal in iron deficiency and abnormal in thalassemia.
- Ethnic background: ethnicity or age does not matter in iron deficiency anemia. Iron deficiency anemia is the most common anemia overall in any age group or gender. Thalassemia is seen in Mediterranean background (e.g., Greeks, Italians) and Asians (e.g., Chinese).
- Ethnic background may not be mentioned in a thalassemia problem or it may be a distractor. Be careful.
- Only B12 deficiency anemia has neurologic symptoms (tingling, numbness).

Exam Tips

- Some questions on iron deficiency anemia may mention a patient's ethnicity (e.g., Italian descent).
- As mentioned before, ethnic background does not matter with iron deficiency anemia. The MCV, ferritin level, and TIBC are what matter.

NERVOUS SYSTEM

Dangerous Headaches

▦ Abrupt onset of severe headache ("thunderclap" headache).
▦ "Worst headache of my life."
▦ First onset of headache after age 50.
▦ Sudden onset of headache after coughing, exertion, straining or sex (exertional headache).
▦ Sudden change in level of consciousness.
▦ Focal neurological signs (e.g., unequal pupil size).
▦ Headache with papilledema (increase ICP secondary to any of the other symptoms).

Rule out these worst case scenarios:

▦ Subarachnoid hemorrhage
▦ Leaking aneurysm
▦ Bacterial meningitis
▦ Increased ICP (intracranial pressure)
▦ Brain abscess
▦ Brain tumor

Temporal Arteritis (giant cell arteritis)

New onset of headaches on one temple that are accompanied by scalp tenderness. It is associated with visual disturbances or blindness of the eye from the affected side. An indurated, reddened and cord-like temporal artery that is tender to touch is found on the same side as the headache. Sedimentation rate is elevated. More common in older adults.

Acute Bacterial Meningitis

Acute onset of high fever, severe headache, stiff neck, and meningismus. Meningococcal disease (discussed under Danger Signals section in Dermatology). Classic purple-colored petechial rashes. Accompanied by nausea, vomiting, and photophobia. Rapid worsening of symptoms progressing to lethargy, confusion, and finally coma. If not treated, it is fatal. This is a reportable disease.

| Fast Facts | **Neurological Testing**

Neurological Exam

Mental Status (frontal lobes)
■ Mini-Mental Exam (orientation, memory, logic speech, etc.)
■ cranial nerve exam

Cerebellar System
■ Romberg test
■ tandem gait

Sensory System
■ vibration sensation
■ pain sensation
■ touch
■ two-point recognition
■ Stereognosis (ability to recognize familiar object through sense of touch only). Place a familiar object (e.g., coin, pen) on the patient's palm (patient's eyes are closed).

Motor exam
Gross and fine motor movements—walking, using hands, jumping, and so forth.

Reflexes
Sides should be compared to each other and should be equal.

Grading Reflexes

0   No response
1+ Low response
2+ Normal or average response
3+ Brisker than average
4+ Very brisk response

Neurological Maneuvers

Both these tests are used to assess for meningeal irritation. Both tests are done with the patient in a supine position. More sensitive tests in children compared with adults.

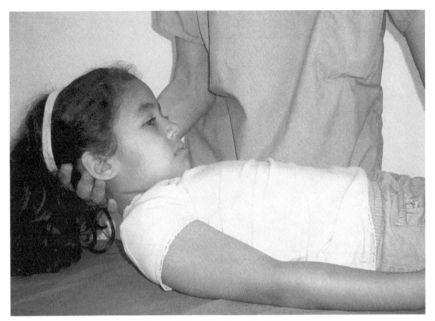

Figure 3.4. Brudzinski Sign

Kernig Sign
Flex patient's hips one at a time, then attempt to straighten the leg while keeping the hip flexed at 90 degrees. Positive: resistance to leg straightening from pain in hamstrings (due to inflammation on lumbar nerve roots).

Brudzinski Sign
Passively flex/bend the patient's neck toward the chest. Positive: patient reflexively flexes the hips and knee to relieve pressure and pain (due to inflammation of lumbar nerve roots).

Cranial Nerve Testing (CN)

Pneumonic "On Old Olympus' Towering Tops, A Finn and German Viewed Some Hops"

The first letter stands for the name of the cranial nerve. The word order corresponds to the sequential numbering of the cranial nerves.

CN 1: On (olfactory)
CN 2: Old (optic)
CN 3: Olympus' (oculomotor)
CN 4: Towering (trochlear)
CN 5: Tops (trigeminal)
CN 6: A (abducens)
CN 7: Finn (facial)
CN 8: And (acoustic)

Table 3.7	Cranial Nerve Testing

Number	Name	Technique
1	Olfactory	Sense of smell (coffee, lemon)
2	Optic	Distance vision, near vision
3, 4 & 6	Oculomotor Trochlear Abducens	EOMs (extraocular muscles), visual fields of gaze
5	Trigeminal 3 branches: V1 (ophthalmic) V2 (maxillary) V3 (mandibular)	Motor portion: clench jaws Sensory portion: corneal reflex/ facial sensation
7	Facial	Puff cheeks, raise eyebrows, smile
8	Acoustic	Hearing test (whisper test), Rinne and Weber tests
9 & 10	Glossopharyngeal Vagus	Gag, symmetrical soft palate, Uvula is midline, voice quality
11	Spinal Accessory	Trapezius muscle atrophy, shoulder shrug
12	Hypoglossal	Tongue fasciculation and deviation Tongue atrophy

CN 9: German (glossopharyngeal)
CN 10: Viewed (vagus)
CN 11: Some (spinal accessory)
CN 12: Hops (hypoglossal)

Exam Tips

- Memorization tips on cranial nerves.
  CN 1: you have one nose
  CN 2: you have two eyes
  CN 8: the number 8 stands for two ears sitting on top of each other
  CN 11: number 11 reminds you of two shoulders shrugging together
- Because cranial nerves are listed only by number on the test (not by name), the correct chronological order is important. Memorize the mnemonic to guide you.
- Herpes zoster infection (shingles) of CN 5 ophthalmic branch can result in blindness.
- Rash at tip of nose and the temple area (rule out shingles infection).
- Memorize "On Old Olympus' Towering Tops, A Finn and German Viewed Some Hops."
- Write down on scratch paper with corresponding cranial nerve "numbers."

Fast Facts **Benign Variants**

Anisocoria
A condition in which the two pupils are not of equal size.

Benign Familial Tremor
A fine tremor of the hand with unknown cause. Tends to run in families.

Fast Facts **Disease Review**

Acute Bacterial Meningitis

A serious and acute bacterial infection of the meninges resulting in increased intracranial pressure (ICP) and damage to the brain. The most common pathogen for all age groups is *neisseria meningitidis. H. influenzae* is more common in infants and children < 6 years of age. Higher risk with otitis media and sinusitis. Patients who recover commonly have some neurologic sequelae.

Classic Case
Described under the Danger Signals section.

Labs
Lumbar puncture: CSF (cerebrospinal fluid) has large numbers of WBCs (purulent). Elevated opening pressure.
Gram stain and C & S of fluid
CBC with differential, electrolytes, etc.

Medications
Infants: ampicillin or 3rd generation cephalosporin
Adults: 3rd generation cephalosporin plus chloramphenicol
Adults over the age of 50: amoxicillin plus 3rd generation cephalosporin
Prophylaxis of close contacts with rifampin or ceftriaxone. This is a reportable disease.

Migraine Headaches (with or without aura)

Migraine headaches with aura (precedes the migraine headache) may present as scotomas (blind spot on visual field) or flashing lights that precede the headache. A positive family history and being female puts one at higher risk (3:1). Migraine headaches can present as abdominal pains in small children.

Classic Case
A female patient complains of a gradual onset of a bad throbbing headache behind one eye along with some photophobia and phonophobia. It is accompanied by

nausea and/or vomiting. She reports that resting in a dark and quiet room with an ice bag on her forehead makes her feel better.

Plan

Neuro exam will be normal. Rest in a quiet and darkened room with an ice pack to the forehead. For nausea, drink ginger ale or chew dry toast. Avoid heavy fatty meals. Avoid precipitating foods or activities such as:

- MSG (monosodium glutamate) in Chinese food, sauces
- alcohol, especially red wine and beer, caffeine, chocolate
- sleep changes, stress, etc.

Abortive Treatment

1) 5-HT-1 Agonists: Sumatriptan (Imitrex)
    - do not start within 2 weeks of taking an MAOI (monamine oxidase inhibitor)
    - do not combine with ergots (e.g., ergotamine/caffeine or Cafergot)
    - for patients over age 40 give first dose in office (theoretical risk of an acute MI)
2) NSAIDs, analgesics (e.g., Extra Strength Tylenol), or narcotics (codeine, hydrocodone)
3) Ergotamine/caffeine (Cafergot)
    - a potent vasoconstrictor
    - do not mix with other vasoconstrictors (triptans, decongestants, etc.)
    - a common side effect is nausea
4) Antiemetics
    - trimethobenzamide (Tigan) IM, supp., PO

Prophylactic Treatment

Beta-blockers: propranolol (Inderal) daily or BID
Tricyclic antidepressants (TCAs): amitriptyline (Elavil) at HS

Contraindications (vasoconstricting drugs)
- Suspected or known CHD (coronary heart disease)
- PVD (peripheral vascular disease)
- Uncontrolled hypertension
- Complex migraine (e.g., basilar/hemiplegic migraine)

Focal Migraines

Also called basilar or hemiplegic migraines. Focal neuro findings with stroke-like signs and symptoms. Resembles a transient ischemic attack (TIA). These patients are at higher risk of stroke. Avoid giving estrogens or any agents promoting clot formation.

Exam Tips

- Distinguish the drugs used for abortive treatment versus prophylaxis.
- Answer options may list the drug class instead of the generic name.

Temporal Arteritis (Giant Cell Arteritis)

A systemic inflammatory process (vasculitis) of the medium and large arteries of the body. If the temporal artery is involved, it is called temporal arteritis. More common in males 50 years of age or older.

Classic Case

A 56-year-old male complains of a headache on his temple along with marked scalp tenderness. Complains of visual disturbances over affected side. May have temporary blindness in affected eye (amaurosis fugax). Physical exam reveals indurated cord-like temporal artery that is tender. Sedimentation rate is elevated.

Plan

- Refer to ophthalmologist stat (or refer to ER). Treated with high dosed prednisone. Carotid biopsy (gold standard).

Complications

Permanent blindness if not diagnosed early (ischemic optic neuropathy).

Exam Tips

- Sedimentation rate is screening test for temporal arteritis (elevated).
- A common case scenario is the person complaining of the worst headache of his life. Best plan is to refer to ER or call 911.

Clinical Tips

- A high index of suspicion is necessary because of serious sequelae.
- Order the sedimentation rate stat.
- Start prednisone in office if you suspect temporal arteritis.
- Refer to ER.

Trigeminal Neuralgia (Tic Douloureux)

A unilateral headache caused by impingement (for example from a tumor) or inflammation of the trigeminal nerve (CN 5). Rare before age 35; peaks at age 60. More common in females.

Classic Case

Older female complains of an onset of severe and sharp shooting pains on one side of her face that is triggered by chewing, eating cold foods, and cold air. The severe lancinating pain lasts a few seconds and only stops when the offending activity ceases.

Plan

- Carbamazepine (Tegretol) or phenytoin (Dilantin). MRI or CT scan. Avoid precipitating factors.

Cluster Headache

A sudden onset of severe "ice-pick" (lancinating pain) headaches behind one eye that occurs several times a day. It is accompanied by tearing, lacrimation, and rhinitis. The attacks happen at the same times daily. Cause is unknown. Resolves spontaneously, but may return in the future in some patients. More common in adult males in their 30s to 40s.

Classic Case

Middle-aged male complains of severe headaches that occur several times a day. He describes them as severe and stabbing "ice pick" pains behind one eye or one temple, accompanied by tearing, a clear runny nasal discharge (rhinitis), and a drooping eyelid (ptosis).

Plan

- Sumatriptan (Imitrex) injection. 100% oxygen @ 7L/ minute

Complications

Higher risk of suicide (males) compared with the other types of chronic headaches.

Muscle Tension Headache

These headaches are secondary to an increase in life stressors that cause the muscles of the scalp to go into spasm. They are bilateral headaches.

Classic Case

An adult patient complains of a headache that is "bandlike," which feels like "someone is squeezing my head." The pain is described as dull in character. The patient admits to increased stress and denies blurred vision and nausea.

Plan

- NSAIDs such as naproxen sodium (Anaprox DS) BID, acetaminophen (Tylenol) QID as needed (PRN). Stress reduction and relaxation techniques. Decrease stressors.

Table 3.8 — Classic Signs and Symptoms: Headaches

Headache	Symptoms	Aggravating Factors
Migraine without aura	Throbbing pain behind one eye Photophobia, Phonophobia Nausea/Vomiting	Red wine, MSG, aspartame, menstruation, stress, etc.
Migraine with aura	Above plus scotoma, scintillating lights, halos, etc.	Foods high in tryptans Teenage to middle-age females
Trigeminal Neuralgia (CN 5)	Intense and very brief; sharp stabbing pain; one cheek (2nd branch CN 5)	Cold food, cold air, talking, touch, chewing Older adults and elderly
Cluster	Severe "ice-pick" piercing pain behind one eye & temple. With tearing, rhinorrhea, ptosis & miosis on one side (Horner's syndrome)	Occurs at same time daily in clusters x weeks to months Middle-aged males
Temporal Arteritis Giant cell arteritis	Unilateral pain, temporal area with scalp tenderness. Skin over artery is indurated, tender, warm, & reddened. Amaurosis fugax (temporary blindness) may occur.	Polymyalgia rheumatica common in these pts (up to 50%). Medical urgency. Older adults and elderly.
Muscle Tension	Bilateral "bandlike" pain, continous dull pain, may last days. May be accompanied by spasms of the trapezius muscles.	Stress Adolescents, adults

Exam Tips

- With the exception of muscle tension headaches that are bilateral, all of the headaches seen on the exam (and notes) are unilateral.
- Muscle tension: bandlike head pain; may last for days
- Migraine: throbbing, nausea, photophobia, phonophobia
- Trigeminal neuralgia (tic douloureux): pain in one side of face/cheek, is aggravated by talking, chewing, cold food, or cold air on affected area.
- Temporal arteritis: indurated temporal artery, pain behind eye/scalp
- Cluster: only HA accompanied by tearing and nasal congestion; severe pain is behind one eye/one side of head. Occurs several times a day. Spontaneously resolves. Seen more in middle-aged males.

Bell's Palsy

Abrupt onset of unilateral facial paralysis that is due to dysfunction of the motor branch of the facial nerve (CN 7). Facial paralysis can progress rapidly within 24 hours. Skin sensation remains intact but tear production on the

Table 3.9	Treatment of Headaches	
Headache	**Acute Treatment**	**Prophylaxis/Other**
Migraine	Ice pack on forehead. Rest in quiet & dark room. Rx: Triptans (Imitrex), Tigan supp. (for nausea) Ultram, NSAIDs, analgesics, narcotics	Tricyclics (TCAs) Beta-Blockers
Temporal Arteritis	Refer to ER or ophthalmologist Stat. Lab: ESR ↑ (Sed rate) (screening lab test) Rx: High dosed steroids	Permanent blindness can result. Temporal artery biopsy is the gold standard.
Cluster	100% oxygen @ 7-10 L/minute per mask. Intranasal 4% lidocaine	May become suicidal. Spontaneous resolution, can reoccur.
Trigeminal Neuralgia	Carbamazepine (Tegretol) or phenytoin (Dilantin). Check serum levels.	Tegretol or Dilantin for several weeks to mos. Watch for drug interactions.
Muscle Tension	NSAIDs, Tylenol, hot bath/ shower, massage, etc.	Stress reduction, yoga, massage, biofeedback

affected side may stop. Most cases spontaneously resolve. Prolonged cases (several weeks) may leave permanent neurological sequelae. Etiology ranges from viral infection of the nerve, an autoimmune process, or pressure from a tumor.

Classic Case

An older adult complains of waking up that morning with one side of his face paralyzed. He has difficulty chewing and swallowing food on the same side and has noticed that he cannot fully close his eyelid.

Plan

■ Rule out stroke, TIA, mastoid infections, bone fracture, Lyme disease, tumor.
■ Corticosteroids at high doses x 10 days (wean).
■ Acyclovir (Zovirax) if herpes simplex suspected.
■ Protect cornea from drying and ulceration with applications of an eye lubricant in the morning and lubricating ointment at bedtime. Patch eye if patient is unable to fully close the eyelid.

Complications

Corneal ulceration
Permanent facial weakness (up to 10%)

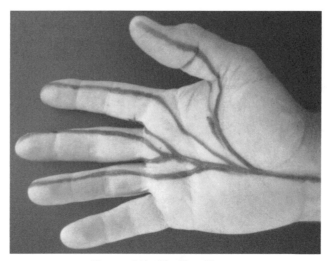

Figure 3.5. Median Nerve

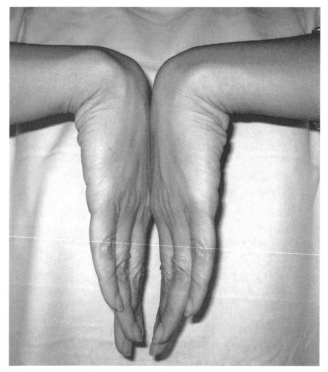

Figure 3.6. Phalen's Sign

Carpal Tunnel Syndrome (CTS)

Median nerve compression that is due to swelling of the carpal tunnel. Commonly caused by activities that require repetitive wrist motion. Can also be due to hypothyroidism.

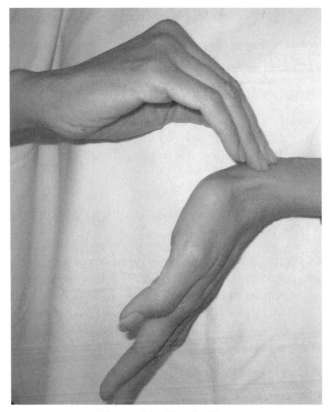

Figure 3.7. Tinel's Sign

Classic Case

Adult patient who uses hands frequently for job (e.g., typing) complains of gradual onset (over weeks to months) of numbness and tingling (paresthesias) on the thumb, index finger, and middle finger areas. Hand grip of affected hand(s) weaker. May complain of problems lifting heavy objects. Chronic severe cases involve atrophy of the thenar eminence (a late sign). History of an occupation or hobby that involves frequent wrist/hand movements.

Tinel's Sign

Tap anterior wrist briskly.
Positive finding: paresthesia or reproduction of symptoms

Phalen's Sign

Full flexion of wrist for 60 seconds.
Positive finding: reproduction of symptoms

Exam Tip

■ There is usually a question on either Tinel's or Phalen's sign.

SEXUALLY TRANSMITTED DISEASES (STDs)

Fast Facts | Danger Signals

Human Immunodeficiency Virus

High-risk factors such as homosexual males, injection drug users, female partners of high-risk males, infants born to infected mothers, and so forth. Early signs include hairy leukoplakia of the tongue, shingles in a healthy adult, lymphadenopathy, and so forth.

Disseminated Gonococcal Disease (disseminated gonorrhea)

Sexually active adult from high risk population (e.g., homeless) complains of petechial skin rashes of hands/soles; swollen, red, and tender joints or one large joint (migratory asymmetrical arthritis) such as the knee. Accompanied by signs of STD (e.g., cervicitis, urethritis). If pharyngitis, will have severe sore throat with green purulent throat exudate that does not respond to usual antibiotics used for strep throat.

Syphilis

Painless chancre in the genitals or mouth that resolves in 2 weeks (first stage). More common in homosexual males and patients of lower socioeconomic status. Organism: treponema pallidum (spirochete)

Fast Facts | Disease Review

STD Screening Recommended by the CDC

All sexually active adolescents and females ages 20 to 24 years.

Risk Factors
- Sexually active single adult with history of multiple sexual partners, especially if with new sexual partner (defined as 3 months or less).
- Inconsistent condom use.

Chlamydia Trachomatis

Obligate intracellular bacteria that infects squamous epithelial cells of the urinary/genital tracts. Chlamydia does not infect pharynx and rectum. Most common bacterial sexually transmitted disease (STD) in this country. Majority of infections are asymptomatic.

Possible Sites of Infection
Both genders: urethritis
Females: cervicitis, endometritis, salpingitis (fallopian tubes), PID
Males: epididymitis, prostatitis
Neonates: conjunctivitis (trachoma), pneumonia

Uncomplicated Infections
Chlamydia (cervicitis, urethritis)

- Azithromycin 1 gm PO single dose
- Doxycycline 100 mg BID × 7 days, possible side effects: abdominal pain, nausea, photosensitivity (avoid sun or use sunscreen)
- Cefixime (Suprax) 400 mg, or Cipro 500 mg or Floxin 400 mg × one dose

CDC prefers DOT (directly observed treatment) × one dose (e.g., azithromycin, ciprofloxacin). No test of cure is necessary for azithromycin or doxycycline.

Pregnant Women
Erythromycin base QID × 7 days. Test of cure 3 weeks after completion of treatment because erythromycin is not as effective as azithromycin or doxycycline.

Neisseria Gonorrhea (GC)

Prevalent in sexually active young adults (below age 24) with multiple sexual partners. Classic signs and symptoms are green-colored penile/vaginal discharge, dysuria, pelvic pain, and dyspareunia (females). More than half of infected patients are asymptomatic.

A Gram-negative sexually transmitted bacteria that infects the urinary and genital tracts, the rectum, and pharynx. High rates of coinfection with chlamydia. If positive for GC, must cotreat for both even if negative chlamydial tests. Unlike chlamydia, GC can become systemic or disseminated if left untreated.

Possible Sites of Infection
Both genders: urethritis, proctitis, pharyngitis
Female: cervicitis, endometritis, salpingitis (fallopian tubes), PID
Males: epididymitis, prostatitis
Children: vaginitis, pharyngitis, proctitis (sexual abuse). More likely to be asymptomatic compared with adults.
Neonates: gonococcal ophthalmia (hospitalize), pharyngitis, scalp abscess

Uncomplicated Infections
Gonorrhea (cervicitis, urethritis, pharyngitis)

- Ceftriaxone 125 mg IM × 1 dose plus co-treat for chlamydia
- Ciprofloxacin (Cipro) 400 mg PO × one dose
- Must co-treat for chlamydia.

Complicated infections
Gonorrhea (acute epididymitis, acute prostatitis, acute proctitis)

- Ceftriaxone (Rocephin) 250 mg IM × one dose
- Must co-treat for chlamydia.

Complicated Infections: Females
Pelvic Inflammatory Disease (PID)
Infection started by GC and/or chlamydia in the cervix; ascends to the fallopian tubes (salpingitis). Infection is mixed with facultative vaginal bacteria, anaerobes, and bacteroids.

Risk Factors
- IUD: the first few months after insertion
- History of PID: 25% reoccurrence
- Multiple partners
- Age 24 or younger

Oral contraceptives reduce the risk of PID (due to thickened mucus plug).

Classic Case
Sexually active teenage to young adult female complains of purulent vaginal discharge, pelvic pain, dyspareunia, and pain on jarring pelvis (heel drop test). History of new male partner (less than 3 months) or multiple sexual partners. Inconsistent condom use.

Bimanual Exam Findings
Cervical motion tenderness, unilateral adnexal pain.
Mucopurulent cervical discharge (may pool in the posterior fornix of vagina).

Jones Criteria: Major criteria for PID
Only one of the following is necessary to diagnose and treat for PID.
1) Lower abdominal tenderness
2) Cervical motion tenderness (CMT)
3) Adnexal tenderness

Labs
Reproductive-age females: rule out pregnancy first.
Gen Probe (use only on urethra and cervix. Do not use on the pharynx and rectum.)
Urine tests for chlamydia and gonorrhea.
Gen-Probe preferred. Mandatory chlamydial cultures with sexual assault (any age).
Gonorrhea (anaerobic cultures) such as the Thayer-Martin or chocolate agar for pharyngeal and rectal areas but can be used for other sites if indicated.
Cultures must be taken for all sexually abused children and sexual assault victims.

Gram Stain: useful for gonorrhea only. Look for Gram-negative diplococci in clusters.

Other STD testing: HIV, syphilis, hepatitis B, herpes type 2

Partners should be tested and treated. No sex until both complete treatment.

Reiter's Syndrome

An immune-mediated reaction secondary to infection with certain bacteria (e.g., chlamydia) that spontaneously resolves. More common in males. Treatment is supportive (e.g., NSAIDs).

Classic Case

A male with current history of chlamydia genital infection (e.g., urethritis) complains of dry, red, and swollen joints that come and go (migratory arthritis in large joints like knee) and ulcers on the skin of the glans penis.

Fitz-Hugh-Curtis Syndrome (Perihepatitis)

Chlamydial and/or gonococcal infection of the liver capsule (not the liver itself) resulting in extensive scarring between the liver capsule and abdominal contents (e.g., colon). Scars look like "violin strings" (seen on laparoscopy). A complication of disseminated GC and/or PID.

Classic Case

Sexually active female with symptoms of PID complains of RUQ (right upper quadrant) abdominal pain and tenderness on palpation. The liver function tests are normal. Treated as a complicated gonorrheal/chlamydial infection (14-day treatment).

Jarisch-Herxheimer Reaction

The sudden massive destruction of spirochetes after a Penicillin G injection causes an immune-mediated reaction that usually resolves spontaneously. Treatment is supportive.

Classic Case

Adult patient complains of severe chills, fever, myalgia, and tachycardia after being treated for syphilis. BP may be high, then falls. Care is supportive.

Exam Tips

- Older and well-known drugs such as doxycycline and ceftriaxone more likely to appear as treatment options.
- GC positive (always cotreat for chlamydia) even if the chlamydia test result is negative.

■ Inverse not true. Positive chlamydia (do not treat for GC unless indicated).
■ Reiter's syndrome (learn signs/symptoms).
■ Erythromycin used for pregnant patients (chlamydia).

Clinical Tips

■ Cure testing not necessary for azithromycin or doxycycline treatment.
■ PID is a clinical diagnosis. Base treatment on the examination of the patient not just on the test results.
■ Chlamydia is a hard organism to culture or to test for. Base decision to treat on patient risk factors and clinical signs or symptoms.
■ Fitz-Hugh Curtis is frequently seen on the test.

Syphilis

Treponema pallidum (spirochete) gets in the body through breaks in the skin or through mucous membrane.

Classic Case
Signs and symptoms dependent on stage of infection.
Primary: painless chancre (heals in 6 to 9 weeks if not treated).
Secondary (> 2 years): condyloma lata (infectious white papules in moist areas that look like white warts); maculopapular rash on palms and soles that is not pruritic.
Latent Stage: asymptomatic
Tertiary (3 to 10 years): neurosyphilis, gumma (soft tissue tumors), aneurysms, valvular damage, and so forth.

Labs
Screening test: RPR or VDRL
Diagnostic test: darkfield exam, FTA-ABS (fluorescent antibody absorption antibody test)
Monitoring treatment response: RPR or VDRL titers (ratio of the decrease in titers used)

Plan
■ Procaine Penicillin G IM (dose depends on stage of disease).
■ Doxycycline BID × 28 days (primary and secondary stages only).
■ Treat sex partner(s).
■ Recheck RPR or VDRL to monitor treatment response (look for at least a fourfold decrease in the pretreatment and posttreatment titers).

Exam Tips

■ Do not confuse condyloma acuminata (genital warts) with condyloma lata.
■ Screening test is RPR or VDRL.

Clinical Tips

■ Use the same serology and lab throughout treatment. If RPR used, continue with it.
■ The most common criterion clinicians use to diagnose PID is cervical motion tenderness.

HIV Infection (Human Immunodeficiency Virus)

Screening: ELISA test (enzyme-linked immunosorbent assay)
    ■ detects antibodies, not viral RNA
    ■ sensitivity/specificity > 99% (too sensitive with higher rates of false positives)
    ■ if positive twice; lab will check Western Blot automatically
Confirmatory Test: Western Blot
    ■ antibody test with high specificity for HIV
Window Period
    ■ weeks to 6 months (<1% up to 36 months)

Diagnostic Tests (a viral RNA test)
PCR (polymerase chain reaction)
    ■ detects viral RNA (actual viral presence)
Viral load
    ■ number of RNA copies in 1 ml plasma. Test measures actively replicating HIV virus, progression of disease, and response to antiretroviral treatment.
P24 antigen
    ■ indicates active HIV replication

Risk Factors
■ sexually active (especially homosexual men)
■ drug use, blood products from 1975 to 1985
■ history of other STDs, multiple partners, homeless, and so forth

Plan
■ Numerous labs are done on work-up to rule out other STDs, immune system function, liver function, electrolytes, urinalysis, etc.
■ Test sex partner(s) for HIV.

Vaccines
■ Annual flu shot
■ Hepatitis B × 3
■ Hepatitis A (anal to oral contact)
■ Td every 10 years

Prophylaxis for PCP (Pneumocystis carinii pneumonia)
If the CD 4 lymphocyte count is <200 cells/uL; prophylaxis for PCP
PCP drugs: TMP-SMX (Bactrim), dapsone or pentamidine by nebulizer

Table 3.10	Sexually Transmitted Diseases: Treatment Guidelines*

Organism	Uncomplicated Infections	Complicated Infections
Chlamydia trachomatis Atypical Bacteria	**Doxycycline 100 mg BID × 7 days or Azithromycin 1 gm × 1 dose** Mucopurulent Cervicitis Urethritis Treat sexual partners **Pregnancy** Erythromycin 500 mg QID × 7 days or Amoxicillin 500 mg TID × 7 days *Test-of-cure (repeat Gen Probe after treatment)*	**Doxycycline 100 mg BID × 14 days** Pelvic inflammatory Disease (PID) Salpingitis, Tubo-ovarian abscess **Males** Epididymitis, Prostatitis
Neisseria Gonorrhea Plus Chlamydia Tx	**Ceftriaxone 125 mg IM × 1 dose plus** **Doxycycline 100 mg BID × 7days** Mucopurulent Cervicitis Urethritis Pharyngitis Proctitis Treat sexual partners **Pregnancy** Treat GC drugs plus chlamydia pregnancy treatment **Doxycycline, Cipro, Floxin are Cat. D: avoid in pregnancy*	**Ceftriaxone 250 mg IM × one dose** **Plus Doxycycline 100 mg BID × 14 days** PID, Salpingitis, Tubo-ovarian abscess **Males** Epididymitis, Epididymo-orchitis Prostatitis *Disseminated GC* Above plus asymmetric arthritis & rash. (Treatment at www.cdc.gov)
Syphilis (spirochete) Treponema Pallidum	**Benzathine Penicillin G 2.4 mU IM × one dose** Early cases, Primary, Secondary or Latent cases < 1 year. Treat sexual partners. *Retreat if clinical signs recur or sustained 4-fold titers RPR/VDRL.* **Pregnancy** Same treatment, may repeat tx after 1 week if during 3rd trimester	**Benzathine Penicillin G 2.4 mU IM weekly × 3 weeks** More than 1 year's duration (latent, indeterminate, cardiovascular, late benign). Maculopapular rash includes palms/soles. Mandatory follow-up for all cases.

*Adapted from Centers for Disease Control, *Sexually Transmitted Disease Treatment Guidelines*, 2006.
All of the above STDs or sexually transmitted infections (STIs) are reportable diseases.

HIV Education

■ Do not handle cat litter (toxoplasmosis).
■ Bird stool contains histoplasmosis spores.
■ Turtles may be infected with salmonella.
■ Do not eat uncooked meat.
■ Safe sex, get partner tested.

Exam Tips

■ PCP prophylaxis when CD4 < 200.
■ Bactrim DS used first, if allergic to sulfa, use pentamidine.
■ Screening test is the ELISA test (tests for antibodies only).
■ Confirmatory test is Western Blot.
■ Example of a diagnostic test is PCR (viral RNA), viral load, etc.
■ HIV-infected pregnant women: start AZT in the 2nd trimester.
■ Hairy leukoplakia of tongue: rule out HIV infection.

HIV Infection: Pregnant Women

With no treatment: 5-25% infants become infected
With breast feeding: transmission rate of 12 to 14%.
Newborns: start treatment with zidovudine (AZT) within first 48 hours
Zidovudine

■ drug of choice for treating pregnant women
■ reduces rate of perinatal transmission by 60%

Start zidovudine during second trimester of pregnancy until delivery.

Condyloma Acuminata (Genital Warts)

Human papilloma virus (HPV) has 70 subtypes (only a few are oncogenic).
Genital Sites: cervix, vagina, external genitals, urethra, anus. Other sites that can be infected are the larynx, nasal mucosa, oral mucosa, conjunctivae.

HIV-positive Women

Higher risk for aggressive HPV disease. Need to have Pap smears every 3 to 6 months to monitor. Higher incidence of cervical cancer.

Pap Smears

■ Cervical cancer screening test is the Pap smear (false-negative rates of up to 18%).
■ Koilocytotic changes (large cell nuclei): may signify human papilloma virus (HPV) infection, test for an infection and refer for a colposcopy.
■ If ASCUS (atypical squamous cells of unknown significance), test for HPV and refer to gyn office.

Colposcope

A specialized microscope for evaluating and treating cervix. It is used to visualize the cervix and to obtain cervical tissue biopsies. A biopsy is the "gold standard" for diagnosing cervical cancer.

Acetowhitening

Areas of white-colored skin (HPV infected skin) on the cervical surface that appear only after acetic acid (distilled vinegar) is swabbed on the cervix. This procedure is done before starting a colposcopic examination and biopsy. HPV-infected skin becomes a bright-white color from the acetic acid exposure.

Medications
- Podofilox (Condylox): self-administered by the patient for external warts only. Podophyllin contraindicated in pregnancy.
- Cryo, bichloracetic, or trichloroacetic acid (caustic acids) done in office.

Herpes Simplex: HSV1 and HSV 2

HSV 1: usually oral infection, sometimes genital.
HSV 2: more likely to be genital infection, can be oral.

Classic Case
May have prodrome (e.g., itching, burning, tingling) on site. Sudden onset of groups of small vesicles sitting on an erythematous base. Easily ruptures and painful. Primary episode more severe and can last up to 2 weeks. Vesicle fluid and crust are contagious.

Plan
- Diagnostic Test: herpes viral culture. Usually diagnosed by clinical presentation.

Initial Infection
Acyclovir (Zovirax) 5x/day × 10 days
Valacyclovir (Valtrex) BID × 10 days
Flare-up: Zovirax or Valtrex × 7 days. Treat as soon as possible; within first 48 hours.

Suppressive Treatment
More than 6 flare-ups per year, consider prophylaxis.

Post-herpetic Neuralgia
Elderly and immunosuppressed at higher risk. Treat with low dose TCAs (e.g., Elavil).

Complications
Post-herpetic neuralgia treated with TCAs (tricyclic antidepressants) such as amitriptyline (Elavil) at bedtime.

Infection of the trigeminal nerve ophthalmic branch (CN 5).
May cause corneal blindness.

Exam Tips

- TCAs used to treat post-herpetic neuralgia (Elavil).
- Acute episode treatment (Valtrex or Zovirax × 10 days).
- CN 5 can damage the cornea, causing blindness.

Lymphogranuloma Venereum (LGV)

Also known as lymphogranuloma inguinale. Painless genital ulcer(s) with multiple enlarged tender inguinal nodes (or buboes). Rare infection.
Organism: *Chlamydia trachomatis*
Treatment: Doxycycline, tetracyclines

WOMEN'S HEALTH: GYNECOLOGY

Fast Facts | Danger Signals

Breast Cancer

Female with a dominant mass on one breast that feels firm to hard and is immobile. Skin changes may be seen such as the "peau d'orange." This is a localized area of skin that resembles an orange peel. Mass is painless with no nipple discharge. Risk factors for breast cancer exist (positive family history, nulliparity, early menarche, etc.).

Paget's Disease of the Breast (ductal carcinoma in situ)

Older female reports a history of a chronic scaly red rash resembling eczema on the nipple (or nipple and areola) that does not heal. The nipple/areolar skin will eventually have crusting, ulceration, and/or bleeding. Some women complain of itching. Nipple discharge and/or a lump may be present. Risk factors for breast cancer exist.

Ectopic Pregnancy

Sexually active female who has not had a period (or had period but light to scant bleeding) in 6 to 7 weeks complains of lower abdominal/pelvic pain or cramping (intermittent, persistent, or acute). If ruptured, pelvic pain worsens and can be

---

* Treatment recommendations for the Sexually Transmitted Diseases section adapted from the CDC's "Sexually Transmitted Disease Treatment Guidelines," 2006.

referred to the right shoulder. Pain worsens when supine or with jarring. If in shock, will be pale, tachycardic, have clammy skin, and may faint. Past medical history of PID, tubal ligation, older age, etc. This is the leading cause of death for women in the United States in the first trimester of pregnancy.

Ovarian Cancer

Older women with complaints of vague symptoms such as low back pain, pelvic pain, abdominal bloating, and/or constipation. If metastases, symptoms depends on area affected. Symptoms may be bone pain, abdominal pain, headache, blurred vision, etc.

Fast Facts | Normal Findings

Menarche

■ Irregular the first year or two after the onset of menarche (not ovulating monthly yet).

Breasts (specialized sweat glands)

■ Pubertal changes start at Tanner Stage II (breast buds).
■ Areola/nipples develop first before other breast tissue (Tanner Stage II).

Cervix

■ Younger girls (before puberty) higher number of glandular cells on the surface.
■ Cells undergo metaplastic changes (transformation zone) during puberty.
■ Most cancers are located in the transformation zone area.

Ovaries

■ Female infants are born with 3 million eggs.
■ Eggs are stored as follicles in the ovaries.

Menstrual Cycle

This example is based on a perfect 28-day menstrual cycle.

Follicular Phase (days 1 to 14)

FSH stimulates the ovaries into making new follicles. As follicles mature, produces estrogen until the end of the cycle. Estrogen stimulates the growth of the endometrial lining. Estrogen is the predominant hormone the first 2 weeks of the menstrual cycle.

Midcycle (day 14): Ovulation

LH is secreted by the anterior pituitary gland that induces ovulation.

Luteal Phase (days 14 to 28)

Progesterone is the predominant hormone. Stabilizes endometrial lining.
After ovulation, corpus lutea is left over. It produces progesterone until the end
of the cycle.

Menstruation

If not pregnant, both estrogen and progesterone fall drastically inducing menses.
The low hormone levels stimulate the anterior pituitary and the cycle starts again.

Menopause

Defined as amenorrhea (no blood or spotting) for 12 consecutive months. Is
caused by physiologic ovarian failure.

■ Mean age 51 years (range 45 to 55 years)
■ FSH >30–35 mIU/ ml (follicle stimulating hormone)

Perimenopause

A transition stage before menopause with classic signs/symptoms of hot flashes,
night sweats, mood changes, insomnia. As ovaries gradually fail, periods become
very irregular and eventually get lighter and disappear.

Fast Facts | Menopausal Body Changes

Ovaries

After several years of menopause, the ovaries are atrophied and a smaller size.
Therefore, a palpable ovary is considered abnormal. Rule out ovarian cancer.
Order an intravaginal/pelvic ultrasound. The CEA 125 is elevated later in ovarian
cancer.

Labia and Vagina

Both become atrophic and thinner with less rugae. The vaginal canal becomes
dry.
    Dyspareunia (painful intercourse) is common. It is treated by lubricants, oral
or topical estrogens.

Urethra and Bladder

These organs atrophy increasing the risk of urinary incontinence and cystoceles.
Cystoceles (prolapsed bladder) are treated by the use of a pessary or by surgery.

Urinary incontinence is treated medically with anticholinergic/antispasmodics (e.g., oxybutynin or Oxytrol), Kegel exercises, pads, fluid limitation, and/or surgical repair.

Hormone Replacement Therapy (HRT) or Estrogen Replacement Therapy (no uterus)

Increased risk of acute MI, thromboembolism, endometrial cancer, and breast cancer.

Recommendations
- Use hormones at the lowest possible dose for the shortest amount of time and only for symptomatic women with moderate to severe symptoms who do not respond to other types of treatment (including alternative medications).
- Evaluate hormone replacement annually.
- Keep menstrual calendar for any episodes of breakthrough bleeding.
- Endometrial biopsy for breakthrough bleeding to rule out uterine cancer.

Fast Facts | Laboratory Procedures

Pap Smears

Screening test only. Diagnostic test is the cervical biopsy (done during a colposcopy).
High false-negative rate of 15 to 40%.
Satisfactory specimen only if both squamous epithelial cells and endocervical cells are present. If endocervical cells are missing, repeat Pap (incomplete).
Endometrial cells
- if present, refer for endometrial biopsy.
ASCUS (atypical squamous cells of undetermined significance)
- check for HPV strain. Oncogenic types must be referred to gyn.
AGCUS (atypical glandular cells of undetermined significance)
- refer for endometrial biopsy.

KOH (potassium hydroxide) Slide

Useful for helping with diagnosis of fungal infections (hair, nails, skin). KOH works by causing lysis of the squamous cells, which makes it easier to see hyphae and spores. KOH is also use for the "Whiff Test" for bacterial vaginosis. A strong fishlike odor is released after one to two drops are added on the slide.

Tzanck Smear

Used as an adjunct for evaluating herpetic infections (oral, genital, skin). A positive smear will show large abnormal nuclei on the squamous epithelial cells.

Gram Stain

Useful for diagnosing gonorrhea in the clinical area. Under high power, the white blood cells are examined for Gram-negative bacteria (neisseria gonorrhea) after the specimen has been stained.

Fast Facts | Oral Contraceptives

Absolute Contraindications

- Past history of thrombophlebitis or thromboembolic disorders (e.g., DVT).
- CVA or CAD (coronary artery disease).
- Migraine with focal aura (e.g., basilar migraines cause TIA-like signs/symptoms).
- Known/suspected cancer of the reproductive system: breast, endometrium, ovary.
- Known or suspected estrogen dependent neoplasia.
- Undiagnosed genital bleeding.
- Cholestatic jaundice of pregnancy.
- Acute or chronic liver disease with abnormal LFT's
  - If acute infection of the liver (e.g., mononucleosis) with elevated LFTs, estrogen is contraindicated.
  - When LFTs are back to normal, can go back on birth control pills.
- Hepatic adenomas or carcinomas.
- Known or suspected pregnancy.
- Hypersensitivity.
- Smoking if over the age of 35 years
  - relative contraindication because women younger than age 35 who smoke can have the pill if no other contraindications exist.

Mnemonic Device
To remember contraindications for oral contraceptives, use "*My CUPLETS.*"

*M*y —Migraines with focal aura
C   CAD or CVA
U   Undiagnosed genital bleeding
P   Pregnant or suspect pregnancy
L   Liver tumor or active liver disease
E   Estrogen dependent tumor
T   Thrombus or emboli
S   Smoking age 35 or older

Relative Contraindications

- Migraine headaches without aura.
- Smoking, if younger than 35 years.

■ Hypertension (uncontrolled by drugs).
■ Fracture or cast on lower extremities.
■ Severe depression.

Exam Tips

■ Problems on absolute versus relative contraindications of birth control pills are designed with answer options that list both a true contraindication and a relative contraindication. For example, a question asking for a relative contraindication may have an answer choice such as: history of a blood clot that resolved (absolute) and migraine headache (relative).
■ Any smoking is an absolute contraindication from age of 35 years and older.

Advantages of the Contraceptive Pill (after >5 years of use)

■ Risk of ovarian cancer decreased by 40%
■ Risk of endometrial cancer decreased by 50%
■ Risk of lower risk of PID and pregnancy (due to thickened cervical mucus plug)
■ Decreased incidence of:

Dysmenorrhea and cramps (decrease in prostaglandins)
Iron deficiency anemia (less blood loss from lighter periods)
Acne and hirsutism (lower levels of androgenic hormones)
Ovarian cysts (due to suppression of ovulation)
Fibrocystic breasts (due to decreased progesterone)

New Prescriptions
There are two methods of starting the first pill pack. Rule out pregnancy first. All patients must use condoms in the first 2 weeks of the menstrual cycle during the first pill pack.

1) "Sunday Start": take first pill on the first Sunday during the menstrual period.
2) "Day One Start": take the first pill during the first day of the menstrual period.

Patient needs follow-up visit in 2 to 3 months to check BP and for side effects, questions, etc.

Oral Contraceptive Pill Problems

Breakthrough bleeding (BTB) and spotting
Term used for menstrual bleeding that occurs out of usual cycle. Oral contraceptive pills contain hormones (estrogen/progesterone) for the first 3 weeks of the pill cycle; the 4th week is hormone-free (when the period occurs).

- If bleeding occurs in the first 2 weeks of the cycle, increase estrogen (or decrease progesterone).
- If bleeding occurs in the last 2 weeks of the cycling, increase progesterone (or decrease estrogen).

NSAIDs can also help decrease bleeding.

Missing Consecutive Days of Oral Contraceptive Pills

Missed 1 day: Take two pills the next day and continue with same pill pack ("doubling up").

Missed 2 consecutive days: Take two pills the next 2 days to catch up and finish the birth control pill pack and use condoms until next pill cycle.

Drug Interactions of Oral Contraceptives

- Anticonvulsants: phenobarbital, phenytoin
- Antifungals: griseofulvin (Fulvicin)
- Certain antibiotics: ampicillin, tetracyclines, rifampin

Pill Danger Signs

Thromboembolic events can happen in any organ of the body. Higher risk with smokers. Advise patient to report or to call 911 if having severe abdominal or chest pains, headaches, visual changes, leg pains, shortness of breath, etc.

Emergency Contraception ("Morning After Pill")

Rule out preexisting pregnancy first. Effective up to 72 hours after unprotected sex. Most effective if taken in first 24 hours.

- Progesterone only (Plan B—levonorgestrel 0.75 mg tabs). Effective up to 89%.
- Estrogen/progesterone birth control pills (e.g., Ovral) in high doses. Effective up to 75%.

Dosing: take first dose as soon as possible (no later than 72 hours after). Take the second dose in 12 hours. Birth control pills cause more vomiting. Prescribe drug for nausea (e.g., Tigan).

If patient vomits within 1 hour, repeat the dose.

Advise patient if she does not have a period in the next 3 weeks, return to rule out pregnancy.

IUD (intrauterine device)

Copper-bearing IUDs such as Copper T 380A can be left in the uterus up to 12 years. Mirena (progestin) is effective for 5 years. Second most commonly used method of contraception in the world (female sterilization is the first).

Contraindications
- Recent infection of the reproductive tract (e.g., cervicitis, PID)
- Suspected or confirmed STD or pregnant
- Uterine or cervical abnormality (e.g., bicornate uterus or two-lobed uterus)
- undiagnosed vaginal bleeding

Increased risk
- Endometrial and pelvic infections (first few months after insertion only)
- Perforation of the uterus
- Heavy or prolonged menstrual periods

Check for missing or shortened string especially after each menses. If the patient or clinician does not feel the string, order a pelvic ultrasound.

Depo Provera (depot medroxyprogesterone)

Each dose by injection lasts 3 months. Check for pregnancy before starting dose. Start in first five days of cycle (day 1-5) because there is less chance of ovulation at this time. There is a 0.03% failure rate.

Risks of Long-Term Use (>5 years)
Increases risk for osteoporosis and weight gain. Women with anorexia nervosa have an even greater risk of osteoporosis and fractures (may already have osteopenia). Recommend calcium with vitamin D and weight-bearing exercises.

All women on Depo Provera for 1 year or longer have amenorrhea because of severe uterine atrophy from lack of estrogen.

Diaphragm With Contraceptive Gel

Latex dome-shaped barrier device. Must be used with spermicidal gel to be effective. Will need additional spermicidal gel/foam inside vagina before every act of intercourse. Do not remove diaphragm while inserting additional vaginal spermicide. Do not remove diaphragm until 6 to 8 hours after last ejaculation. Can leave diaphragm inside the vagina up to 24 hours.

Increased risk for UTIs and toxic shock syndrome (TSS). There is a 20% failure rate.

Condoms

Do not use with any oil-based lubricants, creams, etc. There is a 14% failure rate for male condoms and a 20% failure rate for female condoms.

Exam Tips

- Women who have been in menopause for several years will have ovaries that are not palpable. Uterus is still palpable.

- Contraindications to oral contraceptives (do not confuse a relative with an absolute contraindication).
- If a woman misses 2 consecutive days of the pill, she should take 2 pills next 2 days to finish cycle and use condoms until next cycle starts.
- On the ANCC exam, questions will ask for the best birth control method for a case scenario. Remember the contraindications or adverse effects of the pill, IUD, diaphragms, and condoms.

Clinical Tips

- Do not recommend Depo Provera to women who want to become pregnant in 12 to 18 months. Causes delayed return of fertility.
- It takes up to 1 year for most women to start ovulating; on rare occasions, it can take up to 2 years for some women to be fertile again.

Fast Facts Benign Variants

Supranumerary Nipples

Nipples form a V-shaped line on both sides of the chest down the abdomen. Both sides are symmetrically distributed. Nipples appear like moles that are raised.

Fast Facts Disease Review

Fibrocystic Breast

Monthly hormonal cycle induces breast tissue to become engorged and painful. Attributed to surge of progesterone during the luteal phase (last 2 weeks before menses). Symptoms resolve after menstruation starts.

Classic Case
Adult female complains of tender, bloated, and lumpy breasts 1 to 2 weeks before her menstrual cycle for many years. Relief of symptoms occurs within 1 to 2 days after onset of menses. Denies dominant mass, skin changes, nipple discharge, or enlarged nodes.

Objective Findings
Multiple mobile and rubbery cystic masses on both breasts.
Both breasts have symmetrical findings.
No skin changes (e.g., peau de orange) or nipple discharge.

Plan
- Stop caffeine intake. Take vitamin E and evening primrose capsules daily.
- Wear bras with good support.

■ Refer: patient to gynecologist if there is a dominant mass, skin changes, or a fixed mass.

Polycystic Ovary Syndrome (PCOS)

Hormonal abnormality marked by anovulation, infertility, and excessive androgen production that increases patient's risk for heart disease, breast cancer, and uterine cancer.

Classic Case

Obese teen or young adult complains of excessive facial and body hair (hirsutism 70%), bad acne, and amenorrhea or infrequent periods (oligomenorrhea). Dark thick hair (terminal hair) is seen on the face and beard areas.

Plan

■ Pelvic/intravaginal ultrasound. Enlarged ovaries with multiple follicular cysts. Serum testosterone and androstenedione are elevated. FSH levels normal or low.

Medications

Low-dosed OCs to suppress ovaries
Medroxyprogesterone 10 mg for first 10 days of each month to induce menses
Spironolactone to decrease and control hirsutism
Metformin (Glucophage) to induce ovulation if pregnancy is desired
Weight reduction

Complications

Increased risk for coronary heart disease (CHD), Type 2 diabetes mellitus and breast cancer and endometrial cancer.

Candida Vaginitis

Overgrowth of candida albicans yeast in the vulva/vagina. It results in a large amount of inflammation with symptoms of pruritus, swelling, and redness. The male penis can also get infected (balanitis). Diabetes, HIV, antibiotics make a patient more susceptible.

Classic Case

Adult female presents with complaints of white cheeselike vaginal discharge accompanied by pruritus, burning, redness, and irritation. A large amount of thick white discharge ("curd like") is also seen.

Plan

■ Microscopy or wet mount is the preferred diagnostic test, looking for pseudo-hyphae, spores, and a large number of WBCs.

Medications

Miconazole (Monistat), clotrimazole (Gyne-Lotrimin) are over the counter.
Prescription: Diflucan 100 mg tab × 1 dose, terconazole (Terazol) vaginal cream/suppository.

Exam Tip

- Several questions on different types of vaginitis are on the exam.

Bacterial Vaginosis (BV)

Caused by anaerobic bacterial overgrowth that is due to unknown reasons or develops secondary to pregnancy terminations or Pelvic Inflamatory Disease. Not an STD; therefore sexual partner does not need treatment.

Pregnant women who develop bacteria vaginosis are at higher risk for intrauterine infections and premature labor.

Classic Case

Sexually active female complains of embarrassing unpleasant and fishlike vaginal odor that is worse after intercourse (no condom). Vaginal discharge is copious with thin, milk-like consistency, coats the vaginal walls, color is off-white to gray. There is no vulvar or vaginal redness or irritation.

Plan

Wet Smear Microscopy
Clue cells and very few WBCs. May see Mobiluncus bacteria.
Clue cells: squamous epithelial cells with large amount of bacteria coating the surface that obliterates the edges of the cell.

Whiff test
Apply one drop of KOH (potassium hydroxide) to a cotton swab that is soaked with vaginal discharge.
Positive: a strong "fishy" odor is released.

Vaginal pH
Alkaline vaginal pH > 4.5. Normal vaginal pH is between 4.0 to 4.5 (acidic).

Medications

Metronidazole (Flagyl) BID × 7 days or vaginal gel @ HS (bedtime) × 5 days.
Watch for disulfiram (Antabuse) effect if combined with alcohol (severe nausea, HA, etc).

Clindamycin (Cleocin) cream @ HS × 7 days.

Oil-based creams can weaken condoms.

Sex partners: treatment not recommended by the CDC because vaginosis is not a STD.

Abstain from sexual intercourse until treatment is done.

Trichomonas Vaginitis (Trichomoniasis)

Unicellular protozoan parasite with flagella that infects genitourinary tissue (both males and females). Infection causes inflammation (pruritus, burning, and irritation) of vagina/urethra.

Classic Case

Adult female complains of very pruritic, reddened vulvovaginal area. Copious green and bubbly vaginal discharge. May have dysuria. Sex partner may have same symptoms.

Objective Findings

"Strawberry cervix" from small points of bleeding on cervical surface.

Plan

■ Microscopy Wet Smear (use low power): mobile unicellular organisms with flagella (flagellates) and a large amount of WBCs.

Medications

Metronidazole (Flagyl) 2 gm PO × 1 dose or 500 mg BID × 7 days

Treat sexual partner because this is an STD. Test both for other STDs.

Atrophic Vaginitis

Chronic lack of estrogen in estrogen-dependent tissue of the urogenital tract results in atrophic changes in the genital tract of menopausal women.

Classic Case

Menopausal female complains of vaginal dryness, itching, and pain with sexual intercourse (dyspareunia). Complains of a lot of discomfort with speculum exams (e.g., Pap smears).

Objective Findings

Atrophic labia with decreased rugae; dry, pale pink color to vagina.

Plan

■ Topical estrogens (e.g., Premarin cream). Prolonged vaginal estrogens (if intact uterus) need progesterone supplementation to prevent endometrial hyperplasia.

Table 3.11	Vaginal Infections	
Type	**Signs/Sx**	**Labs**
Bacterial vaginosis anaerobes	"Fishlike" vaginal odor; Profuse milk-like discharge; Not itchy/vulva not red; A *vaginosis*; not vaginitis	Clue cells (large numbers bacteria on cell surface) Whiff test: positive pH: > 4.5 alkaline
Trichomonas vaginitis	"Strawberry cervix"; Bubbly discharge; Vulva/vagina red/irritated	Mobile protozoa with flagella
Candidal vaginitis	Cheesy or curdlike white discharge; Vulva/vagina red/irritated	Pseudohyphae, Spores Numerous WBCs
Atrophic vaginitis	Scant to no discharge; Fewer rugae, color pale; Dyspareunia (painful intercourse)	Atrophic changes on Pap test, can diagnose without labs based on history

Osteoporosis

A gradual loss of bone density secondary to estrogen deficiency and other metabolic disorders. Most common in menopausal females. Other risk groups include

■ patients on chronic steroids (severe asthma, autoimmune disorders, etc.)
■ androgen deficiency, hypogonadism

Bone Density Test Scores
Osteoporosis: T score of −2.5 standard deviation or less
Osteopenia: T scores of between −1.5 to −2.4 standard deviations

Medications/Treatments
1) Weight-bearing exercises several times a week
   ■ swimming is not considered a weight-bearing exercise (good for severe arthritis)
2) Calcium with vitamin D 1200 mg (if on hormone replacement) or 1500 mg per day (if not taking hormone replacement)
3) Bisphosphonates
   Fosamax (Alendronate) 5 to 10 mg/day or 70 mg weekly
   ■ rebuilds bone and stops existing bone loss
   ■ take upon awakening in AM with full glass water on empty stomach
   ■ will cause severe esophagitis or esophageal perforation if lodged in the esophagus

Contraindications: inability to sit upright, esophageal motility disorders, history of PUD or GI

4) SERM class (selective estrogen receptor modulator)

Evista: Category X drug (synthetic estrogen)

■ does not stimulate endometrium or breast tissue growth

■ not for use in premenopausal women (aggravates hot flashes) or with patients with history of venous thrombosis

5) Other hormones

Miacalcin (Calcitonin salmon, derived from salmon)

■ stops bone loss but does not rebuild bone.

■ good choice for relief of bone pain from vertebral fractures

Exam Tip

■ Bone Density Tests: T score > or equal −2.5 standard deviation (osteoporosis)

WOMEN'S HEALTH: PREGNANCY AND CHILDBIRTH

Obstetrics

Fast Facts Danger Signals

Preeclampsia to Eclampsia (Pregnancy Induced Hypertension)

Young primigravida who is at the end of the second to the third trimester complains of new onset of symptoms such as sudden weight gain, blurred vision, headaches, generalized edema and nausea. Edema easily seen on the face, fingers, and feet. Elevated blood pressure and proteinuria. Note: if symptoms occur before 20 weeks, it is not considered preeclampsia or eclampsia

HELLP Syndrome (Hemolysis, Elevated Liver enzymes, and Low Platelets)

Serious but rare complication of preeclampsia. Classic patient is a multipara older than 25 years who is in the third trimester of pregnancy. Complains of severe headaches, edema of the face/hands, abdominal pain, nausea and/or vomiting and fatigue.

Placenta Previa

A multipara who is in the late second to third trimester complains of several episodes of painless vaginal bleeding of bright red-colored blood. Uterus is soft and non-tender. Usually reports history of sexual intercourse preceding the bleeding episode(s). If cervix is dilated or if hemorrhaging, fetus is delivered by C-section.

Treatment is strict bedrest. Intravenous magnesium sulfate if there is uterine cramping. Uterus will reimplant itself if mild. Any vaginal or rectal insertion or stimulation is an absolute contraindication (can precipitate hemorrhage).

Abruptio Placentae

Pregnant woman who is in the late third trimester complains of a sudden onset of a tender and contracted uterus that feels hard (hypertonic) and very painful. Associated with a sudden onset of dark red-colored vaginal bleeding. Up to 20% of women do not have vaginal bleeding (blood is trapped between placenta and uterine wall). If mild, blood is reabsorbed and affected area reimplants. Severe cases cause hemorrhage; fetus must be delivered to save mother's life. Higher risk in females with history of hypertension (before pregnancy) or secondary to abdominal trauma.

Fast Facts Laboratory Testing

Urinalysis

Check protein, leukocytes, nitrite, blood, glucose. Negative protein is normal finding. Proteinuria seen in pregnancy (preeclampsia).

1) Protein (1+ or higher abnormal)
2) If 20 weeks of gestation or more, also rule out pregnancy-induced hypertension or preeclampsia besides renal disease. Order 24-hour urine for protein/creatinine clearance.

Sexually Transmitted Diseases (STDs)

HBsAg (Hepatitis B surface antigen), gonorrhea, chlamydia, rubella titer, HIV, herpes titers

Serum Alpha-fetoprotein (AFP)

Manufactured by the liver of the fetus and mother. Fetus makes the majority of the AFP because of growing liver. Higher levels are seen with multiple gestations.

1) Low AFP
   Down's syndrome (35-year-old female has a 1:200 chance)
   Fetal demise
2) High AFP
   Multiple gestations
   Neural tube defects (risk of 2:1,000 pregnancies)

Prevention with folate 400 mcg. per day (found in leafy green vegetables, fortified cereals)

3) Triple Screen

AFP plus serum hCG and estriol levels increases predictive value of an abnormal AFP screen

Amniocentesis

If age 35 or older or if there is a family history of a genetic disorder (e.g., Tay-Sachs, cystic fibrosis, etc.). Tay-Sachs seen more in Jewish-descent females. Can order test as early as 14–18 weeks.

Human Chorionic Gonadotropin

Manufactured by the chorion by day 8 (develops into the placenta). Urine tests can pick up pregnancy as early as the 2nd week of conception (or by the first missed period).

Doubling Time

An important indicator of the viability of a pregnancy. Useful only in the first trimester; thereafter, it loses its predictive value (do not used after week 12).

- Normal finding: Doubles every 48 hours during the first 12 weeks (first trimester) in a normal pregnancy
- Ectopic pregnancy: Lower values than normal. Values increase slowly and do not double as expected.
- Inevitable abortion: Values start decreasing rapidly. No doubling.

Vaginal Cultures

Group B strep (GBS) at 34–36 weeks. Up to 35% of women have GBS as normal flora in GI tract/vagina. If positive, treat with penicillin G 2.5 million units IV. If penicillin allergic: use clindamycin or erythromycin instead

Fast Facts Drugs and Vaccines During Pregnancy

Most of the drugs used in pregnancy are Category B drugs. There are very few Category A drugs. Because it is unethical to experiment on pregnant women, a large number of drugs are found to be safe only through many years of use by pregnant women.

Category A Drugs

Animal and human data show no risk to pregnant women. Examples are insulin and thyroid hormone.

Category B Drugs

Animal studies show no risk. No human data available.

- Antacids
- Docusate Sodium (Colace). Colace is a stool softener and is approved for pregnant women. It is not a laxative. Avoid laxatives (e.g., Ex-lax, Bisacodyl), especially in the 3rd trimester (may induce labor).
- Analgesics (acetaminophen)

Antibiotics for Pregnant Women

The antibiotics below are category B.

- Penicillins
  amoxicillin (Amoxil), penicillin
- Cephalosporins
  First generation: cephalexin (Keflex)
  Second generation: cefaclor (Ceclor), cefprozil (Cefzil)
  Third generation: ceftriaxone (Rocephin) injections
- Macrolides
  erythromycins (e.g., Emycin, azithromycin, Zithromax)
  All macrolides are category B except for clarithromycin (Biaxin).
  Biaxin is the only macrolide that is a category C. Discuss risk versus benefits.
- Nitrofurantoin
  MacroBid

Use of Anti-Hypertensives with Pregnant Women

Used for women with preexisting hypertension or for moderate-to-severe preeclampsia or eclampsia.

- Methyldopa (Aldomet)
- Hydralazine (Apresoline)
- Labetalol (Normodyne)

Category C Drugs

Adverse effects seen in animal studies. No human data available.

- Sulfa Drugs
  Category C in third trimester because of increased risk of hyperbilirubinemia (hemolysis in utero)
  Trimethoprim-sulfamethoxazole (e.g., Bactrim DS, Septra)

- NSAIDs
  Contraindicated in third trimester because they block prostaglandins. Category B or C (depends on type of NSAID).

Category D Drugs

Evidence of fetal risk. Benefits should outweigh the risk of using the drug.

- ACE Inhibitors and ARBs
  Causes fetal renal abnormalities, renal failure, and hypotension
  Captopril (Capoten) and losartan (Hyzaar)
  Category C in first trimester
  Category D in second and third trimester

- Fluoroquinolones
  Affects fetal cartilage development. A rare side effect is Achilles tendon rupture in athletes. Contraindicated in pregnant or lactating women and children younger than 18 years.
  Ciprofloxacin (Cipro)
  Ofloxacin (Floxin)
  Levaquinolone (Levaquin)

- Tetracyclines
  Stains growing tooth enamel.
  Tetracycline, minocin (Minocycline)

Drugs Contraindicated in the Third Trimester

These are not Category X drugs. They are contraindicated in the third trimester because they can cause hemolysis in utero with resulting hyperbilirubinemia.

- NSAIDs
  blocks prostaglandins
  may cause premature labor

- Sulfa Drugs
  causes hemolysis resulting in hyperbilirubinemia

Category X Drugs

Proven fetal risks outweighs the benefits.

- Accutane (Retinoic acid, a vitamin A derivative)
  Used for severe cystic and nodular acne recalcitrant to treatment.
- Methotrexate (anti-metabolite)
  Used for autoimmune diseases, psoriasis, certain cancers.

- Proscar (anti-androgen)
  Used for BPH and prostate cancer.
- Misoprostol (prostaglandin analogue)
  Used for chronic NSAID users to lessen risk of adverse GI effects such as bleeding.
  Also used as one of the drugs in medical abortions (a component of the "abortion pill").
- Evista (selective estrogen receptor blocker)
  Used for treating osteoporosis.
- All hormonal drugs (natural or synthetic) are category X in pregnancy—
  all forms of estrogens, progesterone, and testosterone.
- Any drug that blocks hormone synthesis or binding
  Depo Lupron is used for infertility, hormone-dependent cancers.

Vaccines

- MMR (mumps, measles, and rubella), oral polio, varicella
- Flu vaccine (2 types)
  Live attenuated influenza virus vaccine (by nasal spray only). Only for healthy persons age 5 to 49 years with no nasal abnormalities. Do not give to pregnant women.
  Inactivated virus (injectable form). Recommended if pregnant in the winter months.
Note: After any live virus vaccine, advise reproductive-age women to use birth control and to wait at least 3 months before becoming pregnant.

Teratogens

Agents that can cause structural abnormalities during pregnancy.

- Alcohol: fetal alcohol syndrome
- Aminoglycosides: deafness
- Cigarettes: intrauterine growth retardation (IUGR), prematurity
- Cocaine: CVAs, mental retardation
- Isotretinoin (Accutane): CNS/ craniofacial/ ear/ cardiovascular defects
- Lithium: cardiac defects (Ebstein's anomalies)

Fast Facts Health Education for Pregnancy

- Prenatal vitamins daily (start 3 months before conception).
- Always wear seatbelt (lap belt below uterine fundus).
- Avoid exercise in hot and humid weather.
- Sex is safe except during vaginal bleeding, incompetent cervix, placenta previa, preterm labor.

- Cat litter or raw beef can cause toxoplasmosis, which can cause congenital infection.
- No raw shellfish, raw meat, uncooked hotdogs (listeria).
- No excessive caffeine (premature labor), smoking (IUGR), alcohol (fetal alcohol syndrome).
- No hot tubs, saunas, or excessive heat.

Weight Gain
- Most weight gained in third trimester (up to 1 lb/week)
- Best weight gain: 20 to 35 lbs.
- For underweight patients: ideal body weight plus 20–35 lbs.
- For obese patients: gain up to 20 lbs.
- After delivery: will lose up to 15–20 lbs in first few weeks.

Fast Facts | Signs of Pregnancy

Positive Signs
- Palpation of fetus by health provider
- Ultrasound and visualization of fetus
- Fetal heart tones (FHT)

    10 to 12 weeks by Doppler/Doptone
    20 weeks by fetoscope/stethoscope

Probable Signs
- Goodell's sign (4 weeks): cervical softening
- Chadwick's sign (6–8 weeks): blue coloration of the cervix and vagina
- Hegar's sign (6–8 weeks): softening uterine isthmus
- Enlarged uterus
- Ballottement
- Urine or blood pregnancy tests (beta hCG)
- "Quickening": the mother feels the baby's movements for the first time. Starts at 16 weeks.

Presumptive Signs
These are the softest and least objective signs. Can be caused by many other conditions besides pregnancy.
- Amenorrhea
- Nausea with/without vomiting (more common in first trimester in the morning, usually disappears by the second trimester).
- Breast changes
- Fatigue
- Urinary frequency
- Slight increase in body temperature

Exam Tips

- Memorize the three positive signs of pregnancy.
- Palpation of fetal movements by the mother is not considered a positive sign of pregnancy.
- Memorize the three "last names" of probable signs.
- Urine/serum pregnancy tests are considered as probable signs (do not confuse as a "positive sign").
- Questions asking for one of the signs will mix them up (mix a positive sign with a probable sign). Make sure that the answer option contains the two signs from the same category.
- This is the reason it is important to memorize the three "positive signs." By the process of elimination, you can rule out (or in) the correct answer choice.

Fast Facts Fundal Heights

12 weeks (3rd month)
Uterine fundus first rises above symphysis pubis.
Fetal heart tones heard by Doppler by 10–12 weeks.

16 weeks (4th month)
Uterine fundus between symphysis pubis and the umbilicus.

20 weeks (5th month)
Uterine fundus at level of the umbilicus.
Fetal heart tones heard with fetoscope or stethoscope by 20 weeks.
From 20 to 35 weeks of gestation, fundal height in cm. = number of weeks gestation. For example, a 24-week gestation fetus should have fundal height between 23 cm and 25 cm.

Size and Date Discrepancy
Defined as a difference of 2 cm (or more) in uterine size from the number of weeks gestation. If present, order an ultrasound for further evaluation.
For example, 30-week gestation with 28 cm. uterus; the uterus is smaller than expected, the fetus is not growing normally. Fetus may have IUGR or other problem.

Fast Facts Physiologic Changes During Pregnancy

Cardiac System

Heart
Displaced upward and to the left in the late second to third trimester.

Plasma Volume
Increases 50% by the end of third trimester.

Physiologic Anemia of Pregnancy
Hemoglobin and hematocrit are decreased because of the hemodilution from increased plasma volume.

Cardiac Output
Increases by 1/3 by last two trimesters.

Systolic Ejection Murmur (95%)
Caused by the increase in blood volume and cardiac output later in pregnancy.

Mammary Souffle
Bilateral continuous murmur from increased blood flow in the mammary vessels.

Blood Pressure (BP)
Decreased systolic and diastolic pressure occurs in the first trimester. Many mothers who are hypertensive before pregnancy can be off prescription anti-hypertensives at this time. By 24 weeks (6 months), BP gradually returns back to pre-pregnancy levels.

Antihypertensives used for pregnant women are Aldomet and Labetalol (beta blocker).

Vena Cava
Compression by enlarged uterus decreases blood return to the brain resulting in orthostatic hypotension. Advise women to lie on the left side and to change positions slowly.

Thyroid
Diffusely enlarged (size up to 15% larger).

GI Tract
Decreased peristalsis from progesterone effects (constipation, heartburn).

Skin Pigmentation
Pigmentary changes from increase in melanocyte-stimulating hormone from higher levels of estrogen. Causes linea nigra (dark pigmented "line" that extends from mons pubis to the umbilicus located midline). Darkening of color of the nipples and areola.

Chloasma (melasma)

Blotchy hyperpigmentation on forehead, cheeks, nose, upper lip seen in pregnant women and in some birth control pill users. Hyperpigmentation of the skin is usually permanent but becomes lighter over time. More common in darker skins (olive skins and darker).

Fast Facts | Naegele's Rule

Used to estimate date of delivery (EDD). Assumes regular 28- to 30-day menstrual cycle. Not as useful for irregular menstrual cycles. Procedure: Subtract 3 months from the month of the last menstrual period (LMP). Then add 7 days to the day of LMP.

Example

A 28-year-old primigravida's last menstrual period was on March 10, 2007. Using Naegele's rule, which of the following dates is correct for her expected date of delivery:

a) November 10, 2007
b) November 17, 2007
c) December 10, 2007
d) December 17, 2007 (correct answer)

How:

1) Subtract 3 months from March = December
2) Add 7 days to date of the LMP; $10 + 7 = 17$.
3) EDD = 12-17-07.

Exam Tip

■ The LMP month on the exam will either be: January (01), February (02) or March (03)

If LMP is:	Expected Date of Delivery (EDD)
January	October
February	November
March	December

Fast Facts | Disease Review

Rh-Negative Women

In Rh-negative mothers with Rh-positive fetuses, the immune system develops isoantibodies against Rh-positive fetal RBCs if not given RhoGAM (gamma globulin against Rh factor). Give RhoGAM for all pregnancies of Rh-negative mothers—even if they terminate in miscarriages, abortion, or tubal or ectopic pregnancies.

RhoGAM (Rh-negative immunoglobulin)

Pooled IgG antibodies prevent isoimmunization in Rh-negative females who have Rh-positive fetus.
Coombs test: detects presence of Rh antibodies against RBCs.

Rh Incompatibility Disease
Rh antibodies in the mother's immune system destroy fetal RBCs causing hemolytic anemia in the fetus (and hyperbilirubinemia). RhoGAM 300 mcg IM first dose is at 28–32 weeks. Give second dose after labor.

Gestational Diabetes

Higher risks are obese females and females with history of delivering macrosomic infants (> 9 lb) or history of gestational diabetes. First line treatment is lifestyle changes. Only 15% require insulin.

Teratogenic effects: CV defects, craniofacial defects, neural tube defects, IUGR, polyhydramnios, and respiratory distress.

Plan
■ All pregnant women: screen at 24–28 weeks of pregnancy. Screen earlier if the patient is high risk.

Labs
Blood sugar measurement 1 hour after 50 gm glucose load.
If blood sugar >140 mg/dL, order 3-hr Glucose Tolerance Test (75 gm glucose load). This is the confirmatory or diagnostic test of choice for gestational diabetes.
Frequent home glucose monitoring (four to five times a day); absolutely no oral antidiabetics used during pregnancy; only insulin is used in pregnant women (if needed).

Urinary Tract Infections (UTI)

Most common organism is E. Coli (Gram-negative). Treat asymptomatic UTIs (or bacteriuria) in pregnant women because they are at higher risk for pyelonephritis (20%). UTIs increase the risk of preterm labor.

Avoid using "3 day" treatment in pregnant women (they are considered as complicated UTIs). Pregnant women should be treated for a minimum of 7 days.

Plan
- Urinalysis: positive nitrites, leukocytes, or blood.
- Repeat urine for culture & sensitivity (C&S) when treatment completed.
- Must document resolution of infection.

Medications
Amoxicillin (Amoxil) TID × 7 days
Cephalexin (Keflex) QID × 7 days
Azithromycin (Z-Pack)
Nitrofurantoin (Macrobid) BID × 7 days

Do not use sulfa drugs (e.g., Bactrim, Macrobid) during the third trimester because of the risk of hemolysis and hyperbilirubinemia.

Spontaneous Abortions

Threatened Abortion
Vaginal bleeding and cramping occur but cervix remains closed.
May be able to salvage the pregnancy.

Inevitable Abortion
Cervix is dilated and unable to stop process. Fetus will be aborted.

Complete Abortion
Placenta and fetus are expelled completely. Cervical os is closed.

Incomplete Abortion
Placental products remain in the uterus (increased risk of endometritis). Cervix remains dilated and bleeding persists, pieces of tissue may be seen at the cervical os.
Treatment: Dilation with curettage (D and C) and antibiotics.

Hypertensive Diseases of Pregnancy

Preeclampsia (Pregnancy-Induced Hypertension)
Triad: hypertension, proteinuria, and edema. Can cause multiorgan failure and death. May start at or after 20 weeks of gestation up to the postpartum period.
Higher risk with young primigravida, multipara older than 35 years of age or prior history of preeclampsia.

Mild Preeclampsia
Defined as BP >140/90 (but less than 160/110) or systolic elevation >30 mm Hg and/or diastolic elevation >15 mm Hg.
Rapid weight gain up to 5 lbs. per week. The only cure is delivery of the fetus.

Placenta Abruptio

Premature separation of a normally implanted placenta from the uterine bed. Usually is due to hypertension, trauma, cocaine use, and so forth.

Plan
- Abdominal ultrasound; bedrest.
- If contractions, give magnesium sulfate (MgSO4) IV.
- Deliver fetus if mother's life is threatened.

Placenta Previa

An abnormally implanted placenta. The placenta implants too low either on top of cervix or on the cervical isthmus/neck. Higher risk if multiparas, fibroids, or history of uterine surgery.

Plan
Abdominal ultrasound only.
- Avoid placing any object in the vagina or rectum because it may cause hemorrhage and fetal distress.
- Avoid any sexual intercourse.
- Bedrest. Close fetal monitoring.
- Perform C-section if mother's life is in danger.
- If contractions, give magnesium sulfate (MgSO4) IV. If mild case, pregnancy can be salvaged and the placenta will reimplant. Perform C-section if mother's life is in danger.

Breast Feeding
If mother has sore nipples, advise her to nurse shorter periods but more frequently and to start nursing on less painful breast.

Initiate "letdown reflex" of milk by massaging/warm shower.

Apply lanolin or breast milk to nipple after nursing to protect from skin breakdown.

Avoid plastic nipple shields.

Avoid poor supporting bras.

Avoid stopping nursing (results in engorgement and interferes with baby "latching" on).

Avoid using soap/alcohol on nipples.

Exam Tip

- If a question describes a mother who complains of sore nipples, do not advise her to stop breastfeeding, to supplement with formula, or to use formula at nighttime feedings. The best answer is to advise the mother that it is a common problem and will resolve.

Breastfeeding Mastitis

Most common in the first two months of breastfeeding. Skin fissures in the nipple(s) allow bacterial entry. Most common organism is Staphylococcus aureus (Gram-positive).

Classic Case
Patient who is breastfeeding a new infant complains of pain and induration of the infected breast. The breast feels warm to the touch. May also have fever and malaise (flu-like symptoms).

Labs
Order C & S of milk.

Medications
Dicloxacillin BID for 7 to 10 days
Can continue to breastfeed on affected breast if no abscess (ultrasound if abscess is suspected).

PEDIATRICS

Fast Facts | Danger Signals

Cryptorchidism (undescended testicle)

Empty scrotal sac(s). One or two testicles may be missing. Testis does not descend with massage of the inguinal area. Infant should be sitting and the exam room should be warm to relax muscles when massaging the inguinal canal. Another option is to examine child after a warm bath.

Increased risk of testicular cancer if testicles are not removed from the abdomen. Surgically corrected within the first year of life if it does not spontaneously descend.

Epiglottitis

Acute and rapid onset of high fever, chills, and toxicity. Child complains of severe sore throat and drooling saliva. Won't eat or drink, muffled voice (hot potato voice) and anxious. Characteristic sitting posture with hyperextended neck with open mouth breathing. Stridor, tachycardia, and tachypnea. Usually occurs between ages 2 to 6. Usually due to *Haemophilus influenzae* type b (75%). Now rare due to the Hib conjugate vaccine. Prophylaxis with rifampin for close contacts. Reportable disease. Epiglottitis can also be caused by staph aureus infection.

Kawasaki Disease/Syndrome

Usually occurs in children younger than 5 years. Onset of high fever (up to 104 F.) and enlarged lymph nodes on the neck. Bright red rash (more obvious on groin area). Conjunctivitis (dry, no discharge), dry cracked lips, "strawberry tongue." Swollen hands and feet.

After fever subsides, skin peels off hands and feet. Treated with high-dosed aspirin and gamma globulin. Resolves within 4 to 8 weeks but may have serious sequelae, such as: aortic dissection, aneurysms of the coronary arteries, blood clots.

Close follow-up with pediatric cardiologist done for several years because effects may not be apparent until child is older (or adult).

Trachoma

Any neonate with acute conjunctivitis presenting within 30 days or less from birth should be tested for chlamydia to rule out chlamydial ophthalmia or trachoma, a highly contagious eye infection that may result in blindness. Make sure sample contains not only exudate, but also conjunctival cells as well. Treated with 14-day course of oral erythromycin QID. Treatment only 80% effective. May need second course. Topical treatment is not effective. Use only systemic antibiotics. Reportable disease.

Chlamydial Pneumonia

In infants with trachoma, also rule out concomitant chlamydial pneumonia. Obtain nasopharyngeal culture for chlamydia. Infant will have frequent cough with bibasilar rales, tachypnea, hyperinflation, and diffused infiltrates on chest X-ray. Treated with erythromycin QID × 2 weeks. Reportable disease.

Gonococcal Ophthalmia

A congenital gonorrhea infection acquired intrapartum. If untreated, may cause rupture of orbital globe and blindness. Hospitalize. Order GC culture of eye exudate (green purulent). Rule out disseminated disease. Treated with high-dose IV or IM ceftriaxone. Reportable disease.

Reye's Syndrome

History of febrile viral illness (varicella, influenza) and aspirin intake (salicylates) in a child. Mortality rate of up to 52%. Five stages of progression.

- Stage 1: persistent vomiting, confusion, lethargy
- Stage 2: hyperactive reflexes, stupor, liver damage starts
- Stages 3-5: cerebral edema, coma, liver damage, seizures, death

Although most cases are in children, disease has been seen in teenagers and adults. This disease is now rare.

Osteomyelitis

More common in infants and children. Favors infected bone/limb area. If on hip, knee, or leg, the patient walks with a limp. Infected bone or joint is red, swollen, warm, and tender to touch. Patient is febrile and irritable. If growth plate infected on the legs, growth is stunted on affected limb.

Sudden Infant Death Syndrome (SIDS)

Unexplained and sudden death in apparently healthy infants younger than 12 months. Higher risk with prematurity, low birth weight, maternal smoking and/or drug use, and poverty. Cause unknown; theories range from central nervous system abnormalities, cardiac arrhythmias, suffocation from soft, thick bedding, etc. To decrease risk, position infants on their side or back. Avoid using thick quilts, soft beds, pillows, and so forth.

Fast Facts Pediatric Skin Lesions

Skin Lesions of Infancy

Erythema toxicum "infant acne"
Small red pustules located on the face, chest, back, and extremities. Lasts from 1 to 2 weeks and resolves spontaneously. Caused by high levels of maternal hormones.

Milia, milaria or "prickly heat"
Multiple yellow or white 1-2 mm papules located mainly on the forehead, cheeks and nose in up to 50% of infants. Most common in neonates and with overheating. Spontaneous resolution.

Seborrheic Dermatitis ("cradle cap")
Excessive thick scaling on the scalp of younger infants. Treated by softening and removal of the thick scales on the scalp with mineral oil left on the scalp for 10 to 15 minutes before shampooing and scrubbing off the scales.

Nevus flammeus or "port wine" stain
Flat, large, dark pink to purple-colored stainlike lesions in irregular shapes and sizes. Large lesion located on half the facial area may be a sign of trigeminal nerve involvement and Sturge-Weber Syndrome (neurological disorder). These lesions can be treated with the pulse-dye laser.

Mongolian spots
Present in up to 80 to 90% of Black, Asian, Hispanic, and Native American infants. Blue to black-colored patches or stains. A common location is the lumbosacral-area (but can be located anywhere on the body). May be mistaken for bruising or child abuse. Usually fades by age 2 to 3 years.

Faun tail nevus

Tufts of hair overlying spinal column usually at lumbosacral area. May be a sign of spina bifida occulta. Order an ultrasound of the lesion to rule out occult spina bifida.

Café au lait spots

Flat, light brown to dark brown spots > 5mm. If six or more spots larger than 0.5 cm. in diameter are seen, rule out neurofibromatosis or Von Recklinghausen's Disease (neurological disorder marked by seizures, learning disorders, etc.). Refer to pediatric neurologist if the spots meet the same criteria to rule out neurofibromatosis.

Vascular Lesions

Strawberry hemangiomas

Raised vascular lesions ranging in size from 0.5 to 4.0 cm. It is a bright red color and feels soft to palpation. It is usually located on the head or the neck. Up to 95% will involute spontaneously by age 5 to 7 years. Watchful waiting is the usual strategy. Can be treated with the pulse-dye laser.

Cavernous hemangiomas

Raised bluish or purple vascular lesions containing numerous AV (atrioventricular) shunts/ other vascular abnormalities. Rarely involutes spontaneously. Order an ultrasound of the lesion to evaluate severity. Oral prednisone can induce spontaneous remission. Surgical repair if large. Refer to pediatrician.

Fast Facts | Screening Tests

Vision Screening

Newborn Vision

- Newborns are nearsighted (20/200 vision); visual acuity becomes 20/20 by age 6 years.
- They can focus best at distance of 24 inches.
- Human face is preferred by newborns.
- Preferred colors are black, red, and white.
- Lacrimal ducts: mature by age 2 to 3 months; newborns do not have tears when crying.

Red Reflex

Screening test for cataracts. Shine light 15 inches away at 15 degrees. Look for symmetrical and round orange glow from both eyes.

Light Reflex Test or Corneal Light Reflex (Hirschberg test)
Screening test for strabismus. Shine light directly on eyes (24 inches away) using a fixation target. Observe for the symmetry of light reflecting from both eyes.

School-age Children
1) Snellen Chart is used for screening central distance vision. Child must have the ability to understand simple instructions and be able to read the alphabet. Can be done as early as age 5 to 6 years.
2) Snellen Picture Chart is used for illiterate preschool children.
3) Ishihara Chart is used for screening color blindness.

Hearing Screening (CN 8 or acoustic nerve)

Newborns: tested electronically by "Auditory Brainstem Evoked Responses."
2 to 3 months: infant orients to voice (prefers female voice).
After 12 months: says a few words, understands simple commands.
Age 4 or older: tested by pure tone audiometry.

Mnemonic Device *(HEARS)* for high-risk factors for hearing loss:
H (hyperbilirubinemia)
E (ear infections that are frequent)
A (Apgar scores low at birth)
R (Rubella, CMV, Toxoplasmosis infections)
S (Seizures)

Laboratory Tests

TSH or Thyroid Stimulating Hormone. This is a mandatory test. Lack of thyroid hormone results in mental and somatic growth retardation. Treated by thyroid hormone supplementation.

PKU (Phenylketonuria)
Federally mandated testing. Severe mental retardation if not treated early. Disorder is an inability to metabolize phenylalanine to tyrosine because of a defect in the production of the enzyme phenylalanine hydroxylase. Perform test only after infant has protein feeding (milk or formula) for at least 48 hours. Higher risk of false negatives if done too early (under 48 hours). Treated by following special diet (phenylalanine-free diet).

Hemoglobin and Hematocrit
Screen in late infancy (9–12 months) for full term, healthy infants.
Healthy babies have enough iron stores to last up to 6 months.
Not screened at birth because it is elevated from maternal RBCs mixed in.

Lead Screening
High-risk children should be screened at age 1 to 2 years.

Fast Facts | Normal Findings

Newborns

Nutrition
Breastfeeding preferred over formula. If formula chosen, start with one fortified with iron.

Breastfeeding
No vitamin supplements or extra fluids (e.g., water, juices) are necessary the first 6 months if breastfeeding and infant is healthy.

Breast milk or formula
Contains 20 calories per ounce.

Colostrum
Secreted first few days and contains large amounts of maternal antibodies. Decreases risk of infections during the first few weeks of life.

Cow's Milk
Avoid cow's milk the first year of life (causes GI bleeding).
Common cause of iron deficiency anemia in babies younger than 12 months.

Solid Foods
Can start at 4 to 6 months. Start with rice cereal (fortified with iron) before other type cereals or food groups.
Introduce one food at a time for 4–5 days (if allergic, easier to identify offending food).

Head Findings
Caput succedaneum is diffused edema of scalp that crosses the midline. Caused by intrauterine and vaginal pressure from prolonged or difficult vaginal labor.

Cephalohematoma
Traumatic subperiosteal hemorrhage. Rule out skull fracture (order radiographs of the skull). Swelling does not cross the midline or suture lines.

Weight Gain and Length
0–6 months: 6–8 ounces per week and 1 inch per month
6–12 months: 3–4 ounces per week and 1/2 inch per month

Birth Weight

Neonates lose up to 10% of body weight but should regain it by 2 weeks of age. They double their birth weight by 6 months. They triple their birth weight by 12 months.

Head Circumference

Increases by 1 cm. per month the first year of life.

Fastest rate of head growth is from 2 to 3 months (head grows up to 2 cm. per month)

First Tooth

5–6 months (lower central incisors). Complete set of teeth by age 2 1/2 years (20 teeth).

First Permanent Teeth

5–7 years old (first molar)

Exam Tips

- Do not confuse questions asking for the "first tooth" with the "first permanent tooth."
- Birth weight doubles at 6 months/ triples at 12 months.
- Head circumference: grows by 1 cm. per month (first 12 months).
- Caput succedaneum crosses midline and cephalohematoma does not (blood blocked by scalp sutures).
- Avoid cow's milk first 12 months of life.
- Breastfeeding: no vitamin supplements or extra fluids (e.g., water, juices) are necessary first 6 months.

Reflex Testing

Moro Reflex (Startle Reflex)

Sudden loud noise will cause symmetric abduction and extension of the arms followed by adduction and flexion of the arms over the body. Disappears by 4 to 6 months.

Placing or Stepping Reflex

Hold baby upright and allow the dorsal surface of one foot to touch the edge of a table. Baby will flex the hip and knee and place the stimulated foot on the tabletop (stepping motion). Absent with paresis and breech births.

Blink Reflex

Eyelids will close in response to bright light. Disappears after 12 months.

Tonic Neck Reflex (Fencing Reflex)

Turning head to one side with jaw over shoulder causes the arm and leg on side where the head is turned to extend. The arm and leg on the opposite side will flex.

Rooting Reflex

Stroking the corner of the mouth causes baby to turn toward stimulus and suck. Disappears by 3 to 4 months.

Exam Tips

- Epsteins's pearls: white papules found on gum line resembles erupting tooth
- Hypospadias: urethral opening under glans/shaft (refer)
- Epispadias: urethral opening on top of glans/shaft (refer)
- Asymmetry of thigh/gluteal folds: rule out congenital hip dysplasia or hip fracture

Fast Facts | Immunizations

MMR (mumps, measles, and rubella)

Live attenuated virus vaccine. Not recommended before the age of 12 months (not effective due to immaturity of immune system). If dose given before 12 months, must be repeated.

Varicella Vaccine

If no reliable history of chickenpox, give anytime after the first birthday.
During 1–12 year old visit: administer if no reliable history (verbal history acceptable) of chickenpox.
Age 12 years or less: needs only one dose.
Age 13 years or older: two doses 1 month apart.
Avoid salicylates × 6 weeks (theoretical risk of Reye's syndrome).
Higher risk with household contacts with immunocompromised health care workers, child in day care or elementary school, prisons.

Influenza Vaccine

It takes 2 weeks to produce antibodies after vaccination. Do not give before age of 6 months because it is not effective (immature immune system).

Two types of flu vaccines:
1. Inactivated vaccine (killed virus)
   Indicated for children from 6 months to 5 years during the flu season, pregnant women, persons age 50 or older, patients with chronic conditions, persons in nursing homes/long-term care facilities
2. Live virus vaccine (live attenuated influenza vaccine or LAIV)

Indicated only for healthy persons ages 5 to 49 years. Administered as a nasal spray.

Forms of DTP Vaccines (diphtheria, tetanus, pertussis)

DTaP (diphtheria, tetanus, acellular pertussis) is the only form used in this country. Fewer side effects compared to older DTP form.

Indicated only for children younger than age 7 years. Of all childhood vaccines, pertussis has the most adverse effects.

DT is for infants/children younger than age 7 years unable to tolerate pertussis component.

Td is for children age 7 years or older and adults.

Side Effects: DTP or DTaP
- Advise parent to give acetaminophen or ibuprofen every 4 to 6 hours × 1 to 2 days after.
- Fever (defined as 100.4° F) in up to 50% of patients.
- Swelling and/or redness at injection site in up to 50% of patients.
- Irritability in up to 50% of patients.
- Acute encephalopathy: 1 in 110,000

A vaccine "superfund" exists to care for children with serious sequelae from vaccinations. A portion of the price of each bottle of vaccine sold in this country goes toward this fund. If it is proven that a child has been permanently damaged from a vaccine (e.g., brain damaged), the child's healthcare for a lifetime is paid for by the fund.

True Contraindications
- Persistent inconsolable crying lasting > 3 hours (within 48 hr of dose)
- Fever equal or > 105° F (within 48 hr of dose)
- Seizures (within 3 days of dose)
- Hypotonic and hyporesponsive (shocklike) state within 48 hours after dose
- Encephalopathy
- Anaphylaxis

Not Considered Contraindications to DTP/ DTaP Vaccination
- Family history of seizures
- Family history of SIDS (sudden infant death syndrome)
- Fever less than 105° F from prior DTaP vaccination

Exam Tips
- Learn contraindications of vaccines and at what ages not to give the vaccine.

| Table 3.12 | Childhood Immunization Schedule* |

Vaccine	Birth	2 Mos.	4 Mos.	6 Mos.	12 Mos.	15 Mos.	18 Mos.	4–6 yrs.Preschool
Hepatitis B (3 doses)	One	Two		Three				
DTaP (5 doses) Diphtheria, tetanus, accelular pertusis		One	Two	Three		Four		Five *Do not use after age 7 yrs (use Td)*
Hib (3 doses) Hemophilus influenza type B		One	Two	Three				*Do not give after age 7 yrs*
IPV (Polio) (3 doses) Inactivated Polio		One	Two					Three
MMR (2 doses) Live virus measles, mumps, rubella				*Contra. younger 12 mos.*	One			Two *Do not give before age 12 months*
Varicella *(1 dose)				*Contra. younger 12 mos.*	One			*Do not give before age 12 months *After age 13, needs 2 doses*
PCV (3 doses) Pneumococcal Conjugate Vac.		One	Two	Three				*Do not give after age 7 yrs*
Influenza				Start 6 mos.	High risk only	Asthma HIV, etc.		*Do not give before age 6 months*

*Adapted from Centers for Disease Control *Recommended Childhood Immunization Schedule*, 2006. This table is a simplified version; it is for the certification exams only. Do not use for clinical practice.

- Only vaccine at birth is Hepatitis B. If HBsAg positive mother, give HBIG (Hep. B immunoglobulin).
- Do not give Hib, PCV, DTaP vaccines after age 7 years. Use Td (tetanus) at age 7 or older.

Primary Series of Vaccination: Missing or Not Done

After 7th birthday (never been vaccinated) these patients only need these four vaccines:

1) Td (3 doses primary, then every 10 years)

2) IPV (3 doses)

3) Hepatitis B (3 doses)

4) MMR (2 doses)

Fast Facts Growth and Development

Newborns

Strong primitive reflexes (e.g., Moro, rooting, fencing, blink, etc.).
Head lag.
Pasty yellow stool after each feeding (especially if breastfed).
Eats every 2 to 3 hours or nurses from 8 to 10 times a day.
Newborns do not have tears when crying. Tear ducts do not mature until age 2 months.
Sleeps 16 hours per day.
Report: high-pitched cry, "cat-like" cry, floppy.

6 Months Old

Fine motor
- Palmar grasp of objects.
- Reaches for toys using palmar grasp.

Gross motor
- Sits up without support.
- Rolls over well.

Language
- Babbles consonants.
- Report failure to follow objects past midline (180 degrees), poor eye contact

9 Months Old

Fine motor
- Pincer grasp starts

Gross motor
- Pulls self up to stand
- Crawls and "cruises"
- Bears weight well

Language
- Non-specific "mama," "dada"
- "Stranger anxiety"

Report absence of babble, inability to sit alone, strong primitive reflexes such as the Moro (startle reflex), fencing (tonic neck reflex)

12 Months Old

Gross motor
- Stands independently
- Walks independently
- Waves "bye bye"

Language
- Knows at least 2 to 4 words
- Specific "mama," "dada"
- Knows first name
- Growth rate slows down

Labs: check for anemia, lead poisoning if high-risk
Report absence of weight bearing, inability to transfer objects hand to hand.

2 Years Old

Fine motor
- Stacks 6 cubes
- Imitates horizontal and vertical lines
- Feeds self

Gross motor
- Goes up stairs using same foot
- Runs

Language
- Speaks in 2 to 3 word sentences (intelligible only to family)
- Understands simple commands
- Knows first name

Others

- Has "security blanket" or other transitional objects
- Can start with toilet training

3 Years Old

Fine motor
- Copies a circle (but not a cross)

Gross motor
- Pedals a tricycle
- Walks up stairs with alternating feet

Table 3.13 Growth & Development

	Characteristics	Abnormal
Neonate	Strong reflexes. Minimum of: BMs × 6 /day; Voids × 8/day	Jaundice at birth (hemolysis) High-pitched cry. Irritable. "Floppy." Poor reflexes.
3rd month	Supports head well. Smiles. Good eye contact.	Inability to hold head up. Avoids eye contact.
6th month	Sits up without support. Rolls front to back. Says "bye bye."	Lack of babbling. Inabililty to turn head past midline (180 degrees).
9th month	Pincer grasp (fine motor). Separation anxiety starts. Recognizes mom.	Missing pincer grasp. Infantile reflexes strong.
1 year	Supports own weight. Walks with hands held.	Unable to support own weight.
2 years	Walks. Runs. Climbs stairs using hand rails. Speech mostly understood by family. Transitional objects such as blanket/toy.	Unable to speak 2 word "sentences." Does not understand simple commands. Unable to speak in consonants.
3 years	Speaks 3-word sentences; understood by strangers. Rides tricycle. Draws a circle. Plays with other kids. Knows gender.	Unable to speak 3 word sentences. Speech hard to understand. Unable to understand simple commands.
4 years	Rides bicycle. Draws a cross. Knows some alphabet, numbers. Draws person with 3 parts.	Unable to speak in full sentences. Inability to skip, run, hop. Cannot put on clothes without help. Unable to play with other kids.

Language
- Speaks in full sentences; can be understood by strangers
- Knows full name, age, sexual identity

Others
- Toilet training in progress or done.

4 Years Old

Fine motor
- Can copy a cross. Draws a person with two parts.

Gross motor
- Rides a bicycle. Hops on one foot.
- Dresses with little assistance.

Safety Education

■ Choking: remove objects smaller than 2 inches (coins, nuts, carrots, hot dogs, balloons).

■ Safest place in the car for infant/child < 12 years of age is in the middle of the back seat.

■ Infants up to 20 lbs. should be in rear-facing seats.

■ Kids between 40 to 100 pounds need booster seats in the back of the car until the shoulder harness fits correctly over shoulders.

Fast Facts Disease Review

Physiologic Jaundice

A transient unconjugated (indirect) hyperbilirubinemia that usually resolves within one week. Bilirubin (breakdown product from old RBCs) damages the brain and the nerves (neurotoxic). Physiologic jaundice starts after 24 hours (when levels are higher than 5 mg/dl). Jaundice first appears on the head and progresses downward.

Evaluate
Jaundice at birth or within first day of life (fetal bleeding or hemolysis before birth). Bilirubin level increases too rapidly (> 5mg/day) or if levels greater than 15 mg/dL.

Plan
■ Phototherapy if bilirubin level > 15mg/dL. Light used is from the white to blue spectrum (not red or other color). Converts bilirubin into a water-soluble form so that it is excreted in the urine.

Complications
Kernicterus: high levels of unbound bilirubin in circulation damages infant's central nervous system (CNS).

Physiologic Anemia of Infancy

Physiologic and temporary shutdown of erythropoietin production of the kidneys. The lowest level (nadir) is at 6 to 8 weeks of life. Erythropoietin production re-starts spontaneously and stimulates the bone morrow to produce red blood cells.

Congenital Lacrimal Duct Obstruction

Also known as congenital nasolacrimal duct obstruction. Failure of the tear duct to open at birth. Thin membrane blocks the entrance of nasolacrimal duct causing tear blockage.

Classic Case

An infant's mother reports persistent tearing in both eyes with mucoid discharge. Occasional episodes of crusty yellow to green-colored eye discharge (secondary bacterial infection). Spontaneously resolves.

Plan

▪ Lacrimal Sac Massage: Place finger on lacrimal sac and massage downward toward mouth. Repeat several times a day.

Infant Colic (rule of 3's)

The goal when evaluating an infant with colic is to rule out conditions causing pain and/or discomfort, infections, environment, and formula "allergy."

▪ Crying and irritability lasting a total of 3 hours a day in an infant younger than 3 months.
▪ Occurs more than 3 days in a week and crying last more than 3 hours a day.
▪ Crying usually occurs at the same time each day. Usually resolves by 3 to 4 months.

Coarctation of the Aorta

Congenital narrowing of a portion of the aorta. Usually involves the descending aorta. Compare radial and femoral pulses simultaneously.

Screening

Take BP measurements of arm and thigh.

Normal finding: systolic BP higher in legs than in arms.

Abnormal: a delay or change in amplitude of pulses or systolic BP higher in arms than in thighs.

Abdominal Tumors: Malignant Tumors

Neuroblastoma

Tumor of the adrenal medulla. Most common presentation is a hard, smooth abdominal mass.

Abdominal mass is fixed, firm, irregular, and frequently crosses the midline.

Most are diagnosed in children less than 4 years.

Wilms Tumor (nephroblastoma)

Asymptomatic abdominal mass that extends from the flank toward the midline. Higher incidence in Black, female children. Peak age is 2 to 3 years.

Exam Tips

- Lacrimal duct massage.
- Physiologic anemia: lowest level of hemoglobin and hematocrit (nadir) is from 6 to 8 weeks.
- Wilms tumor (crosses midline). Congenital tumor of the kidneys.

Pediatric Orthopedics

Causes of Intoeing ("Pigeon-toe")

Metatarsus Adductus (kidney-shaped feet). Most common cause of intoeing. Caused by the tight muscles and ligaments inside the uterus (intrauterine forces). Kidney-shaped feet that can be moved into anatomic position. Most cases resolve once infant starts ambulating regularly. Special stretching exercises and massage done several times daily to stretch ligaments. Benign.

Internal Tibial Torsion

Tibia is rotated toward the middle of the body (internal rotation) causing "knock-knees." Seen commonly in toddlers. Most will spontaneously resolve by preschool years. Benign.

Talipes Equinovarus "clubfoot"

A rigid deformity that is corrected surgically by casting involving the foot and ankle. A medial rotation of the tibia with flexion of the ankle along with an inversion of the forefeet.

Congenital Hip Dysplasia

Ortolani Test

The femoral head slips off the acetabulum during abduction when the hip is rotated through its full range of motion. Examiner's hands should feel femoral head as it slips off acetabulum. Will hear an audible "click." If test is positive, refer to orthopedics.

Barlow's Test

Examiner attempts to dislocate hip by gently pressing down the head of the femur. If abnormal, the hip will dislocate (sublux) backward with the gentle pressure. If test is positive, refer to orthopedics.

Summary of Rashes

Roseola Infantum: Herpes Virus 6

Abrupt onset of high fever (103-106° F) lasting 1 to 5 days. During fever, child appears well. After high fever disappears (defervescence), maculopapular rash appears.

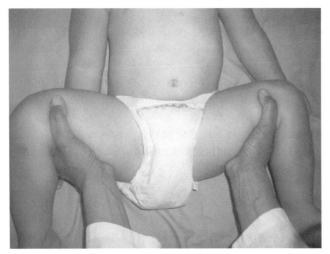

Figure 3.8. Ortolani Maneuver

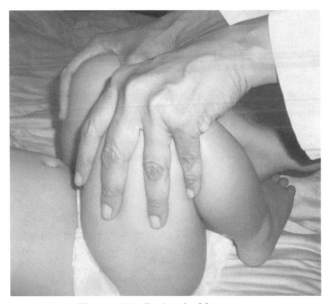

Figure 3.9. Barlow's Maneuver

By day 3 to 4, profuse maculopapular rash appears mainly on the chest and abdomen. Duration: 7 days.

Fifth Disease (Erythema Infectiosum)
Human Parvovirus B 19. Rash has three stages:
1) "Slapped cheek" appearance (or an erythematous rash with circumoral pallor).
2) Lace-like maculopapular rash the next day on arms and legs.
3) Rash may recur for 2 to 3 weeks if aggravated by sunlight or heat.

Duration: 5 to 10 days.

Varicella (Chickenpox)

Infection from the herpes zoster virus. Transmitted by respiratory droplets and through touching crusted lesions, then touching mucous membranes or inhaling particles.

Classic rash starts as a red macule, than becomes vesicular, ruptures and gets crusty. Lesions are very pruritic and generalized. Infectious from 24 hours before onset of rash until all lesions crusted.

Secondary infection possible (due to staph or strep).

Can be severe/ fatal in adults and immunocompromised patients.

Medications

Acyclovir (80mg/kg) divided in 4 doses for children older than 12 years and other high-risk patients such as newborns, HIV-infected, chronic pulmonary or skin disorder, etc. Do not use salicylates for fever; use Tylenol instead. VZIG (varicella-zoster immune globulin) – for high-risk patients with exposure to varicella (e.g., pregnant women, newborns, HIV).

Scarlet Fever

Strep throat accompanied by a generalized rash. Caused by strep pyogenes. Child with sore throat accompanied by a diffused erythematous rash. Skin starts to peel (desquamation) on the hands and feet.

Strawberry tongue. Sandpaper-like rash (not seen in Kawasaki disease).

No conjunctivitis (as seen in Kawasaki disease).

Medications

Penicillin QID × 10 days

Kawasaki Disease

Starts with fever up to 104°F or higher lasting > 5 days. Then rash appears mostly on trunk/ perineal area. Dry cracked lips and a strawberry tongue. Erythema of palms and soles that desquamates. Must have at least one large cervical node (1.5 cm). Bilateral dry conjunctivitis. Etiology: unknown.

Complications

Coronary arteries inflamed and damaged (20%)

Aneurysms, MI, arrhythmias, CHF, CAD

Differential DX: scarlet fever, viral exanthems, juvenile RA

Refer for hospitalization

Needs cardiologist for follow-up for several years after infection because of higher risk of cardiac sequelae.

Pediculosis Capitis (lice)

Infestation by pediculosis or head lice. Easily transmitted through close contact, combs, and hats. Child will keep scratching scalp until it becomes excoriated. Look for small red papules (bites) and tiny oval shiny white nits on hair shafts

Table 3.14	Childhood Rashes
Fifth Disease or Erythema Infectiosum	Rash has 3 stages: 1st "Slapped cheek" 2nd Lace-like arms & legs 3rd Rash reappears if overheated/ sunlight
Roseola infantum	Child appears & behaves normally despite high fever. When fever gone, rash appears.
Impetigo	"Honey-colored" crusted lesions. Fragile bullae. Pruritic.
Measles	Koplik's spot
Varicella	Generalized rash in different stages; new lesions crop daily. Papules = vesicles = pustules = crusts. Pruritic. Very contagious.
Scarlet fever	"Sandpaper" rash with sore throat. Strawberry tongue not specific (but also seen in Kawasaki Disease).
Kawasaki Disease	Bright red & swollen skin palms and soles = desquaminates. Strawberry tongue. Bright red conjunctivitis (no exudate or dry).
Pediculosis Capitis or Head Lice	Ovoid white nits on hair hard to dislodge. Red papules that are very itchy on scalp.
Molluscum contagiosum	Smooth round papules 5 mm size. Central umbilication with white plug.
Scabies	Located in interdigital webs of hands, waist, axillae, penis, etc. Very pruritic, especially at night.

that are hard to dislodge. Wood's light will reveal shiny white nits (darkened room).

Medications
Permethrin 1% Cream Rinse (Nix-OTC)
Nit removal: fine-toothed comb
Soak brushes and combs in Nix/Rid shampoo or hot water
Discard infested clothes
   Lindane 1% shampoos out of favor because of neurotoxic effects. Contraindicated in infants, toddlers, or any patient with neuro or seizure disorder.

Cutaneous Larva Migrans
Dog or cat hookworm larva
   Very pruritic rashes that are erythematous, serpiginous lesions that advance 1 cm. per day. Location: soles of feet, buttocks, hands, upper thighs.

Medications

Thiabendazole (Mintezol) 0.25 g–1.5 g orally B.I.D. × 2 days. (Dosage is calculated based on weight of patient.)

Molluscum Contagiosum: Poxvirus

White-to-tan colored smooth, waxy, dome-shaped papules with umbilication. No pruritus or inflammation. Self-limiting and clears in 6 months. If located on the genital area on child: rule out STDs, sexual abuse. Lesions can be treated by cryo, and so forth.

Review of Viral Rashes

- Measles: Koplik's spots
- Rubella: fetal birth defects, but mild illness to child (also known as 3-day measles).
- Erythema Infectiosum (fifth disease): slapped cheek appearance.
- Roseola: high fever up to 106°. Despite very high fever, child appears well.
- Pityriasis rosea: "Christmas-tree pattern" or Herald patch.

ADOLESCENCE

Fast Facts Danger Signals

Testicular Torsion

Sudden onset of unilateral testicular pain that increases in severity; the pain radiates to abdomen or the groin. Associated with severe nausea and vomiting. Ischemic changes result in a firm swollen scrotal sac and testicular tenderness.

Urinalysis: negative for WBCs. Doppler ultrasound to check for blood flow to the affected testicle. Testicle not functional after 24 hours if not repaired. If repaired within the first 6 hours, about 80% are salvaged. Refer to ER. This is a surgical emergency.

Perthes Disease

Affects mostly children between the ages of 2 to 12 years. Child limps and complains of pain in the affected hip and/or groin. Pain may be referred to the knee. Rare disease.

Sequelae: leg shortening, fractures of the hip, early onset of arthritis of the hip.

Suicidal and/or Homicidal Teenager

Teen (especially males) with active suicidal plan or homicidal plan using lethal method such as a gun or hanging. Previous history of suicide attempts. Children and teenagers on an SSRI are at higher risk. Avoids socializing, is a loner, is angry, has poor grades, altered sleep patterns.

Fast Facts Normal Findings

Puberty

The time period in life when secondary sexual characteristics start to develop (Tanner Stage II). Girls' ovaries start producing estrogen and progesterone. Boys' testes start producing testosterone. All of these changes result in reproductive capability.

Adolescence

Defined as the onset of puberty until sexual maturity.
Most common cause of death during this period is motor vehicle crashes.
Most common bacterial STD is Chlamydia trachomatis.

Girls

Puberty starts at age 8 years
  - precocious puberty if starts before age 8 years
  - delayed puberty if no breast development by age 13 years

Growth Spurt
Majority of somatic changes occur between the ages of 10 to 13 years
  - Majority of skeletal growth occurs before menses. Afterward, growth slows down markedly.
  - Girls start their growth spurts 1 year earlier than boys.
Timeline for growth: Breast development begins → peak growth → menarche

Table 3.15 Tanner Stages

Stage	Girls	Boys	Pubic Hair
I	Prepuberty	Prepuberty	None
II	Breast bud	Testes enlarge Scrotum ruggae ↑	Few straight, fine hairs
III	Breast & areola one mound	Penis lengthens	Darker, coarse, starts to curl
VI	Breast & areola secondary mound	Penis widens	Thicker, curly, darker, coarse
V	Adult pattern	Adult pattern	Adult pattern inner thigh

Menarche

- Average age is 11.8 years (ranges from 10 to 15 yrs).
- When Tanner Stage II starts (breast bud stage), girls start menses within 1 to 2 years.

Boys

Puberty starts at age 9 years

- precocious puberty if starts before age 9 years
- delayed puberty if no testicular growth by age 14 years

Growth Spurt

Majority of somatic changes occur from age 10 to 14 years

- boys' growth spurt is 1 year later than girls'.

Spermarche

- defined as the first ejaculation in males
- average age is 13.4 years

Tanner Stages

Boys
Stage I: prepuberty
Stage II: testis begins to enlarge/ increased rugation of scrotum
Stage III: penis elongates
Stage IV: penis thickens
Stage V: adult pattern

Girls
Stage I: prepuberty
Stage II: breast bud (onset of thelarche or breast development)
Stage III: breast tissue and areola are in one mound
Stage IV: areola/ nipples form a secondary mound
Stage V: adult pattern

Pubic Hair (both genders)
Stage I: prepuberty
Stage I: sparse growth of straight hair that is easily counted
Stage III: hair starts to curl and gets darker
Stage IV: hair curly but not on medial thigh yet like in adult. Hair is coarser.
Stage V: adult pattern, hair spreads to medial thigh and lower abdomen

Exam Tips

- Pneumovax vaccine: give only to high risk adolescent × one dose (if healthy).
- Annual flu vaccine: given starting in November of each year.

Table 3.16	Immunizations: Pre-adolescents (>age 10), Adolescents, & Adults*
Vaccine	**Immunizations**
Hepatitis B	Total 3 doses over 6 months
MMR # 2	Give 2nd dose (if needs to catch up)
Varicella	If no reliable history of chickenpox administer after age 12 months. After age 13 years, need 2 doses.
Tetanus	Every 10 years (teens usually due for booster by age 14 to 16 years)
Hepatitis A	High risk groups (homosexuals), endemic areas (certain areas of Southwest U.S., Latin America, Africa, Asia)
Influenza	Annually if high-risk (congenital heart disease, asthma, etc.) 2 types: inactivated and live virus (nasal)
Polio	Catch up if did not receive total of 3 doses as an infant. Need 3 doses (lifetime).
Meningococcal	For all college freshmen living in dormitories. Meningococcal conjugate vaccine (MCV4)

*Adapted from *Centers for Disease Control Recommended Immunization Schedule*, 2006. This table is a simplified version and is designed for studying for the certification exams only. Do not use this table as a guideline for clinical practice.

- All college freshmen living in dormitories: high risk of meningococcal infection.
- Meningococcal conjugate vaccine (MCV4) is recommended.
- Vaccine Adverse Event Reporting System (VAERS): Program to report clinically adverse events.
- Live Attentuated Influenza Virus (LAIV) nasal: indicated only for healthy persons 5–49 years of age.
- Children < age 8 receiving flu vaccines first time: need 2 doses (separated at least 2 weeks for inactivated virus injections and at least 6 weeks for nasal spray LAIV).
- High risk (flu): HIV, asthma, heart dz, sickle cell, cystic fibrosis, diabetes, etc. Household members/health workers of infants/all ages with above diseases also need vaccination.

Fast Facts Laboratory Tests

Elevated Alkaline Phosphatase

Elevated during puberty and teenage years during growth spurts because of excess production from growing bone.

Fast Facts | Legal Issues

Right to Consent and Confidentiality

Minors can give consent without a parent or guardian for the following:

- contraception
- diagnosis and management of pregnancy
- treatment for STDs

Emancipated Minor Criteria

These minors may give full consent as an adult without parental involvement:

- married
- parent or pregnant
- enlisted in the armed forces

Other Issues

Gunshot wounds, stab wounds, and child abuse (actual or suspected abuse) must be reported to the authorities.

Exam Tips

- Secondary sexual development (or puberty) starts at Tanner stage II, not Stage I.
- Puberty ends at Tanner stage V (adult).
- Only Tanner stage II to stage IV need to be memorized for the exam.
- There is no need to memorize pubic hair changes.

Fast Facts | Disease Review

Gynecomastia

Excessive growth of breast tissue. Most cases resolve spontaneously. Normal in up to 40% of pubertal boys (peaks at age 14). Seen in neonates from maternal hormones that resolve when hormones are gone.

Classic Case
Adolescent male is brought in for a visit by a parent for complaint of enlarged breasts (one may be larger), may be tender to palpation. Child is embarrassed and scared about breast changes.

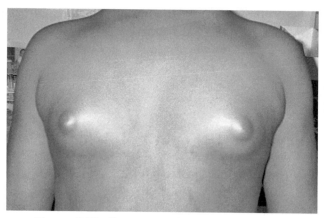

Figure 3.10. Gynecomastia (11-year-old boy)

Objective
Round rubbery and mobile mound (disc-like) under the areola of both breasts. Skin has no dimpling, redness, or changes. If mass is irregular, fixed or hard, order a sonogram.

Plan
- Evaluate for Tanner stage (check testicular size, pubic hair, axillary hair, body odor)
- Rule out serious etiology (testicular or adrenal tumors, brain tumor, hypogonadism, etc.)
- Check for drug use: both illicit and prescription (e.g., steroids, cimetidine, antipsychotics)

Pseudogynecomastia
Seen more in obese males. Enlarged breast is due to excessive adipose tissue and not true gynecomastia.

Delayed Puberty

If girl does not develop a breast bud (Tanner Stage 2) by age 14 or if a male does not have testicular development by age of 15 years, it is considered as delayed puberty.

Labs
Check hormone levels (e.g., gonadotropins, estrogen, progesterone, DHEA, FSH, TSH).
X-ray of the hand is used for estimating "bone age."

When the long bone epiphyses (growth plates) close, then the growth spurt has ended and skeletal growth is finished.

Karyotyping to rule out genetic disorders such as Klinefelter's (boys) or Turner's (girls).

Klinefelter's Syndrome

Chromosomal abnormality. These males have an extra X chromosome. Normal males have the "XY" pattern. These males have the "XXY" (45, XXY) or "XXXy" chromosomal pattern. Diagnosis in utero is by amniocentesis.

Classic Case
Tall and thin male with lack of secondary sexual characteristics such as small testes/penis, gynecomastia, sparse body hair such as in genitals, face, axillae. Sterile.

Turner's Syndrome

Chromosomal abnormality. These females have only one "X" chromosome (45, X or 45, X0) instead of the normal female pattern of "XX" (45, XX). Diagnosis in utero is by amniocentesis.

Classic Case
These females are short with a webbed neck, low set eyes and ears. Chest diameter is wider than normal. Amenorrhea and sterile.

Idiopathic Scoliosis

Lateral curvature of the spine. More common in girls (80% of patients).
Screening test: Adam's Forward Bend Test or the Forward Bend Test.
Painless and asymptomatic. Scoliosis is more likely to progress if it occurs in the beginning of the growth spurt.

Classic Case
Pubertal to young teen complains that one hip or shoulder is higher than the other. No complaints of pain.

Adam's Forward Bend Test
Bend forward with both arms hanging free. Look for asymmetry of spine, scapula, thoracic and lumbar curvature. Also known as the Forward Bend Test.

Scoliosis Parameters
Curves less than 20 degrees: Observe and monitor for changes in spinal curvature.
Curves of 20 to 40 degrees: Bracing (e.g., Milwaukee Brace).

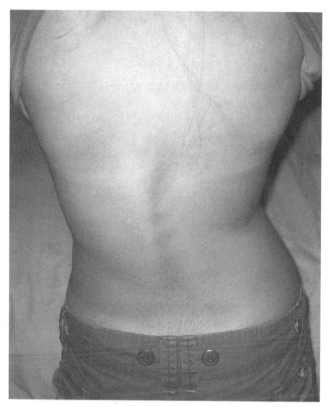

Figure 3.11. Scoliosis

Curves greater than 40 degrees: Surgical correction with Harrington rod used on spine.

Exam Tips

▪ There is always a question on this disorder.
▪ Curves less than 20 degrees are monitored for worsening.
▪ Screening exam is the Forward Bend Test.

Osgood-Schlatter Disease

Microtears of the patellar tendon that are due to overstress or overuse of the quadricep muscles of the knees. Repetitive stress and trauma from excessive traction to the patellar tendon. More common in boys from ages 10 to 17 years. More common during growth spurts especially in males.

Classic Case

More common in teenage males who are physically active and play sports that stress the quadriceps muscle (e.g., basketball, soccer). Complaints of tender bony mass over the anterior tubercle of one (or both) knees. Aggravated by activities that stress knees such as jumping.

Medications
Tylenol or NSAID for pain, avoid sports and excessive exercise.
Lateral X-rays of knees (optional). Diagnosed clinically.
Avoid excessive stress or physical activity of the knees for 1 to 2 years.
Spontaneous resolution from a few weeks to a few months. Casting, intralesional steroid injections rarely needed.

Exam Tip

■ Scoliosis question on treating 10 degree curve (observe for worsening).

GERIATRICS

Fast Facts | Danger Signals

Temporal arteritis (giant cell arteritis)

Temporal headache (one sided) with tenderness or induration over temporal artery; may be accompanied by visual loss in one eye.

Cerebrovascular Accident (CVA)

Sudden onset of neurological deficit that worsens within hours. Deficits may include blurred vision, slurred speech, one-sided upper and/or lower extremity weakness, confusion, and so forth. Signs and symptoms dependent on location of infarct.

Actinic Keratosis (precursor of squamous cell carcinoma)

Small rough pink-to-reddish lesions that do not heal. Located in sun-exposed areas such as the cheeks, nose, back of neck, arms, chest, and so forth. More common in light-skinned individuals. Squamous cell precancer skin lesions. Diagnostic method of choice is the biopsy. Small number of lesions can be treated with cryo. Larger numbers with wider distribution treated with 5-FU cream.

Fractures of the Hip

Acute onset of limping and guarding affected limb. Inability or difficulty bearing weight. Hip pain; may be referred to the knee. Unequal leg length. Affected leg is abducted (turned away from the body). History of osteoporosis or osteopenia. Fractures of the hip are a major cause of morbidity and mortality in the elderly. Up to 20% of elderly with hip fractures die from complications (e.g., pneumonia).

Exam Tips

■ Actinic keratosis: precursor of squamous cell cancer. Memory tip: the letter "C" in ACTINIC is a reminder for CANCER.

■ Do not confuse this with seborrheic keratosis, which is benign (common mistake).

| Fast Facts | **Normal Findings** |

Skin Findings

Thinner epidermis, dermis, and subcutaneous layers
Less fat, less elasticity (less collagen), slower wound healing
Sebaceous glands hypertrophy

Seborrheic keratoses

Soft, wart-like skin lesions that appear "pasted on." Mostly seen on the back/trunk. Benign.

Senile purpura

Bright purple-colored patches with well-demarcated edges. Located on the dorsum of the forearms and hands. Lesions eventually resolve over several weeks. Benign.

Lentigines

Also known as "liver spots." Tan-to-brown-colored macules on the dorsum of the hands and forearms from sun damage. More common in light skin. Benign.

Arcus senilis (corneal arcus)

Opaque white ring at the periphery of the cornea. Develops gradually and is not associated with visual changes. Cataracts: opacity and stiffening of the lens of the eye(s).
Test: Red reflex (reflection is opaque versus orange-red glow).

Presbycusis (sensorineural hearing loss)

High frequency hearing is lost first (speaking voice is high frequency). Degenerative changes of the ossicles, fewer auditory neurons, and atrophy of the hair cells resulting in sensorineural hearing loss.

Cardiac

Elongation and tortuosity (twisting) of the arteries. Thickened intimal layer of arteries resulting in increased systolic BP from increased vascular resistance (isolated systolic hypertension). Mild increase of left ventricular muscle is normal.

Baroreceptors less sensitive to changes in position. Decreased sensitivity of the autonomic nervous system. Blunted BP response; higher risk of orthostatic hypotension.

S4 heart sound a normal finding in the elderly if not associated with heart disease.

Lungs

Less elasticity and cilia. Peak expiratory flow decreased. Residual volume increased. Total lung capacity remains unchanged.

Liver

Liver size and function decreased. The enzyme systems (e.g., cytochrome P450) less active. Slower metabolism of drugs. Cholesterol levels increased.

Renal function

GFR (glomerular filtration rate) starts to decrease starting at the age 40. By age 70, up to 30% of renal function is lost. Decreased renal blood flow. Reduced clearance of drugs.

Musculoskeletal system

Kyphosis: compression fractures of vertebrae (osteoporosis). Osteoporosis and osteopenia. Osteoarthritis (DJD).

Gastrointestinal System (GI)

Less hydrochloric acid, decreased sensitivity of taste buds. Decreased efficiency absorbing nutrients from the small intestines. Increased risk of colon cancer (age >50 years is greatest risk factor).

Endocrine

Increased levels of insulin along with mild peripheral insulin resistance. Fat is redistributed mostly in the abdomen and the thighs.

Sex hormones

Males: testes active for the entire life cycle. Less testosterone production.

Females: estrogen and progesterone production cease due to ovarian failure (menopause). Adipose tissue is able to synthesize very small amounts of estrogen.

Hematology

Increased risk of iron and folate deficiency anemia as a result of decreased efficiency of the GI tract.

Immune system

Immune system activity slightly decreased.

Risk Factors: Falls in the Elderly

■ Frailness, dementia, poor eyesight, and/or poor lighting.
■ Use of area rugs; poor fit to shoes or slippers.
■ Certain medications can cause sedation and/or confusion.

Drugs: Higher Risk of Adverse Effects in Elderly

Diphenhydramine (Benadryl): sedation/confusion in elderly.

Benzodiazepines: confusion, dizziness, ataxia resulting in falls, etc.

Hypnotics: avoid long-acting (e.g., Halcion). Prefer shorter duration (e.g., Ambien).

Narcotics: start at lower doses; lasts longer in the elderly.

Beta blockers: depression and slowing.

Amitriptyline or Elavil (tricyclic antidepressants): confusion, delirium, hallucinations.

Digoxin (warfarin sodium): high doses cause visual changes, fatigue, depression.

Muscle relaxants (Soma, Skelaxin, Norflex): drowsiness, confusion, delirium.

Exam Tips

■ Delirium is reversible; dementia is irreversible.
■ Reversible causes for delirium: high fever, infections, metabolic derangements, certain drugs, dehydration, etc.
■ Irreversible causes for dementia: Alzheimer's disease, CVAs, severe chronic B12 deficiency, Parkinson's disease, etc.
■ Do not confuse reversible versus irreversible causes of dementia/delirium on the exam.
■ Presbycusis is a sensoneural. This type of hearing loss starts with high frequencies such as the spoken voice.
■ Memorize the Arcus seniles or corneal arcus description.

Clinical Tips

▨ Prescribe shorter-acting drugs such as Xanax (half-life of 4 hours) versus Valium (can last 12 hours).
▨ Never give elderly Benadryl, especially those with dementia.

Fast Facts | Screening for Dementia

Mini-Mental Exam (MME)

A brief screening exam to assess for dementia. Low scores are seen in dementia, delirium, schizophrenia. Five subject areas are tested.

1) Orientation
   ▨ Date, day of the week, state, county, home address, etc.
2) Attention and Calculation
   ▨ Serial 7's (ask patient to subtract 7 from 100 and so on).
   ▨ Spell "world" (or another word) backwards.
3) Recall
   ▨ Name 3 objects. Ask patient to repeat names after 5 minutes (short-term memory).
4) Write a sentence
   ▨ Tell the patient to write a sentence such as "I am going to the doctor."
5) Copy a design
   ▨ Examiner draws a square or a triangle and asks the patient to copy the design.

Clock Drawing Test

Quick method for assessing dementia. If abnormal, screen with MME. Instruct patient to draw a clock and mark it with the hands showing a certain time.

Exam Tip

▨ A question will ask you to identify the MME "activity" that is being performed. You are being tested for your ability to apply the concepts of the MME.

Sample question:
A nurse practitioner instructs a patient to copy a square (or spell world backwards, subtract 7 from 100, etc.). Which of the following tests is being performed:

a) MMPI (or Minnesota Multiphasic Personality Inventory; for personality testing)
b) CAGE (for alcohol abuse screening in primary care)
c) MME
d) Beck's Inventory (a depression screening tool)

The correct answer is option C or the MME.

Fast Facts | Disease Review

Dementia

An irreversible disorder with gradual and insidious onset. Global intellectual decline. Short-term memory is usually one of the early signs of the disorder. At the end stage, patient is usually incoherent to nonverbal, unable to ambulate, eat, or perform self-care.

In Alzheimer's disease (the most common cause of dementia), terminal stage is approximately 10 year from onset.

Etiology

Alzheimer's disease (most common cause of dementia in this country)
Stroke or cerebrovascular accident (CVA)
Parkinson's disease (up to 20% become demented)
AIDS dementia

Medications

Start as early as possible on Cognex, Eldepryl, or Tacrine (hepatotoxicity risk).
Gingko Biloba (increases CNS blood circulation). Antioxidants.
Supportive. No cure but medications can delay progression.

Delirium

A reversible process that has an acute and dramatic onset and is temporary. Duration is usually brief (hours to days). Acute decline in mental status. Excitable, irritable, and combative. Patient is incoherent and disoriented.

Etiology

Fever
Shock
Drugs, alcohol
Dehydration

Plan

- Remove and/or treat illness, metabolic derangement, and so forth.

"Sundowning"

Seen in both delirium and dementia. Starting at dusk/sundown, the patient becomes very agitated, confused, and combative. Symptoms resolve in the morning. Commonly recurs.

Plan

- Avoid quiet and dark rooms. keep patient in a well-lit room with a radio, TV or clock. Familiar surroundings important. Do not move furniture or change décor.

- Avoid drugs that affect cognition (antihistamines, sedatives, hypnotics, narcotics).

Exam Tip

- Parkinson's Disease patients have cogwheel rigidity with "masked facies."

Alzheimer's Disease (AD)

Accumulation of neurofibrillary plaques/tangles causes permanent damage to brain. The median survival time after diagnosis is 10 years.

Three A's: Aphasia, Apraxia, Agnosia:

Aphasia (difficulty verbalizing)

Apraxia (difficulty with gross motor movements such as walking)

Agnosia (inability to recognize familiar objects and people)

Classic Case

An early symptom is short-term memory loss that the patient attempts to hide by confabulation. After 10 years (terminal stage), the patient is usually nonverbal/incoherent, incontinent, wheelchair-bound, and needs total care.

Medications

Selegiline (Eldepryl): start during the early stages of dementia; slows down disease process.

Gingko Biloba: increases blood circulation of the brain and helps with memory.

Tacrine (Cognex): start early; must monitor liver enzymes periodically.

Plan

- Most patients with Alzheimer's are taken care of at home by a family member or caregiver. Fecal incontinence is a major reason a patient is placed in a nursing home by the family.

Complications

Death usually from an overwhelming infection such as pneumonia and sepsis. Hip fractures are also a common cause of death (from complications).

Parkinson's Disease

Progressive neurodegenerative disease (marked decrease of dopamine receptors). More common after 60 years of age. Depression common (up to 2/3 of all patients).

Classic Signs

An elderly patient complains of a gradual onset of motor symptoms such as cogwheel rigidity, pill-rolling tremor, and difficulty initiating voluntary movement. Walks with slow shuffling gait. Generalized muscular rigidity with masked facies. Up to 20% have dementia.

Plan

■ Rule out other causes of dementia that are reversible (e.g., B12 deficiency, heavy metals, neurosyphilis, drug effects, tumors that are resectable, etc.).

Medications

Levodopa-carbidopa (Symmetrel) BID
Selegiline (Eldepryl) daily

Complications

Frequent falls may result in fractures of the face, hips, etc.

Clinical Tip

■ Eldepryl is a specialized MAO inhibitor. Do not combine with an SSRI. Increases risk of serotonin syndrome (see Mental Health section).

MEN'S HEALTH

Fast Facts Danger Signals

Testicular Torsion

Male teenager awakens with a sudden onset of severe unilateral scrotal pain associated with nausea and vomiting and abdominal pain. May be spontaneous or associated with physical activity or trauma. More common in the left testicle. Higher risk with "bell clapper deformity" present in up to 12% of males. Salvage rate of 100% if corrected within the first 6 hours and 0% if done after 24 hours.

Testicular Cancer

Sensation of heaviness or aching with one testicle larger and/or tender. Testicular cancer can present as a new onset of a hydrocele (from tumor pressing on vessels). Usually painless and asymptomatic until metastasis. More common in White males ages 15 to 30 years. Rare in African Americans.

Prostate Cancer

Low back pain, rectal area/perineal pain or discomfort accompanied by obstructive voiding symptoms such as weaker stream and nocturia. May be asymptomatic. More common in Black men, positive family history of prostate cancer, age > 50 years.

Priapism

Continuous penile erection of at least 4 hours or longer unrelated to sexual desire or stimulation. May have recently taken drugs for erection dysfunction (ED) either oral or intracavernous form and/or have a history of sickle cell anemia or other blood clotting disorder, spinal cord injury (especially quadriplegia), medications (e.g., antipsychotics, cocaine). A medical emergency.

Fast Facts | Normal Findings

Spermatogenesis

Sperm production starts at puberty and continues for the entire lifetime of the male. Sperm are produced in seminiferous tubules of the testes. Sperm production takes 64 days (about 3 months).

Ideal temperature (for sperm production) is from 1 to 2 degrees lower than core body temperature.

Prostate Gland

Heart shaped gland that grows throughout the life cycle of the male. Produces PSA (prostate specific antigen) and prostatic fluid. Prostatic fluid (alkaline pH) helps the sperm survive in the vagina (acidic pH). Up to 50% of 50-year-old males have BPH (benign prostatic hypertrophy).

Testes

Oval-shaped gland that feels rubbery and has a smooth surface. The left testicle usually hangs lower than the right.

Epididymis

Sits like a cap on the upper pole of the testes. Located on top and the sides of each testicle in a posterior lay.

Cremasteric reflex

The testicle is elevated toward the body in response to stroking the ipsilateral inner thigh (or the thigh on the same side as the testicle).

Transillumination: Scrotum

Useful for evaluating testicular swelling, mass, or bleeding.
Direct a beam of light behind the scrotum.

Serous fluid inside scrotum = brighter red glow (e.g., hydrocele).
Blood or mass = dull or no glow may indicate a tumor (cancer).

Fast Facts   Disease Review

Testicular Cancer

Most common from of cancer in White males ages 15 to 30 years. (Rare in Black males).

Classic Case
Young adult male complains of nodule, sensation of heaviness or aching, one larger testicle, tenderness in one testicle. May present as a new onset of a hydrocele (from tumor pressing on vessels). Usually painless and asymptomatic until metastasis.

Objective Findings
Affected testicle feels "heavier" and more solid.
May palpate a hard, fixed nodule (most common site is the lower pole of the testis); 20% will have concomitant hydrocele.

Labs
Ultrasound of the testicle may reveal a solid mass.
Gold standard of diagnosis: testicular biopsy.
Refer to urologist. Surgical removal (orchiectomy).

Prostate Cancer

Most common cancer in older males (but lung cancer causes the highest mortality).

Objective Findings
Hard fixed nodule or indurated area on the prostate gland on an older male that is painless.
Indurated area or nodule on digital rectal exam (DRE)
Elevated PSA > 4.0 ng
Diagnostic test: biopsy. Screening test: PSA level with DRE

Plan
- Most cancers not aggressive and slow-growing. Watchful waiting by urologist
- Serial PSA (every 4 to 6 months) and sonograms
- Surgery: high risk of impotence
- Drug therapy with antiandrogens (Proscar), hormone blockers (e.g., Lupron), etc.

Blue Dot Sign (testicular appendage torsion)

Torsion of testicular appendage can present with a "Blue Dot sign." Signs and symptoms may mimic testicular torsion. A testicular appendage is a benign polyp-like soft mass that is attached to the surface of a testicle(s) or the epididymis.

NOT an emergent condition since the testicle itself is not involved. Treated with analgesics.

Classic Case
A male child complains of gradual onset of localized pain in one testicle accompanied by an indurated and tender blue-colored mass (Blue Dot sign) underneath scrotal skin. No voiding or obstructive symptoms.

Objective Findings
A round and tender blue-to-purple-colored mass located underneath the testicular skin (blue dot sign). Does not cause the entire testicle to swell (compared to testicular torsion).

Benign Prostatic Hypertrophy (BPH)

Also known as benign prostatic hyperplasia. Seen in 50% of males older than age 50 (up to 80% of males older than 70 years of age). Rarely seen in males younger than age 40 years.

Classic Case
Older male complains of gradual onset of urinary obstructive symptoms such as dribbling, decreased force of stream, post-void dribbling, urinary retention and frequency. Nocturia very common.

Objective Findings
PSA (prostate specific antigen) is mildly elevated (norm ranges from 0–4 ng/ml). Enlarged prostate that is symmetrical in texture and size (rubbery texture).

Plan
▪ Gold standard test: transurethral prostate biopsy

Medications
Alpha-adrenergic antagonist: terazosin (Hytrin).
Anti-androgen: finasteride (Proscar).
Herbal: Saw Palmetto (does not work for everybody).

Exam Tip

▪ Proscar is a category X drug. Teratogenic. Should not be touched with bare hands if reproductive-age female.

Chronic Prostatitis

Gradual onset of symptoms such as frequency, burning, dribbling, and nocturia. May be asymptomatic. More common in older males. Caused by Gram-negative bacteria such as E. Coli, pseudomonas, klebsiella, proteus mirabili. If STDs, rule out neisseria gonorrhea (Gram-neg.) and chlamydia trachomatis (atypical bacteria).

Classic Case
Older male with history of frequency, burning sensation for weeks to months. Gradual onset. May complain of suprapubic discomfort or perineal discomfort. If prostate enlarged, will complain of nocturia and weaker stream, and dribbling.

Objective Findings
Prostate may feel normal or "boggy" upon palpation. Not tender.

Plan
- Urine and prostatic fluid cultures—uses three tubes: urethra, bladder, and prostate (obtained after prostatic massage). Send for culture and STD testing.

Medications
Ofloxacin (Floxin) or Bactrim DS PO BID × 12 weeks (3 months).

Exam Tips
- Learn to distinguish between chronic prostatitis and acute prostatitis.
- Chronic: gradual onset; prostate can feel normal (older males).
- Acute: sudden onset; prostate is swollen and very tender (younger males).
- Proscar is a Category X drug.
- Blue dot sign is not emergent (compared to torsion) on the exam.

Clinical Tip
- Most boys with torsion of a testicular appendage do not manifest the blue dot sign.

Acute Bacterial Epididymitis

Bacteria ascends up the urethra (urethritis) and reaches epididymis causing an infection. Found in sexually active males < 35 years old; more likely caused by STD (chlamydia, GC). In older males (> 35 years) it is usually caused by Gram-negative bacteria (E. coli).

Classic Case
Adult male complains of systemic symptoms such as fever, chills and anorexia accompanied by unilateral testicular pain. Markedly tender and indurated epididymis. Urethral discharge especially if gonorrheal (green color). Color and amount depend on organism. Also complains of voiding symptoms such as dysuria and frequency.

Positive Prehn's Sign: relief of pain with scrotal elevation

Labs
CBC: leukocytosis with shift to the left
UA: leukocytes (pyuria), blood (hematuria), nitrites

Medications
If high-risk, treat for gonorrhea and/or chlamydia × 21 days. Treat sex partner.
Ofloxacin (Floxin) or ciprofloxacin (Cipro) BID × 21 days.
Bactrim DS BID for × 21 days.
Stool softeners (e.g., docusate sodium or Colace).
Analgesics or NSAIDs for pain and fever (e.g., Tylenol, ibuprofen, naproxen).
Bedrest if severe, or hospitalize for IV antibiotics.
Scrotal elevation and scrotal ice packs.

Acute Prostatitis

Acute infection of the prostate. Infection ascends up urinary tract. May be secondary to untreated urethritis, cystitis, or epididymitis. Usually caused by STDs in sexually active younger males (< 35 years old) and by Gram-negative bacteria (E. coli) in older males.

Classic Case
Adult male complains of acute onset of fever, chills, and malaise accompanied by suprapubic or perineal pain/discomfort, low back pain, dysuria, and frequency. Pain on defecation, especially if constipated.

Objective Findings
Gently examine prostate. Do not vigorously massage, can result in bacteremia. Prostate is extremely tender and warm to touch.

Labs
Urine before and post prostatic massage for C & S.
Urine or Gen-Probe test for gonorrhea and chlamydia.

Medications
Ofloxacin (Floxin), ciprofloxacin (Cipro) or Bactrim DS BID × 21 days.
Treat sex partner.

Erectile Dysfunction (ED)

Inability to produce an erection firm enough to perform sexual intercourse. Caused by vascular insufficiency, neuropathy (diabetics), medications (SSRIs, beta-blockers), smoking, alcohol, hypogonadism. May be psychological causation or mixture of physical and psychological.

Organic Cause

Inability to have an erection under any circumstances. Due to neurovascular or vascular damage.

Psychological Cause

Early morning erections or can achieve a firm erection with masturbation.

Medications

Sildenafil citrate (Viagra) 25/50/100 mg. Take one dose 1/2 to 1 hour before sex. Use only one dose every 24 hours.
Other forms of treatment: intracavernous injections (Caverject).

Contraindications
■ Concomitant nitrates. Recent post-MI, post-CVA, major surgery, or any condition where exertion is contraindicated.

Complications
Priapism: penile erection lasting > 4 hours is emergent condition. Refer to ER.

Other Conditions

Peyronie's disease

Crooked penile erection (may be painful). Palpable hard plaques beneath skin of penile shaft. Surgical correction an option if vaginal penetration problematic.

Balanitis

Candidal infection of the glans penis; more common in uncircumcised men.

Phimosis

Foreskin cannot be pushed back from the glans penis due to edema; usually seen in neonates.

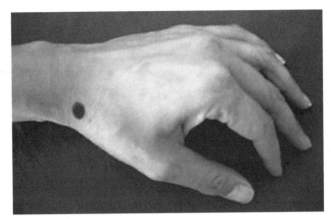

Figure 3.12. Navicular Space

Varicocele

Varicose veins in scrotal sac (feels like "bag of worms"). New onset varicocele can signal testicular tumor (20%).

MUSCULOSKELETAL SYSTEM

Fast Facts | Danger Signals

Navicular Fracture

Acute wrist pain on deep palpation of the anatomical snuffbox that occurs after a history of trauma (e.g., falling forward with hyperextension of the wrist to break the fall).

Hip Fracture

History of slipping or falling. Anterior groin and thigh pain. Pain may radiate to the knee. Affected leg shorter. External rotation of the hip/leg (abduction). More common in elderly people with osteoporosis.

Pelvic Fracture

History of significant or high-energy trauma such as a motor vehicle accident or elderly with history of osteoporosis. Signs and symptoms depend on degree of injury to pelvis and other pelvic structures such as nerves, blood vessels, and pelvic organs. May complain of difficulty in ambulation, pain with hip movement, bladder and/or fecal incontinence, etc. Severe hemorrhage can result in shock. May be life threatening.

Fast Facts   Normal Findings

Joint Anatomy

Synovial fluid: thick serous clear fluid that provides lubrication for the joint (cloudy synovial fluid can be indicative of infection; order C & S).
Synovial space: space between two bones (the joint) filled with synovial fluid.
Articular cartilage: the cartilage lining the open surfaces of bones in a joint.
Ligaments help stabilize joints; muscles attach to joints by their ligaments.
Bursae: present on anterior and posterior areas of a joint; act as padding. Filled with synovial fluid.

Benign Variants

Genu recurvatum: hyperextension or backward curvature of the knees
Genu varum: bowlegs
Genu valgum: knock-knees

Exam Tip

■ To remember valgum, think of gum stuck between the knees (knock-knees). Opposite is valgus or bowlegs.

Fast Facts   Exercise and Injuries

Injuries and Exercise

Inflammation of the joints: injuries, sprains, arthritic exacerbations, inflammatory disorders
Within the first 48 hours, acutely inflamed joints should not be exercised in any form (not even isometric exercises).
No heat of any form is allowed (e.g., hot showers or tub baths, hot packs)
No active range of motion (ROM) exercises.
   ■ if done too early, will cause more inflammation and damage to the affected joints

RICE Mnemonic

Within the first 48 hours after musculoskeletal trauma, follow these rules:
Rest: avoid using injured joint or limb.
Ice: cold packs on injured area (e.g., 20 minutes on; 10 minutes off, etc.) from BID to QID for first 48 hours.
Compression: use an ACE bandage over joints to decrease swelling and provide support. Joints that are usually compressed are the ankles and the knees.
Elevation: prevents or decreases swelling. Avoid weight-bearing on affected joint.

Isometric Exercise

Useful during the early phase of recovery before regular active exercise is performed.

Defined as the controlled and sustained contraction and relaxation of a muscle group.

Less stressful on joints than regular exercise.

Usually done first before active exercise post injury.

Non-weightbearing exercise
- spares weight on joints. Swimming is a good example.

Weightbearing exercise
- walking, jogging
- only weightbearing exercise helps build bone
- recommended for osteoporosis (e.g., walking, biking)

Fast Facts | Orthopedic Maneuvers

Always test both extremities. Use the normal limb as the "baseline" for comparison.

Drawer Sign

A test for knee stability (also can be done on ankles).

McMurray Sign

Positive if damage to the meniscus.

Lachman Sign

A test for knee stability (more specific for the anterior cruciate ligament).

Table 3.17 | Orthopedic Maneuvers

Name	Purpose	Positive Results
Drawer	Knee stability	Affected knee: more laxity (compared to normal knee). Both knees must be tested on all these maneuvers.
Lachman	Knee stability	More specific for ACL tears (anterior cruciate ligament). Affected knee: more laxity.
McMurray	Meniscus tears	Knee locks up. Unable to fully extend affected knee.

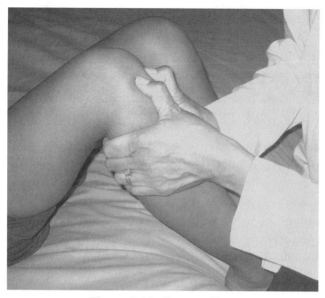

Figure 3.13. Drawer Sign

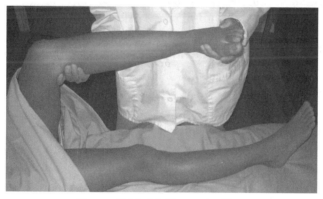

Figure 3.14. McMurray's Sign

MRI (magnetic resonance imaging)

Best for soft tissue injuries such as tendons and cartilage.

X-rays (radiographs)

Best for bone injuries such as fractures.

Orthopedic Terms

Abduction (varus): movement is going away from the body.
Adduction (valgum): movement is going toward the body.

Carpal (carpo): refers to the bones of the hands and the wrist.

Tarsal (tarso): refers to bones of the feet or the ankle.

Fast Facts | Disease Review

Degenerative Joint Disease (DJD or Osteoarthritis)

Arthritis occurs when the cartilage covering the articular surface of joints becomes damaged. Risk factors: older age, overuse of joints, and positive family history.

Goal of treatment
- Pain relief, preserve joint mobility and function
- Strengthen supporting muscles (decreases stress over joints)
- Decrease stress on the affected joint(s)

Classic Case
Early morning joint stiffness with inactivity of shorter duration compared to rheumatoid arthritis (RA) symptoms that can last hours to days.

Absence of systemic symptoms: not a systemic inflammatory illness like RA.

Large weight-bearing joints such as hips and knees commonly affected.

Heberden's Nodes (DIP)

Bony nodules on the distal interphalangeal joints (DIP).

Bouchard's Nodes (PIP)

- Bony nodules on the proximal interphalangeal joints (PIP)

Plan
- Mild analgesics if pain but no inflammation (acetaminophen/Tylenol)
- If inflammation present: shorter-acting NSAIDs preferred (ibuprofen, naproxen)
- If high risk for stomach ulcers, COX-2 inhibitors: celecoxib (Celebrex)
- Exercise only after acute inflammation is gone. For example, knee-strengthening (quadriceps) exercises will reduce stress on knees.

Exam Tips

- Heberden's and/or Bouchard's nodes have appeared many times on the exam. Memorize the location of each. The following may help: Heberden's: the "den" ending on the word is the letter "D" for DIP joint. By the process of elimination, Bouchard's is on the PIP joint.

- Types of treatment methods used for DJD: NSAIDs, analgesics, steroid injection on inflamed joints (NO systemic/oral steroids compared to RA), surgery (e.g., joint replacement).
- Do not confuse DJD treatment with treatment for RA.
- Treatment for RA includes all of DJD treatment methods plus systemic steroids, antimalarials (Plaquenil), and antimetabolites (methotrexate).

Rheumatoid Arthritis (RA)

Systemic autoimmune disorder that is more common in women (8:1). Mainly manifested through multiple joint inflammation and damage. Patients are higher risk for other autoimmune disorders (e.g., Graves' disease, pernicious anemia, etc.).

Classic Case
Adult female complains of gradual onset of symptoms over months with daily fatigue, low-grade fever, generalized body aches, and myalgia. Complains of generalized aching joints that usually involve the fingers/hands and wrist. Morning stiffness lasts longer than DJD's with painful, warm, and swollen joints.

Objective Findings
Joint involvement is symmetrical with more joints involved compared to DJD. Most common joints affected: hands, wrist, elbows, ankles, and shoulders. Morning stiffness last longer compared to DJD. Rheumatoid nodules present (chronic disease).

Labs
Sedimentation rate: elevated
CBC: mild microcytic or normocytic anemia common
Rheumatoid Factor: positive in 75 to 80% of patients
Radiographs: bony erosions, joint space narrowing, subluxations (or dislocation)

Plan
- Refer to rheumatologist for aggressive systemic management.

Medications
NSAIDs (e.g., ibuprofen, naproxen sodium) and analgesics
Steroids: systemic oral doses (e.g., methylprednisone or Medrol Dose Pack)
Plaquenil (an antimalarial), gold salts, etc.
Methotrexate (DMARD or Disease Modifying Agent for Rheumatoid Disease)
Surgery: joint replacement such as the hip, knees

Complications
Uveitis (refer to ophthalmologist stat).
Scleritis, vasculitis, pericarditis, etc.

Exam Tips

■ Uveitis: refer to ophthalmologist for treatment (high dose steroids).
■ Drug class question: Plaquenil is an antimalarial.

Gout

Deposition of uric acid crystals inside joints and tendons from excess production or low excretion of purine crystals (byproduct of protein metabolism). High levels of uric acid crystallize in joints with predisposition for first joint of great toe. More common in middle-aged males > 30 years.

Classic Case

Middle-aged male presents with painful, hot, red, and swollen metatarsophalangeal joint of great toe (podagra). Patient is limping from severe pain on weight bearing on affected toe. History of previous attacks on the same site. Precipitated by alcohol, meats, or seafood. Chronic gout has tophi (small white nodules full of urates on ears and joints).

Labs

Uric acid level: elevated (>7mg/dl). During acute phase, the first goal is to provide pain relief. Only two types of NSAIDs are most effective (narcotics do not work as well).

Acute Phase

■ Indomethacin (Indocin) BID or naproxen sodium (Anaprox DS) BID PRN.
■ If no relief, combine with colchicine 0.5mg, 1 tab every hour until relief or until diarrhea occurs.
■ After acute phase, wait at least 4 to 6 weeks before initiating maintenance treatment.

Maintenance

■ Allopurinol (Zyloprim) daily for years to lifetime. Check CBC (affects bone marrow).
■ Probenecid (a uricosuric) lowers uric acid.

Low Back Pain

Very common disorder with a lifetime incidence of 85%. Usually caused by soft tissue inflammation with muscle spasms, sciatica, herniated disc (usually on L5 – S1) and arthritic changes of the spine. Often seen in elderly with osteoporosis or in patients on chronic long-term steroids.

Further evaluation is recommended for patients having

■ History of significant trauma
■ Suspect cancer metastases

- Osteomyelitis
- Fracture (elderly with osteoporosis, chronic steroid use)
- New onset of back pain in patient >50 years old
- History of spinal stenosis (ankylosing spondylitis)
- Symptoms worsening despite usual treatment
- Herniated disc: common site is at L5 to S1 (buttock/ leg pain)

Labs
MRI: best method for diagnosing a herniated disc.

Plan
- NSAIDs (naproxen sodium); warm packs.
- Muscle relaxants if associated with muscle spasms (causes drowsiness; warn patient).
- Abdominal and core strengthening exercises after acute phase.
- No bedrest except for severe cases only (if possible, limit to 24 hours).

Complications

Cauda Equina Syndrome
Acute pressure on a sacral nerve root results in inflammatory and ischemic changes to the nerve. Sacral nerves innervate pelvic structures such as the sphincters (anal and bladder), and the sensory nerves. Considered a surgical emergency. Needs sacral spine decompression to avoid permanent nerve damage. Refer to ER. Symptoms are bowel or bladder incontinence and saddle anesthesia. The name cauda equina means "horse tail." Sacral nerves when spread out straight appear like a horse's tail.

Exam Tip

- Recognize signs and symptoms so you are able to diagnose cauda equina syndrome on the exam.

Clinical Tip

- The innervation of the bladder and anal sphincter comes from the sacral nerves.

Acute Musculoskeletal Injuries

R.I.C.E (acronym for rest, ice, compression, elevation)
- Cold is best first 48 hours post injury.
- 20 minutes per hour × several times/ day (frequency varies).
- Rest and elevate affected joint to help decrease swelling.
- Compressed joints as needed. Use ACE bandage (most common joints compressed are knees and ankles). Helps with swelling and provides stability.
- NSAIDs (naproxen BID, ibuprofen QID) for pain and swelling PRN.

Tendonitis (all cases)

Microtears on a tendon(s) causes inflammation resulting in pain. Usually caused by repetitive microtrauma, overuse, or strain. Follow RICE mnemonic for acute injuries.

Supraspinatus Tendonitis
Common cause of shoulder pain. Also called cuff tendonitis. Due to inflammation of the supraspinatus tendon.

Classic Case
Complains of shoulder pain with certain movements. The movements that aggravate the pain are arm elevation and abduction (reaching to the back pocket). There is local point tenderness over the tendon located on the anterior area of the shoulder.

Epicondylitis

Common cause of elbow pain. Lateral epicondyle tendon pain (tennis elbow) or medial epicondyle tendon pain (golfer's elbow).

Sprains

Grade III (complete rupture of ligaments)
Refer these patients to an orthopedic specialist:

- Inability to ambulate
- Resists any foot motion
- Marked edema
- Severe pain
- Large amount of bruising

Meniscus Tear (of knees)

The meniscus is the cartilaginous lining between joints. Tears on the cartilage result from trauma and/or overuse.

Classic Case
Complains of locking of the knee(s). Patient may limp. Complains of knee pain and difficulty walking and bending the knee. Unable to fully extend affected knee. Best test: MRI (magnetic resonance imaging). Refer to orthopedic specialist for repair.

Ruptured Baker's Cyst (bursitis)

Bursae are protective synovial sacs over joints that contain synovial fluid. When inflamed, synovial fluid production increases, causing swelling or bursitis.

Classic Case
Physically active patient who jogs complains of ball-like mass that is soft and smooth behind one knee. Pressure pain or asymptomatic. If cyst ruptures, will cause an inflammatory reaction resembling cellulitis on the area such as redness, swelling, and tenderness.

Objective Findings
A Baker's cyst resembles a golf ball in the middle of the popliteal fossa. If it is ruptured, synovial fluid is released into the surrounding tissues, causing an inflammatory reaction. The area becomes inflamed and tender.

Plan
- RICE (rest, ice, compression, and elevation)
- Large bursa drained with syringe #18 needle. Synovial fluid a clear golden color.
- If cloudy synovial fluid, order C & S to rule out infection.

Exam Tips

- X-ray of knee does not show meniscal injury or any joint cartilage.
- Best test for joint injuries is the MRI.
- Remember the signs of a meniscus tear (joint locks up).
- Carpals or carpo... (bones of the hand).
- Tarsals or tarso... (bones of the foot).

MENTAL HEALTH

Fast Facts Danger Signals

High Risk of Suicide

- Elderly White males (especially after death of a spouse).
- Past history of attempted suicide.
- Family history of suicide.
- Plan to use a gun or lethal weapon.
- Females make more attempts (but are not as successful).
- Males have a higher success rate.

Fast Facts | Disease Review

Major Depression

Also known as unipolar depression (vs. bipolar depression). Attributed to dysfunction of the neurotransmitters serotonin and norepinephrine. Genetic component.

Diagnosis

At least 5 or or more of the following must be present for 2 weeks or longer:

- Depressed mood. In children and adolescents, depression can present as irritability.
- Anhedonia: loss of interest in activities that previously gave the patient pleasure.
- Weight: unintentional loss of > 5% of body weight or failure to gain weight in children.
- Fatigue: lack of energy almost daily.
- Feelings of guilt and worthlessness.
- Cognition: difficulty of concentration and poor short-term memory.
- Altered sleep (hypersomnia or insomnia).
- Altered appetite (anorexia or increased appetite).
- Recurrent thoughts or fantasies of suicide.

Evaluation

Immediate goal is to assess for suicidal or homicidal ideation. Check history of previous suicide or homicidal attempts, illicit drugs, bipolar disorder (patient and family). Rule out organic causes such as hypothyroidism, anemia, autoimmune disorders, etc.

Plan

- First line: selective serotonin reuptake inhibitors (SSRIs)
- Second line: tricyclic antidepressants (TCAs)
- Psychotherapy (plus antidepressants works better than either method alone).
- After initiation, follow-up in 2 weeks to check for compliance and side effects.

Alcoholism

Compulsive desire to drink ethyl alcohol (ETOH) despite personal, financial, social consequences.

Levels > 0.8% is illegal. Females metabolize ETOH slower than males.

Labs

GGT (gamma glutamyl transaminase): lone elevation (or with ALT or AST) is a sign of occult alcohol abuse.

AST/ALT Ratio: ratio is 2.0 or higher more likely with ETOH abuse.

Cage Test

Quick screening test for identification of ETOH abuse/ alcoholism.

Positive finding of at least 2 (out of 4) highly suggestive of alcoholism.

C: Do you feel the need to cut down?

A: Are you annoyed when your spouse/friend comments about your drinking?

G: Do you feel guilty about your drinking?

E: Do you need to drink early in the morning? (an eye-opener)

Examples of some quotes using CAGE:

C: "I would like to drink less on the weekends"; "I only drink a lot on weekends."

A: "My wife always nags me about my drinking"; "My best friend thinks I drink too much."

G: "I feel bad that I don't spend enough time with the kids because of my drinking."

E: "I need a drink to feel better when I wake up in the morning."

Delirium Tremens

Delirium, confusion, hallucinations, delusions, tachycardia, hypertension, grand mal seizures. Considered a medical emergency. Refer to ER.

Plan

- Benzodiazepines (Librium, Valium), antipsychotics if needed (e.g., Haldol)
- Vitamins: Thiamine 100 mg IV, folate and multivitamins with high caloric diet
- Refer to Alcoholics Anonymous (12-step program), therapist

Korsakoff's Syndrome

A complication of chronic alcohol abuse. A potentially permanent CNS (central nervous system) disorder that results in dementia. Chronic thiamine deficiency damages the brain permanently. May recover with intensive thiamine supplementation if intervention done in the early stages.

Exam Tips

- Alcoholics Anonymous (AA) is one of the most successful methods for recovering alcoholics. They are a group of people meeting on a regular basis to share issues.
- AA is based on a 12-step program with belief in a "higher power."
- Support group for family is called Al-Anon.
- Support group for teen children is called Ala-teen.
- One glass of wine or one beer per day is not alcohol abuse.
- Cirrhosis increases risk of liver cancer.

Anorexia Nervosa

Onset usually during adolescence. Irrational preoccupation and intense fear of gaining weight. Severe food restriction or binge-eating and purging. Some examples of purging are by using laxatives, vomiting, and excessive daily exercise.

Complications

Marked weight loss (>15% of body weight)

Amenorrhea (no menses × 3 consecutive months or more)

Lanugo (increased lanugo especially in the back and shoulders)

Osteoporosis from prolonged estrogen depletion and low calcium intake. Stress fractures.

Cardiomyopathy. Death usually due to cardiac cause or suicide.

Exam Tips

▨ Recognize how anorexic patients present (lanugo, peripheral edema, amenorrhea, weight loss >15% of body weight)

▨ Increased risk of osteoporosis or osteopenia

▨ Low albumin level

Fast Facts Psychotropic Drugs

Selective serotonin reuptake inhibitors (SSRIs)

First line treatment for

    ▨ major depression, OCD (obsessive-compulsive disorder)

    ▨ GAD (generalized anxiety disorder), panic disorder, social anxiety disorder

    ▨ premenstrual dysphoric disorder (or PMS)

Medications

Fluoxetine (Prozac)—longest half-life of all SSRIs (may last up to 4 weeks).

Sertraline (Zoloft), paroxetine (Paxil; has the shortest half-life).

Side Effects

Sexual dysfunction, loss of appetite, anxiety, insomnia, tremor

Avoid use with anorexic patients and undernourished elderly (depresses appetite more).

Contraindications

▨ Avoid SSRIs within 14 days of a MAOI (serotonin syndrome)

▨ Be careful in prescribing drug to patients with anorexia nervosa (can worsen anorexia).

Tricyclic Antidepressants (TCAs)

Not used as first line treatment for depression. May cause a fatal arrhythmia if patient overdoses (suicide attempt).
Imipramine (Tofranil), amitriptyline (Elavil), and nortriptyline (Norpramine).

Monoamine Oxidase Inhibitors (MAOIs)

Rarely used (for refractory depression not responsive to multiple drugs).
Example: phenelzine (Nardil), tranylcypromine (Parnate)
Contraindications
- Do not combine with SSRI or tricyclic antidepressants
- Wait at least 2 weeks before initiating (high risk of serotonin syndrome)
- Avoid foods with high tyramine: aged cheese, red wine, chocolate, fermented food such as beer, etc.

Acute Serotonin Syndrome

Agitation, confusion, muscle rigidity, very high fever, and myoclonus. Can be fatal. Treatment is supportive.

Smoking Cessation

Bupropion (Wellbutrin is classified as an atypical antidepressant) is used for depression and smoking cessation (Zyban). It can be used with nicotine products such as gums, nasal sprays, etc.

Contraindications
- seizures
- hypertension
- CHF and so forth

Nicotine Patches

Do not use with other nicotine products (e.g., gum, inhaler) because patient will overdose with nicotine (affects the heart from overstimulation).

Benzodiazepines

Tranquilizer action is potentiated by alcohol, psych drugs, hypnotics, etc. For elderly patients, Xanax is a better choice because it has a shorter half-life compared to Valium, which can last up to 12 hours.

Examples
- Alprazolam (Xanax) 0.25 to 6 mg TID (lasts about 4 hours)
- Diazepam (Valium) 2 to 10 mg BID (last about 12 hours)

Illicit Drugs

Cocaine (stimulant)
Nasal perforation if chronic use, tachycardia, euphoria, hyperactivity, hypertension, chest pain (preexisting CAD, can have acute MI, CVA).

Amphetamines (stimulants)
Preferred treatment of ADHD (attention deficit hyperreactivity disorder) and ADD (attention deficit disorder). Signs of overdose are tachycardia, euphoria, hyperactivity, hypertension, chest pain (preexisting CAD, can have acute MI, CVA).

Examples
- Adderall
- Dexedrine

Marijuana (depressant)
Feelings of well-being, very relaxed, lack of anxiety, nausea relief (cancer patients).

Exam Tips

- A list of drugs is given and you are asked to pick out the SSRI (suffix "ine") such as fluoxetine, sertraline, fluvoxamine, etc.
- Diazepam is used for patients in acute alcohol withdrawal and/or delirium tremens.
- Foods that interact with MAOIs are important to remember because they are a safety issue.
- TCAs: herpetic neuralgia, migraine headache prophylaxis (not acute treatment).
- Learn the criteria for the diagnosis of a major depressive episode.
- Lone elevation of GGT indicates occult alcoholism.
- Lanugo is also seen in girls with anorexia nervosa.
- Anorexics are at higher risk for osteoporosis and lower levels of albumin.
- A question on the CAGE concept may ask for the "most likely" or "least likely" person to become an alcoholic.

Clinical Tips

- Patients starting to recover from depression may commit suicide (from increase in psychic energy).
- If patient is potentially suicidal, be careful when refilling or prescribing certain medications that may be fatal if overdosed (e.g., benzodiazepines, hypnotics, narcotics, amphetamines, TCAs, etc.). Give the smallest amount and lowest dose possible.
- SSRI overdose very rarely causes death (vs. TCAs).
- TCAs are good choice for patients who are depressed and have insomnia.

Abuse: All Types

Abusive behaviors are multifactorial. Abuse may include physical, emotional, sexual and/or neglect. It can happen at any age and during pregnancy (higher risk).

A common finding is a delay in seeking medical treatment for the injury. The pattern of the injuries is inconsistent with the history. Elderly who are most likely to be abused are older than 80 years old and/or frail. Children with mental, physical, or other disabilities, and male children are more likely to be abused.

Factors That Increase Likelihood of Child Abuse
- Increased financial strain
- Job loss or job stress
- Low educational attainment
- Stepchild
- Abuser has a history of being abused as a child

Physical Exam
- Another health provider (witness) should be in the same room during the exam.
- Interview victim without abuser in the same room.
- Visual evidence of trauma via Polaroid camera to document all injuries.
- Look for spiral fractures (greenstick fracture), multiple healing fractures especially in rib area, burn marks with pattern, welts, etc.
- Look for signs of neglect (underweight, dirty clothes, dehydration, etc.).
- Sexual abuse/rape cases: chlamydial and GC cultures (must also use cultures in addition to the Gen Probe); HIV, hepatitis B, syphilis, herpes type 2. Genital, throat, and anal area culture and STD testing must be done.

Plan
- Prophylactic treatment against several STDs (with parental consent for minors).
- Health care professionals must report actual or suspected child abuse.

Good Communication Concepts
- State things objectively. Do not be judgmental. Example: "You have bright red stripes on your back," instead of "It looks you have been whipped on the back."
- Open-ended questions are preferred.
- "How can I help you?" instead of "What type of object was used to hurt your back?"
- Do not reassure patients (stops patients from talking more about their problems).
- "We will make sure you get help," instead of "Don't worry, everything will be fine."

- Let the patient ventilate his/her feelings. Do not discourage them from talking.
- "Why don't you tell me why you feel so sad?"
- Validate feelings. "Why do you feel that way?" instead of "I would feel angry too if someone hit me."

Exam Tips

- There will always be a few questions on abuse (especially the ANCC exam). The abuser is described as a controlling person who does not want the "abused" person out of sight.
- The abuser answers all the questions for the patient.
- In abuse cases, interview couple separately.
- Any answer choice that reassures patients is wrong.
- Judgmental responses are always wrong.
- Delaying an action (e.g., waiting until the patient feels better, etc.) is always wrong.
- Use these rules to help rule out the obvious incorrect answer options.

PROFESSIONAL ISSUES

Nursing Practice

Reimbursement

Today, nurse practitioners (NPs) can be reimbursed directly by Medicare, Medicaid, Champus, and some insurance plans. Medicare reimburses NPs 85% of the usual and customary fee that is paid to a physician for the same visit.

Statutory Authority

Another term used for this concept is "legal authority." Elected officials (legislature) vote on a bill (e.g., Nurse Practice Act). Bills that pass become law and have statutory authority.

Nurse Practice Act

Each state has a "Nurse Practice Act." The Nurse Practice Act gives nurses the legal right to practice. It has statutory authority and is legally enforceable.

Nurse Practitioner (NP) Practice

The legal authority for NP practice is granted through the Nurse Practice Act. Each state has its own version of the Nurse Practice Act. The right to practice is not derived from the federal government, the AMA, or the Department of Health.

Board of Nursing (BON)

An official governmental agency of the state whose main job is the enforcement of the Nurse Practice Act of the state. Another prominent role is the granting of licensure to nurses. Inversely, it can also revoke licenses and discipline nurses.

Standards of Practice (American Nurses Association, 1996)

This document lists nursing standards of practice in a generic manner and is meant to be used on a national level. It contains "authoritative statements" that are used to evaluate and measure the nursing "quality of practice, service, or education."

Nurse Practitioner Role

Requirements for Nurse Practitioner Practice

A nurse practitioner must meet the *minimal* educational requirements as required by the state's (of practice) Nurse Practice Act.

Collaborative Agreement

A written document between a physician and nurse practitioner outlining the nurse practitioner's role and responsibility to the clinical practice. It must be signed by both and is usually submitted to the board of nursing. Agreements must be reviewed periodically. Each state board has its own criteria on how the collaborative agreements should be written and when they are to be reviewed.

Title Protection

Professional designations such as registered nurse (RN) or nurse practitioner are protected by law and cannot be used by anyone who does not meet the educational criteria for a nurse. Laws such as this help protect the public from unlicensed "nurses."

Clinical Guidelines

Clinical guidelines are written by expert panels and/or specialty organizations (e.g., the American Heart Association or the American Cancer Society). They are evidence based and act as treatment guidelines. A few examples of diseases with treatment guidelines are hypertension, hyperlipidemia, and pneumonia.

Nurse Practitioner Role

Loretta C. Ford, PhD, RN, and Henry K. Silver, MD, introduced NP role in 1965
First nurse practitioners were pediatric NPs.

A huge shortage of primary care physicians in rural areas was one of the driving forces for the development of this role. The University of Colorado started its first class in 1978 and was the first one to develop and start a nurse practitioner (NP) program in the country.

Budget Reconciliation Act of 1989 (HR 3299)

The first time nurse practitioners are reimbursed directly by Medicare. Only board-certified pediatric and family nurse practitioners were allowed as primary providers as long as they practiced in designated "rural" areas.

Case and Risk Management

Case Management (case managers)

The process of monitoring patients who have certain high-cost or chronic conditions to help third party payers and/or hospitals best manage the health care costs associated with the condition. Case management is very useful for third party payers and hospitals.

Risk Management

A system of monitoring and assessing for high-risk areas and procedures. If high-risk areas are identified, interventions are done to minimize the chances of the event happening in the future. Risk management helps reduce the risk of adverse events to the health facility or an organization and minimizes the risk of lawsuits.

Utilization Review (UR)

The process of evaluating the appropriateness of inpatient hospitalization. Proof of the medical necessity for the patient's hospitalization is done mainly through chart reviews. If the reviewer and payor (e.g., insurance company) do not agree with the decision for the hospitalization, the claim can be denied, resulting in denial of payment to the health facility.

Accreditation

A nongovernmental entity may grant accreditation. It is voluntary. If the health facility meets the accrediting agency's criteria (or standards), then it can earn certification (they usually expire every few years and must be renewed). A well-known accrediting organization is the Joint Commission. Accreditation demonstrates to the public that the health facility has gone beyond the normal requirements and has "excelled" in its class.

Legal Health Issues

The following are legally binding documents. They are signed before witnesses and must be notarized in order to be valid. The patient must be mentally competent.

Power of Attorney for Health

A person (the proxy) designated by a patient to make his future health care decisions in the event that he becomes mentally incompetent.

Power of Attorney

This role of the proxy is broader and encompasses not only health care, but also any decisions that must be made for the patient in order to manage his or her affairs (e.g., finances).

Advanced Directive or Living Will

A written document that lists the patient's preferences for treatment (or nontreatment) in the event that he or she becomes mentally incompetent. The Living Will is a type of advanced directive.

Living Will

Written instructions listing the patient's preferences for treatment or nontreatment. Ideally, nurses and other health providers should discuss the document when the patient is admitted (if mentally competent). Health care providers for the patient and family members ideally should be made aware of the patient's decision.

Informed Consent

Patient must be mentally competent to give informed consent (e.g., not demented, not on pain medications or any drugs affecting cognition, etc.) and should be at least 18 years of age. Emancipated minors are allowed to sign consents without the parent's signature.

The patient is informed of the following and given an opportunity to ask questions:

- Purpose of the procedure/treatment
- Success rate or failure for the suggested treatment or procedure
- Alternative(s) to the suggested procedure/treatment
- Risk versus benefits of the procedure such as adverse events, anesthesia risk, etc.
- Prognosis and success rate

A mentally competent patient has the right to refuse treatment. The patient's decision along with the rationale and the staff's actions regarding the decision must be documented on the patient's chart.

Ethical Concepts (for Nurses)

- Beneficence (the duty to help others)
- Non-malfeasance (the duty to avoid harm to others)
- Confidentiality (the right to keep records private)
- Accountability (the nurse is responsible for her actions)
- Human dignity (respect for the patient)
- Compassion

Public Health Policy

Medicare Part A
Automatic at age 65 years if the patient paid Medicare taxes (deducted from pay-checks or other forms of payment when younger). Pays for:

- Inpatient hospitalizations
- Skilled nursing facilities (not custodial, long-term care, or nursing homes)

Medicare Part B
Patient must sign up and pay a monthly premium to become eligible for Part B. Pays for

- Outpatient care (80%; patient pays 20%).

Medicare Part B: Medically necessary service or supplies (outpatient)
- Outpatient physician visits, labs, X-rays
- Durable medical equipment (wheelchairs, walkers, etc.)
- Skilled nursing visits
- Mammograms/colonoscopy after age 50
- Rehab

Medicare
Does not pay for

- Routine care (routine PE, glasses, dental, etc.)
- Custodial nursing homes (do not confuse with skilled nursing facilities)

Title XIX of the Social Security Act (Medicaid)
A federal and state matching program (means that a state must match what the federal government allocates for its Medicaid programs). Medical assistance to low income persons, the disabled, blind, or members of families with dependent children.

- Pays for health care, nursing home, prescription drugs.
- Providers must agree to accept Medicaid payment in full and not collect from the patient or beneficiaries.

Theoretical Concepts

Health Belief Model (Becker, 1972)
The person who feels susceptible to the disease and believes that he will benefit from changing his behavior is more likely to perform the healthier behavior.

Self-Efficacy Theory (Alfred Bandura, 1970s)

A person who believes that he can succeed in performing an action (or has feelings of self-efficacy) that will result in a positive outcome is more likely to perform the healthier behavior.

Systems Theory

All parts of a system are interrelated and dependent on each other. If one part of the system is damaged or dysfunctional, the rest of the system is also affected.

Family Systems Theory

Derived from the Systems Theory. Families develop at a different rate. If one family member is dysfunctional, the rest of the family is affected negatively. For example, if a member has poor coping or communication skills, the entire family becomes dysfunctional.

Health Care Organizations

HMO (Health Maintenance Organization) and PPO (Preferred Provider Organization)

Physicians and health care providers are paid a monthly fee for each patient enrolled in their panel. This is called the "capitation fee." The fee is paid monthly and does not depend on the number of times the patient is seen.

HMO (Health Maintenance Organization)

Patients are assigned to a primary care provider (PCP). Patients must get authorization for services or specialist visits from the PCP office.

PPO (Preferred Provider Organization)

Patient does not need authorization to visit specialists. Patients are encouraged to utilize "preferred providers." Patients can see physicians who are "out of network" but the cost is higher for the patient.

Practice Questions

SECTION A

1

A 72-year-old woman has been on hydrochlorothiazide 12.5 mg for many years to control her Stage II hypertension. Her blood pressure (BP) at this visit is 168/96. She is currently complaining of pain on her right hip and on both knees. She has increased her dose of ibuprofen (Motrin) from 400 mg three times day (TID) to 800 mg TID. She is still in pain and would like something stronger. Which of the following statements is the best explanation of the effects of ibuprofen (Motrin) on her disease?

a) it increases the chances of adverse effects to her health
b) it inhibits the effect of renal prostaglandins and blunts the effectiveness of the diuretic
c) it prolongs the therapeutic effects of hydrochlorothiazide and other diuretics
d) none of the statements are true

2

All of the following are infections that affect mostly the labia and vagina except?

a) bacterial vaginosis
b) candidiasis
c) trichomoniasis
d) *Chlamydia trachomatis*

3

The nurse practitioner would test the obturator and iliopsoas muscle to evaluate for?

a) cholecystitis
b) acute appendicitis
c) inguinal hernia
d) gastric ulcer

4

Treatment for mild preeclampsia includes all of the following except?

a) bedrest except for bathroom privileges
b) close monitoring of weight and blood pressure
c) close follow-up of urinary protein, serum creatinine, and platelet count
d) a prescription of methyldopa (Aldomet) to control blood pressure

5

All of the following services are covered under Medicare Part A except?

a) inpatient hospitalizations
b) medicines administered to a patient while hospitalized
c) nursing home care
d) surgeons

6

A 28-year-old student is seen in the school health clinic with complaints of a hacking cough that is productive of small amounts of sputum and a runny nose. He does not take any medications, denies any allergies, and has no significant medical history. Physical examination reveals a low-grade temperature of 99.9 degrees Fahrenheit, respirations of 16/min, a pulse of 90 beats per minute, and diffused fine crackles in the base of the lungs. A chest radiograph (X-ray) shows diffuse infiltrates on the lower lobe of the right lung. The total white blood cell count is 10,500 /uL. What is the most likely diagnosis?

a) streptococcal pneumonia
b) mycoplasma pneumonia
c) acute bronchitis
d) Legionnaire's disease

7

A 39-year-old migrant worker presents to the clinic 2.5 days after a purified protein derivative (PPD) test. What minimum size of induration would be considered positive for this patient?

a) 3 mm
b) 5 mm
c) 10 mm
d) 15 mm

8

All of the following are correct statements regarding a durable power of attorney's role except?

a) their decisions are legally binding
b) it can be used in other areas of the patient's life such as financial issues
c) they can decide for the patient who is on life-support when it can be terminated
d) the patient's spouse has a right to override the durable power of attorney's decisions

9

All of the following are true statements regarding Munchausen syndrome except:

a) it is considered a mental illness
b) the patient has a medical illness that causes an anxiety reaction and denial
c) the patient fakes an illness in order to gain attention from health care providers
d) the patient has an inconsistent medical history along with a past history of frequent hospitalizations

10

Which of the following antihypertensive medications should the nurse practitioner avoid when treating patients with emphysema?

a) calcium channel blockers
b) angiotensin-converting enzyme (ACE) inhibitors
c) beta blockers
d) diuretics

11

A 30-year-old chef complains of pruritic hives over her chest and arms but denies difficulty swallowing or breathing. She reports a family history of allergic rhinitis and asthma. Which of the following interventions is most appropriate?

a) perform a complete and thorough history
b) prescribe an oral antihistamine such as dipenhydramine 25 mg. PO QID
c) give an injection of epinephrine 1:1000 intramuscularly stat
d) call 911

12

Which of the following findings is most likely in young primigravidas with pregnancy-induced hypertension?

a) abdominal cramping and constipation
b) edema of the face and the upper extremities
c) shortness of breath
d) dysuria and frequency

13

Which of the following symptoms is associated with B12 deficiency anemia?

a) spoon-shaped nails and pica
b) an abnormal neurological exam
c) a vegan diet
d) tingling and numbness of both feet

14

A second triple screen on a 35-year-old primigravida reveals abnormally low levels of the alpha fetoprotein and estriol and high levels of human chorionic gonadotropin. Which of the following interventions is the best choice for this patient?

a) order an ultrasound
b) order a computed tomography (CT) scan of the abdomen
c) order a 24-hour urine for protein clearance
d) assess for a history of illicit drug or alcohol use

15

All of the following are true statements about diverticula except?

a) diverticula are located in the colon
b) a low-fiber diet is associated with the condition
c) most diverticula in the colon are infected with Gram-negative bacteria
d) supplementing with fiber such as psyllium (Metamucil) is recommended

16

Patients who are diagnosed with gonorrhea should also be treated for which of the following infections?

a) chancroid
b) *Chlamydia trachomatis*
c) herpes genitalis
d) PID (pelvic inflammatory disease)

17

Kyphosis is a late sign of?

a) old age
b) osteopenia
c) osteoporosis
d) osteoarthritis

18

A 35-year-old primigravida who is at 28 weeks of gestation is expecting twins. You would expect her alpha fetoprotein (AFP) values to be?

a) normal
b) higher than normal
c) lower than normal
d) none of the above

19

Which of the following antihypertensive medications has beneficial effects to an elderly White female with osteoporosis?

a) calcium channel blockers
b) angiotensin-converting enzyme (ACE) inhibitors
c) beta blockers
d) diuretic

20

The Lachman maneuver is used to detect which of the following?

a) knee instability
b) nerve damage of the knee due to past knee injuries
c) the integrity of the patellar tendon
d) tears on the meniscus of the knee

21

When an adolescent male's penis grows more in length than width, which of the following Tanner stages is he classified at?

a) Tanner Stage II
b) Tanner Stage III
c) Tanner Stage IV
d) Tanner Stage V

22

Fetal TORCH infections can cause microcephaly, mental retardation, hepato-splenomegaly, and intrauterine growth retardation. The acronym TORCH stands for?

a) *Toxoplasma gondii*, other infections, rubella, cytomegalovirus, and herpes
b) toxic shock syndrome, ocular infections, rubella, cytomegalovirus, and herpes zoster
c) tetanus, ophthalmic infections, roseola, cancer, and head abnormalities
d) toxins, other infections, roseola, candidiasis, and head abnormalities

23

Human papilloma virus (HPV) infection of the larynx has been associated with?

a) laryngeal neoplasia
b) esophageal stricture
c) cervical cancer
d) metaplasia of esophageal squamous cells

24

Mr. Brown is a 65-year-old carpenter complaining of morning stiffness and pain in both his hands and right knee upon awakening. He feels some relief after warming up. On exam, the nurse notices the presence of Heberden's nodes. Which of the following is most likely?

a) osteoporosis
b) rheumatoid arthritis
c) degenerative joint disease
d) Reiter's syndrome

25

What does a positive posterior drawer sign in a 10-year-old soccer player signify?

a) an abnormal knee
b) instability of the knee
c) a large amount of swelling on the knee
d) an injury of the meniscus

26

A multigravida who is at 28 weeks of gestation has a fundal height of 30 cm. Which of the following is the best recommendation for this patient?

a) advise the mother that her pregnancy is progressing well
b) order an ultrasound of the uterus
c) refer her to an obstetrician for an amniocentesis
d) recommend bedrest with bathroom privileges

27

A multigravida who is at 34 weeks of gestation wants to know at what level her uterine fundus should be. The best answer is to advise the mother that her fundus is?

a) midway between the umbilicus and the lower ribs
b) at the level of the umbilicus
c) from 33 to 35 cm
d) from 32 to 34 cm

28

Which of the following laboratory tests is used in primary care to evaluate renal function?

a) electrolyte panel
b) creatinine
c) alkaline phosphatase
d) blood urea nitrogen (BUN) to creatinine ratio

29

All of the following are false statements regarding acute gastritis except?

a) chronic intake of nonsteroidal anti-inflammatory drugs (NSAIDs) can cause the disorder
b) chronic lack of dietary fiber is the main cause of the disorder
c) the screening test for the disorder is the barium swallow test
d) the gold standard to evaluate the disorder is a colonoscopy

30

Signs and symptoms of depression include all of the following except?

a) anhedonia and changes in appetite
b) decreased energy and irritability
c) apathy and low self-esteem
d) apraxia and fatigue

31

Which of the following is an accurate description of eliciting for Murphy's sign?

a) upon deep inspiration by the patient, palpate firmly in the right upper quadrant of the abdomen below the costovertebral angle
b) bend patient's hips and knees at 90 degrees, then passively rotate hip externally, then internally
c) ask the patient to squat, then place the stethoscope on apical area
d) press into the abdomen deeply, then release it suddenly

32

A 28-year-old multipara who is at 32 weeks of gestation presents to your office complaining of a sudden onset of small amounts of bright red vaginal bleeding. She has had several episodes and appears anxious. On exam, her uterus is soft to palpation. Which of the following is most likely?

a) placenta abruptio
b) placenta previa
c) acute cervicitis
d) molar pregnancy (hydatidiform mole)

33

Epidemiologic studies show that Hashimoto's disease occurs most commonly in?

a) middle-aged to older women
b) smokers
c) obese individuals
d) older men

34

A 48-year-old woman is told by a physician that she is starting menopause. All of the following are possible findings except?

a) hot flashes
b) irregular menstrual periods
c) severe vaginal atrophic changes
d) cyclic mood swings

35

A 63-year-old patient with a 10-year history of poorly controlled hypertension presents with a cluster of physical exam findings. Which of the following indicate target organ damage commonly seen in hypertensive patients?

a) pedal edema, hepatomegaly, and enlarged kidneys
b) hepatomegaly, AV nicking, bibasilar crackles
c) renal infection, S3, neuromuscular abnormalities
d) glaucoma, jugular vein atrophy, heart failure

36

A 30-year-old primigravida is diagnosed with a possible threatened abortion. The result of the urine pregnancy test is positive. Which of the following statements is true regarding a threatened abortion?

a) vaginal bleeding and cramping are present, but the cervix remains closed
b) vaginal bleeding and cramping are present along with a dilated cervix
c) the fetus and placenta are all expelled
d) the products of conception and the placenta remain inside the uterus along with a dilated cervix

37

A 30-year-old female who is sexually active complains of a large amount of milk-like vaginal discharge for several weeks. A microscopy slide reveals a large amount of squamous epithelial cells that have blurred margins. There are very few white blood cells seen. The vaginal pH is at 6.0. What is most likely?

a) trichomonas infection
b) bacterial vaginosis
c) candidal infection
d) a normal finding

38

The pap smear result on a 20-year-old sexually active student who uses condoms inconsistently shows a large amount of inflammation. Which of the following is the best follow-up action?

a) call the patient to return to the clinic so she can get tested for a possible cervical infection

a) treat the patient with metronidazole vaginal cream over the phone
b) call the patient and tell her she needs a repeat pap smear in 6 months
c) advise her to use a Betadine douche at bed time × 3 days

39

While performing a pap smear on a postmenopausal patient, several areas of flat white skin lesions that are irregularly shaped are found on the patient's labia. The patient reports that the lesions are extremely itchy and have been present for several years without much change. Which condition is best described?

a) chronic scabies infection
b) lichen sclerosus
c) chronic candidal vaginitis
d) a physiologic variant found in some older women

40

The heart sound S2 is caused by?

a) closure of the atrioventricular valves
b) closure of the semilunar valves
c) opening of the atrioventricular valves
d) opening of the semilunar valves

41

A pelvic exam on a woman who is 12 weeks pregnant would reveal that her uterus is located at which of the following areas?

a) between the umbilicus and the suprapubic bone
b) just rising above the suprapubic bone
c) between the suprapubic bone and the xiphoid process
d) between the umbilicus and the xiphoid process

42

All of the following are covered under Medicare Part B except?

a) persons age 65 years or older
b) durable medical equipment
c) mammograms annually starting at age 50
d) anesthesiologist's services

43

All of the following patients are at higher risk for suicide except?

a) a 66-year-old White male whose wife of 40 years recently died
b) a high school student with a history of bipolar disorder
c) a depressed 45-year-old female with family history of suicide
d) a 17-year-old teen who has only one close friend in school

44

A 70-year-old male patient complains of a bright red spot in his left eye for 2 days. He denies eye pain, visual changes, or headaches. He has a new onset of cough from a recent viral upper respiratory infection. The only medicine he is on is Bayer aspirin one tablet a day. Which of the following is most likely?

a) corneal abrasion
b) acute bacterial conjunctivitis
c) acute uveitis
d) subconjunctival hemorrhage

45

Which of the following is appropriate follow-up for this 70-year-old patient?

a) referral to an optometrist
b) referral to an ophthalmologist
c) advise the patient that it is a benign condition and will resolve spontaneously
d) prescribe an ophthalmic antibiotic solution

46

Jason, an 8-year-old with type 1 diabetes, is being seen for a 3-day history of frequency and nocturia. He denies flank pain and is afebrile. The urinalysis result is negative for blood and nitrites but is positive for a large amount of leukocytes and ketones. He has a trace amount of protein. Which of the following is the best test to order initially?

a) urine for culture and sensitivity
b) 24-hour urine for protein and creatinine clearance
c) 24-hour urine for microalbumin
d) an intravenous pyelogram

47

All of the following are not recommended for the outpatient treatment of mild preeclampsia except?

a) severe sodium restriction
b) restrict fluid intake to less than 1 liter per 24 hours
c) Aldomet (methyldopa) 250 mg PO (orally) BID
d) bedrest on the left side with bathroom privileges

48

The best test for diagnosing congenital glaucoma is which of the following?

a) fluorescein staining
b) tonometry
c) Snellen vision exam
d) the refractive index

49

Rocky Mountain spotted fever is caused by the bite of the?

a) mosquito
b) tick
c) insect
d) flea

50

All of the following are false statements about atopic dermatitis except?

a) contact with cold objects may exacerbate the condition
b) it does not have a linear distribution
c) it is associated with bullae
d) the lesions have vesicles that are full of serous exudate

SECTION B

51

A mother brings in her 4-year-old daughter who just started attending preschool. She tells the nurse practitioner that her child is complaining of burning and itching in both eyes along with a runny nose. During the physical exam, the child's eyes appear injected bilaterally. The throat is red and her inferior nasal turbinates are swollen. Which of the following is most likely?

a) herpes keratitis
b) corneal ulcer
c) viral conjunctivitis
d) bacterial conjunctivitis

52

A sexually active woman is complaining of amenorrhea and vaginal spotting. On exam, her left adnexa is tender and cervical motion tenderness is positive. Which test should the nurse practitioner initially order?

a) flat plate of the abdomen
b) complete blood count (CBC) with white cell differentials
c) urine pregnancy test
d) pelvic ultrasound

53

A toddler with congenital heart disease is seen for a 1 week history of facial and lower extremity edema accompanied by shortness of breath. The child's mother reports that the child's appetite has been poor. The chest X-ray reveals that the child has congestive heart failure (CHF). Which of the following heart sounds are found in these patients?

a) S1 and S2
b) S1, S2, and S3
c) S1, S2, and S4
d) Still's murmur and S4

54

A 53-year-old crossing guard complains of twisting his right knee while working that morning. The knee is swollen and tender to palpation. The nurse practitioner diagnoses a Grade II sprain. The initial treatment plan includes which of the following?

a) application of cold packs the first 24 hours followed by applications of low heat at bedtime
b) elevation of the affected limb and intermittent applications of cold packs for the next 48 hours
c) rechecking the knee in 24 hours and isometric exercises
d) the application of an ACE bandage to the affected knee

55

Erythromycin 200 mg with sulfisoxazole 600 mg suspension (Pediazole) is contraindicated in which of the following conditions?

a) G6PD deficiency anemia
b) lead poisoning
c) beta thalassemia minor
d) B12 deficiency anemia

56

The mother of an 11-year-old boy with sickle cell anemia calls on the phone complaining that her son woke up because of a painful penile erection that will not go away. The nurse practitioner's most appropriate intervention is?

a) insert a Foley catheter and measure the child's intake and output for the next 24 hours
b) insert a Foley catheter to obtain a specimen for a urinalysis and urine for C & S (culture and sensitivity)
c) recommend an increase in the child's fluid intake
d) recommend immediate referral to the ER

57

A positive Coombs test on an Rh-negative pregnant woman means?

a) the mother has autoantibodies against Rh-positive red blood cells (RBCs)
b) the fetus has autoantibodies against maternal RBCs
c) the mother does not have Rh factor against fetal RBCs
d) the fetus does not have RBC autoantibodies

58

Folic acid supplementation is recommended for women who are planning pregnancy in order to?

a) prevent renal agenesis
b) prevent anencephaly
c) prevent kidney defects
d) prevent heart defects

59

All of the following are possible causes for secondary hypertension except?

a) acute pyelonephritis
b) pheochromocytoma
c) renovascular stenosis
d) coarctation of the aorta

60

Fitz-Hugh-Curtis syndrome is associated with the following infection?

a) syphilis
b) *Chlamydia trachomatis*
c) herpes genitalis
d) lymphogranuloma venereum

61

A nursing home resident reports to his physician that his previous roommate was recently started on tuberculosis treatment. A Mantoux test and chest X-ray are ordered for the patient. What is the minimum size of induration considered positive for this patient?

a) 3 mm
b) 5 mm
c) 10 mm
d) 15 mm

62

In small children with acquired immunodeficiency syndrome (AIDS), which of the following vaccines is contraindicated?

a) diphtheria and tetanus (Td)
b) hepatitis B and mumps
c) varicella
d) Td and oral polio

63

A 44-year-old female who is undergoing treatment for infertility complains of not having a menstrual period for a few months. The night before, she started spotting and is now having cramp-type pains in her pelvic area. Her blood pressure (BP) is 160/80, the pulse rate is 110, and she is afebrile. Her labs reveal a mild anemia with mild leukocytosis. On pelvic exam, the uterine fundus is found above the symphysis pubis. The cervical os is dilated at 3 cm. Which of the following is most likely?

a) inevitable abortion
b) threatened abortion
c) incomplete abortion
d) acute pelvic inflammatory disease

64

A 14-year-old female who is sexually active is brought in by her mother for an immunization update. According to the mother, her daughter had one dose of Hepatitis B vaccine. Which of the following vaccines would you administer at this visit?

a) Td and Hepatitis B
b) DTaP (diphtheria, tetanus, acellular pertussis) and Hepatitis B
c) Hepatitis B only
d) MMR (measles, mumps, rubella) and Td

65

An Rh-negative pregnant woman with negative rubella titers should be vaccinated at what time period in pregnancy?

a) she can be vaccinated at any time in her pregnancy
b) during the second trimester
c) during the third trimester
d) during the postpartum period

66

Medicare Part B will pay for all of the following services except?

a) outpatient physician visits that are medically necessary
b) durable medical equipment
c) outpatient laboratory and radiology tests
d) eyeglasses and routine dental care

67

Which of the following is used to screen for color blindness in a 7-year-old boy?

a) Snellen chart
b) Ishihara chart
c) Cover/uncover test
d) Red reflex

68

A 67-year-old retired clerk presents with complaints of shortness of breath and weight gain over a 2-week period. A nonproductive cough accompanies her symptoms. The lung exam is positive for fine crackles in the lower lobes with no wheezing. The exam is positive for egophony. Which of the following conditions is most likely?

a) acute exacerbation of asthma
b) left-heart failure
c) right-heart failure
d) chronic obstructive pulmonary disease

69

Which of the following drugs is most likely to relieve the patient's symptoms?

a) atenolol (Tenormin)
b) trimethoprim/sulfamethoxazole (Bactrim DS)
c) furosemide (Lasix)
d) hydrocodone/ guaifenesin syrup (Hycotuss)

70

A patient has recently been diagnosed with migraine headache with aura. She wants advice on what she should eliminate from her diet to reduce her risk of headaches. The best response is to advise this patient to avoid?

a) foods with aspartame (Equal) because they can trigger migraines
b) foods with monosodium glutamate because they promote diuresis
c) foods with garlic because they promote hypertension
d) foods with nitrates because they do not induce flushing

71

A patient with a history of mitral valve prolapse (MVP) is requesting prophylaxis before her dental surgery. Which of the following would you prescribe this patient?

a) amoxicillin a half hour before and 2 hours after the procedure
b) amoxicillin 1 hour before the procedure
c) amoxicillin 1 hour before and 3 hours after the procedure
d) prophylaxis is not recommended for this patient

72

Koplik's spots are associated with?

a) poxvirus infections
b) measles
c) Kawasaki's disease
d) Reye's syndrome

73

Stella, a new mother, complains to you that she has been feeling irritable and jittery almost daily for the past few months. She complains of frequent palpitations and more frequent bowel movements along with weight loss. Her BP is 160/70, her pulse is 110, and she is afebrile. All of the following conditions should be considered in the differential diagnosis for this patient except?

a) mitral regurgitation
b) Graves disease
c) generalized anxiety disorder
d) illicit drug use

74

An elderly patient with a productive cough and fever is diagnosed with pneumonia. All of the following organisms are capable of causing community-acquired pneumonia except?

a) haemophilus influenzae
b) mycoplasma pneumoniae
c) treponema pallidum
d) streptococcus pneumoniae

75

Human chorionic gonadotropin (hCG) is produced by the?

a) placenta
b) hypothalamus
c) anterior pituitary
d) ovaries

76

The majority of serum alpha fetoprotein is produced by the?

a) fetal liver
b) mother's liver
c) placenta
d) fetal neural tube

77

Stella works in the housekeeping department of a hospital. She presents to the employee health clinic with a complaint of a needlestick to her left thumb. The needle was in one of the garbage bags from the emergency room. The patient had a little bleeding which stopped spontaneously. Which of the following is the next step?

a) order an enzyme-linked immunosorbent assay (ELISA) test as soon as possible
b) recommend a tetanus booster in 1 week
c) offer the patient Hepatitis B immunoglobulin
d) order a chest X-ray

78

An elderly woman has been on digoxin (Lanoxin) for 10 years. Her electrocardiograph (EKG) is showing a new onset of atrial fibrillation. Her pulse is 64/min. She denies syncope and dizziness. Which of the following interventions is most appropriate?

a) order an electrolyte panel and a digoxin level
b) order a serum thyroid-stimulating hormone (TSH), digoxin level, and an electrolyte panel
c) order a serum digoxin level and decrease her digoxin dose in half while you wait for results
d) discontinue the digoxin and order another 12-lead EKG

79

You note the following result on a routine urinalysis of a 37-year-old primigravida who is at 30 weeks of gestation. Leukocyte = trace, nitrite = negative, protein = 2 +, blood = negative. Her weight has increased by 5 lbs. during the past week. Which of the following is most likely?

a) HELLP syndrome
b) pregnancy-induced hypertension (preeclampsia)
c) eclampsia of pregnancy
d) primary hypertension

80

The nurse practitioner who suspects that one of her hypertensive patients has Cushing's syndrome would expect to find which of the following laboratory results?

a) hyponatremia
b) hypoglycemia
c) elevated serum cortisol levels
d) decreased urine 17-ketosteroids

81

The first teeth to erupt during infancy are which of the following?

a) first molars
b) second molars
c) incisors
d) canines

82

The positive signs of pregnancy include?

a) palpation of the fetus and auscultation of the fetal heart tones by the nurse practitioner
b) palpation of the fetus and a positive quantitative serum pregnancy test

c) fetal heart tones and a positive quantitative serum pregnancy test
d) fetal heart tones and feeling of movement of the baby by the mother

83

Chadwick's sign is characterized by?

a) softening of the cervix
b) blue coloration of the cervix and vagina
c) softening of the uterine isthmus
d) nausea and vomiting during the first trimester of pregnancy

84

A college student has recently been informed that he has an HPV (human papil-loma virus) infection on the shaft of his penis. Which of the following may reveal subclinical lesions on the penile skin?

a) perform a KOH (potassium hydroxide) exam
b) scrape off some of the affected skin and send it for a culture and sensitivity
c) apply acetic acid to the penile shaft and look for acetowhite changes
d) order a serum herpes virus titer

85

Carol M. is a 40-year-old bank teller who has recently been diagnosed with obsessive-compulsive disorder by her therapist. Her symptoms would include?

a) ritualistic behaviors that the patient feels compelled to repeat
b) attempts to ignore or suppress the repetitive behaviors, which increase anxiety
c) frequent intrusive and repetitive thoughts and impulses
d) all of the above

86

Which of the following medications is indicated for the treatment of obsessive-compulsive disorder?

a) paroxetine (Paxil CR)
b) haldoperidol (Haldol)
c) lorazepam (Xanax)
d) imipramine (Elavil)

87

You would advise an 18-year-old female student who has been given a booster dose of MMR at the college health clinic that?

a) she might have a low grade fever during the first 24 to 48 hours
b) she should not get pregnant within the next 3 months
c) her arm will be very sore on the injection site in 24 to 48 hours
d) her arm will have some induration on the injection site in 24 to 48 hours

88

Jean, a 68-year-old female, is suspected of having Alzheimer's disease. Which of the following is the best initial method for assessing the condition?

a) computed tomography scan of the brain
b) Mini Mental Exam
c) obtain a history from the patient and family members
d) EEG (electroencephalography)

89

A 55-year-old woman who has type 2 diabetes is concerned about her kidneys. She has a history of three urinary tract infections within the past 8 months. She denies dysuria and frequency at this visit. Which of the following is the best initial course to follow?

a) recheck the patient's urine and order a urine for culture and sensitivity
b) order an IVP (intravenous pyelogram)
c) advise the patient to follow up with a urologist
d) evaluate the patient for a possible kidney infection

90

A nurse practitioner is giving dietary counseling to a male alcoholic who has recently been diagnosed with folic acid deficiency anemia. Which of the following foods should the nurse practitioner recommend to this patient?

a) tomatoes, oranges, and bananas
b) cheese, yogurt, and milk
c) lettuce, beef, and dairy products
d) spinach, liver, and whole wheat bread

91

The ELISA and Western Blot test are both used to test for HIV. Which of the following statements is correct?

a) it is a test to detect viral RNA
b) it is a test to detect antibodies against the HIV
c) it is a test to detect viruses
d) it is a diagnostic test for the AIDS virus

92

Hegar's sign is considered a?

a) positive sign of pregnancy
b) probable sign of pregnancy
c) presumptive sign of pregnancy
d) problem in pregnancy

93

When the nurse practitioner is palpating a woman who is at 20 weeks of gestation, she should be able to feel the uterine fundus at what level?

a) just rising above the level of the pubic symphysis
b) between the pubic symphysis and the umbilicus
c) at the level of the umbilicus
d) above the level of the umbilicus

94

A 67-year-old female with a 50 pack/year history of smoking presents for a routine annual physical examination. She complains of being easily short of breath and is frequently fatigued. Physical examination reveals diminished breath sounds, hyperresonance, and hypertrophied respiratory accessory muscles. Her CBC results reveal that her hematocrit level is slightly elevated. Her pulmonary function test (PFT) results show increased total lung capacity. What is the most likely diagnosis for this patient?

a) bronchogenic carcinoma
b) COPD (chronic obstructive pulmonary disease)
c) chronic bronchitis
d) congestive heart failure

95

Your patient of 10 years, Mrs. Leman, is concerned about her most recent diagnosis. She was told by her dermatologist that she has an advanced case of actinic keratosis. Which of the following is the best explanation for this patient?

a) it is a benign condition
b) it is a precancerous lesion and needs to be followed up with her dermatologist
c) apply hydrocortisone cream 1% BID for 2 weeks and most of it will go away
d) it is important for her to follow up with an oncologist

96

Patient confidentiality is breached when?

a) medical information is given to a spouse
b) records are subpoenaed
c) reports are sent to the Public Health Department
d) records are released to insurance companies

97

A 25-year-old woman's last menstrual period was 6 weeks ago. She is complaining of nausea with vomiting in the morning and fatigue. Her breasts feel bloated. The nurse practitioner suspects that she is pregnant. Her symptoms would be considered?

a) positive signs of pregnancy
b) probable signs of pregnancy
c) presumptive signs of pregnancy
d) possible signs of pregnancy

98

A 55-year-old male patient describes to you an episode of chest tightness in his substernal area that radiated to his back while he was jogging. It was relieved immediately when he stopped. Which of the following conditions does this best describe?

a) angina pectoris
b) acute myocardial infarction
c) gastroesophageal reflux disease
d) acute costochondritis

99

Which of the following would you recommend to this 55-year-old patient?

a) start an exercise program by starting with walking instead of jogging
b) consult with a cardiologist for further evaluation
c) consult with a gastroenterologist to rule out acute cholecystitis
d) take ibuprofen (Advil) 600 mg for pain every 4 to 6 hours PRN

100

Carol, a 73-year-old patient, complains of episodic vertigo, slight confusion, and weakness that last nearly an hour each time. Movement does not worsen the vertigo. She "rests" and her symptoms subside, but she is puzzled because the weakness "jumps from side to side" sometimes on the right and sometimes on the left of her body. Her symptoms suggest?

a) benign paroxysmal positional vertigo
b) Ménière's disease
c) TIA (transient ischemic attack)
d) CVA (cerebrovascular accident)

SECTION C

101

All of the following measures have been found to help lower the risk of osteoporosis except?

a) drinking organic juice
b) eating low-fat dairy foods
c) performing weight-bearing exercises
d) vitamin D supplementation

102

A 28-year-old male nurse of Hispanic descent reports a history of a cold that resolved 2 weeks ago except for a dry cough and pain over his right cheek which worsens when he bends down. The patient denies fever. He tells the employee health nurse practitioner that he is very allergic to both cephalexin (Keflex) and erythromycin. The vital signs show that the patient's temperature is 99.2 degrees Fahrenheit, a pulse of 72 beats per minute and a respiratory rate of 12 breaths per minute. Which of the following conditions is most likely?

a) acute sinusitis
b) acute bronchitis
c) fever secondary to the previous viral URI (upper respiratory infection)
d) Munchausen's syndrome

103

A 38-year-old multigravida who is at 32 weeks of gestation calls the family nurse practitioner complaining of bright red vaginal bleeding. There is no watery discharge. She complains that her uterus feels hard and is very painful. Which of the following conditions is most likely?

a) placenta previa
b) placenta abruptio
c) a molar pregnancy
d) an ectopic pregnancy

104

The Jarisch-Herxheimer reaction is best described as?

a) an immune-mediated reaction precipitated by the destruction of a large number of spirochetes due to an antibiotic injection
b) severe chills and elevated blood pressure
c) caused by infection with either the *Chlamydia trachomatis* or gonorrheal infection of the liver capsule
d) associated with certain viral illnesses

105

During a breast exam of a 30-year-old nulliparous female, the nurse practitioner palpates several rubbery mobile areas of breast tissue. They are slightly tender to palpation. Both breasts have symmetrical findings. There are no skin changes or any nipple discharge. The patient is expecting her menstrual period in 5 days. Which of the following would you recommend?

a) referral to a gynecologist for further evaluation
b) tell her to return 1 week after her period so her breasts can be rechecked
c) advise the patient to return in 6 months so that you can recheck her breasts
d) schedule the patient for a mammogram

106

When evaluating the blood pressure on both the arms and legs of an infant who has a diagnosis of coarctation of the aorta, which of the following is the correct finding?

a) the blood pressure is higher in the arms than in the legs
b) only the diastolic blood pressure is higher in the legs than in the arms
c) the blood pressure is higher in the legs than the arms
d) the blood pressure is lower in both arms than in the legs

107

Which of the following should you expect to find on a wet mount slide of a patient diagnosed with bacterial vaginosis?

a) Tzanck cells
b) a large amount of leukocytes and epithelial cells
c) a large amount of bacteria coating the squamous cells and very few leukocytes
d) epithelial cells and a small amount of blood

108

A 40-year-old woman is in the office complaining of palpitations and some light-headedness for the past 6 months. These are random episodes. The nurse practitioner notices a midsystolic click with a late systolic murmur that is best heard in the apical area during auscultation of the chest. You would suspect?

a) atrial fibrillation
b) sinus arrhythmia
c) mitral stenosis
d) mitral valve prolapse

109

Your 35-year-old patient is being worked up for microscopic hematuria. All of the following are differential diagnoses of microscopic hematuria except?

a) kidney stones
b) bladder cancer
c) acute pyelonephritis
d) renal stenosis

110

During a routine physical exam of an elderly woman, a triangular thickening of the bulbar conjunctiva on the temporal side is noted to be encroaching on the cornea. She denies any eye pain or visual changes. Which of the following is most likely?

a) corneal arcus
b) pterygium

c) pinguecula
d) chalazion

111

Mr. Jones, who has been on pravastatin (Pravachol) 20 mg at bedtime for the past few months, complains of lately feeling extremely fatigued. The patient also noticed that his urine is a darker color during the past 2 weeks. Which of the following is the best treatment plan to follow?

a) discontinue his Pravastatin and order a liver function profile
b) continue the Pravastatin but on half the dose
c) schedule him for a complete physical exam
d) schedule him for a liver function profile

112

Jane, a young primigravida, reports to you that she is starting to feel the baby's movements in her uterus. This is considered to be which of the following?

a) presumptive sign
b) probable sign
c) positive sign
d) possible sign

113

A 14-year-old teen is worried that she has not started to menstruate like most of her friends. During the gynecological examination, the nurse practitioner tells the mother, who is in the room with the patient, that her daughter is starting Tanner Stage II. What are the physical exam findings during this stage?

a) breast buds and some straight pubic hair
b) fully developed breast and curly pubic hair
c) breast tissue with the areola on a separate mound with curly pubic hair
d) no breast tissue and no pubic hair

114

The Phalen test is used to evaluate?

a) inflammation of the median nerve
b) rheumatoid arthritis
c) degenerative joint changes
d) chronic tenosynovitis

115

Physiologic anemia of pregnancy is due to?

a) an increase in the cardiac output at the end of the second trimester
b) a physiologic decrease in the production of RBCs in pregnant women

c) an increase of up to 50% of the plasma volume in pregnant women
d) an increase in the need for dietary iron in pregnancy

116

All of the following are implicated in causing chronic cough except?

a) chronic bronchitis
b) allergic rhinitis
c) acute viral upper respiratory infection
d) gastroesophageal reflux disease

117

Which of the following is a true statement regarding the effect of aspirin on platelet function?

a) the effect on platelets is reversible
b) the effect on platelets is reversible and lasts only 1 week
c) it has a minimal effect on platelet function
d) the effect on platelet function is irreversible and lasts 15 to 20 days

118

All of the following agents are used to control the inflammatory changes seen on the lungs of asthmatics except?

a) albuterol inhaler (Proventil)
b) triamcinolone (Azmacort)
c) montelukast (Singulair)
d) cromolyn sodium inhaler (Intal)

119

Rovsing's sign is associated with which of the following?

a) an acute abdomen such as during a ruptured appendix
b) knee instability
c) damage to the meniscus of the knee
d) acute cholelithiasis

120

Which of the following is contraindicated in the care of pregnant women with placenta previa?

a) echocardiogram
b) intravaginal ultrasound
c) abdominal ultrasound
d) pelvic ultrasound

121

A patient is positive for anti-HCV (hepatitis C virus antibody). What is the next step to further evaluate this patient?

a) refer the patient to a gastroenterologist
b) order a hepatitis C PCR (polymerase chain reaction) test
c) order a hepatitis B comprehensive panel
d) the patient is immune to hepatitis C and no further testing is indicated

122

A 62-year-old female complains of chronic severe low back pain. She also reports mild episodes of fecal incontinence and numbness to her lower legs over the past week. You would suspect which of the following?

a) fracture of the lower spine
b) a herniated disc
c) cauda equina syndrome
d) ankylosing spondylitis

123

A 40-year-old White female with a BMI (body mass index) of 32 complains of colicky pain on the right upper quadrant of her abdomen that gets worse if she eats fried food. During the physical exam, the nurse practitioner presses deeply on the left lower quadrant of the abdomen. After releasing her hand, the patient complains of pain on the right side of the lower abdomen. What is the name of this finding?

a) rebound tenderness
b) Rovsing's sign
c) Murphy's sign
d) Psoas test

124

Which of the following viral infections is associated with occasional abnormal forms of lymphocytes during an acute infection?

a) cytomegalovirus (CMV)
b) Epstein-Barr virus (EBV)
c) human papilloma virus (HPV)
d) Coxsackie virus

125

A faun tail nevus is a sign for which of the following?

a) Down syndrome
b) infantile scoliosis
c) congenital heart disease
d) spina bifida

126

Jenny, a 21-year-old, complains to you of a 1 week episode of dysuria, frequency, and a strong odor to her urine. This is her second episode of the year. What is the most appropriate follow-up for this patient?

a) order a urinalysis and urine for culture and sensitivity (C&S) and treat the patient with antibiotics
b) order a urine C&S and hold treatment until you get the results from the lab
c) treat the patient with a 7-day course of antibiotics and order a urine for culture and sensitivity (urine C&S) now and after she completes her antibiotics
d) treat the patient with a stronger drug such as ofloxacin (Floxin) for 10 days

127

Café-au-lait spots look like tan-to-light brown stains that have irregular borders. They can be located anywhere in the body. Which of the following is a correct statement?

a) they are associated with neurofibromatosis or von Recklinghausen's disease
b) they may be considered as precancerous after a biopsy
c) they are more common in darker skinned children
d) they are associated with Wilson's disease

128

During the eye exam of a 50-year-old hypertensive patient who is complaining of an onset of a severe headache, you find that the borders of the disc margins on both eyes are blurred. What is the name of this clinical finding?

a) normal optic disc
b) optic neuropathy
c) papilledema
d) hypertensive retinopathy

129

A high school teacher complains of a dry cough for the past 6 weeks. It worsens when he is supine. He has episodes of heartburn, which he self-treats with an over-the-counter (OTC) antacid. He chews mints for his "bad breath." Which of the following is a possible cause for this patient's cough?

a) asthma
b) gastroesophageal reflux
c) pneumonia
d) chronic postnasal drip

130

The red reflex is elicited by shining a light in the eyes of the infant at an angle with the light about 15 in. away. The nurse practitioner is screening for

a) cataracts

b) strabismus
c) blindness
d) the blinking response

131

A 44-year-old patient with Down syndrome starts to develop impaired memory and difficulty with his usual daily life routines. He is having problems functioning at the job that he has done for the past 10 years. The physical exam and routine labs are all negative. The vital signs are normal. His appetite is normal. The most likely diagnosis is?

a) tic douloureux
b) a stroke
c) Alzheimer's disease
d) delirium

132

Which of the following findings is associated with the chronic use of chewing tobacco?

a) cheilosis and xerostomia
b) glossitis
c) a geographic tongue
d) leukoplakia and oral cancer

133

Which of the following is recommended treatment for erythema migrans or early Lyme disease?

a) doxycycline (Vibramycin) 100 mg PO BID × 21 days
b) ciprofloxacin (Cipro) 250 mg PO BID × 14 days
c) erythromycin (E-mycin) 333 mg PO TID × 10 days
d) dicloxacillin 500 mg PO BID × 10 days

134

Nurse practitioners and clinical nurse specialists derive their legal right to practice from?

a) the Nurse Practice Act of the state where they practice
b) the laws of the state where they practice
c) the Medicare Bill
d) the Board of Nursing from the state where they practice

135

You are checking a 75-year-old woman's breast during an annual gynecological exam. The left nipple and areolar are scaly and reddened. The patient denies pain and pruritis. She has noticed this scaliness on her left nipple for the past 8 months. Her dermatologist gave her a potent topical steroid, which she used twice a day for 1 month. The patient never went back for the follow-up. She still has the rash and wants an evaluation. Which of the following is the best intervention for this patient?

a) prescribe another potent topical steroid and tell the patient to use it twice a day for 4 weeks
b) order a mammogram and refer the patient to a breast surgeon
c) advise her to stop using soap on both breasts when she bathes to avoid drying up the skin on her areola and nipples
d) order a sonogram and fine needle biopsy of the breast

136

The following children are considered at higher risk for tuberculosis (TB) except?

a) a child who has recently been diagnosed with leukemia
b) an infant whose family is homeless
c) a child who was born in Japan
d) a Hispanic child with asthma who is using a steroid inhaler

137

During a sports physical exam of a 14-year-old high school athlete, the nurse practitioner notices a split of the S2 component of the heart sound during deep inspiration. She notes that it disappears upon expiration. The heart rate is regular and no murmurs are auscultated. Which of the following is correct?

a) this is an abnormal finding and should be evaluated further by a cardiologist
b) a stress test should be ordered
c) this is a normal finding in some young athletes
d) an echocardiogram should be ordered

138

Mrs. J. L. is a 55-year-old female with a body mass index (BMI) of 24 and a history of asthma. She has hypertension that has been under control with hydrochloro-thiazide 12.5 mg PO daily. Her total cholesterol is 230 g/dl. How many risk factors for coronary heart disease (CAD) does she have?

a) one risk factor
b) two risk factors
c) three risk factors
d) four risk factors

139

A common side effect of metformin (Glucophage) therapy is?

a) weight gain
b) lactic acidosis
c) hypoglycemic episodes
d) gastrointestinal problems

140

While doing a cardiac exam on a 45-year-old male, you note an irregular rhythm with a pulse rate of 110 beats per minute. The patient is alert and is not in distress. What is the most likely?

a) atrial fibrillation
b) ventricular fibrillation
c) cardiac arrhythmia
d) first degree right bundle branch block

141

The following are patients who are at high risk for complications due to urinary tract infections. Who does not belong in this category?

a) a 38-year-old diabetic patient with a HbA1C of 7.5%
b) a woman with a history of rheumatoid arthritis who is currently being treated with a regimen of methotrexate and low-dose steroids
c) a 21-year-old woman who is under treatment for two sexually transmitted infections
d) pregnant women

142

A 68-year-old woman with hypertension and diabetes is seen by the nurse practitioner for a dry cough that worsens at night when she lies in bed. She has shortness of breath, which worsens when she exerts herself. The patient's pulse rate is 90/min and regular. The patient has gained 6 lbs. over the past 2 months. She is on a nitroglycerine patch and furosemide daily. The best explanation for her symptoms is?

a) kidney failure
b) congestive heart failure
c) ACE inhibitor-induced coughing
d) thyroid disease

143

A nurse practitioner is doing a funduscopic exam on a 35-year-old female during a routine physical exam. He notices that she has sharp disc margins and a yellowish-orange color in the macular area. The ratio of veins to arteries is 3:2. What is the next most appropriate action?

a) advise the patient that she had a normal exam
b) advise the patient that she had an abnormal exam
c) refer the patient to the emergency room
d) refer the patient to an ophthalmologist

144

During a sports physical, you note that the vision of an 18-year-old male athlete is 20/30 in both eyes. Which of the following statements below is true?

a) the patient can see at 20 ft. what a person with normal vision can see at 30 ft.
b) the patient can see at 30 ft. what a person with normal vision can see at 20 ft.
c) the patient cannot engage in contact sports
d) the patient needs to be referred to an ophthalmologist

145

Carol, a 30-year-old type 2 diabetic, is on regular insulin and Lente insulin in the morning and in the evening. She denies changes in her diet or any illness but recently started attending aerobic classes in the afternoon. Because of her workouts, her blood sugars have dipped below 50 mg/dL very early in the morning. Her fasting blood sugar before breakfast is now elevated and higher than normal. Which of the following is best described?

a) Somogyi phenomenon
b) Dawn phenomenon
c) Raynaud's phenomenon
d) insulin resistance

146

A 40-year-old female is positive for anti-hepatitis C virus (HCV). Which test is appropriate for follow-up?

a) HCV RNA
b) HCV antibodies
c) HCV core antigen
d) Hepatitis C surface antigen

147

When the nurse practitioner is evaluating a patient for intermittent claudication, she would first?

a) order a venogram
b) order T.E.D. anti-embolism stockings
c) check the ankle and brachial blood pressure before and after exercise
d) check the pedal and posterior tibial pulses

148

All of the following drugs can interact with theophylline (Theo-24) except?

a) erythromycin
b) montelukast (Singulair)
c) phenytoin sodium (Dilantin)
d) cimetidine (Tagamet)

149

You note a high-pitched and blowing pansystolic murmur in a 70-year-old male. It is Grade II/VI and is best heard at the apical area. Which of the following is most likely?

a) ventricular septal defect
b) tricuspid regurgitation
c) mitral regurgitation
d) mitral stenosis

150

The cover/uncover test is a screening tool for?

a) color blindness
b) strabismus
c) visual acuity
d) cataracts

SECTION D

151

The mother of a 4-week-old infant is concerned that her infant's eyes are crossed for a few seconds occasionally. The nurse practitioner would?

a) recommend referral to a pediatric ophthalmologist
b) advise the mother that this is a normal finding in infants up to 2 months of age
c) recommend multivitamin supplements should be given to the infant daily
d) educate her on how to patch the infant's eye every 4 hours

152

All of the following are factors important in determining the peak expiratory flow volume except?

a) weight
b) height
c) age
d) gender

153

You are reviewing a pap smear report on a 25-year-old female. Which of the following cells should be on a pap smear to be classified as a satisfactory specimen?

a) clue cells and endometrial cells
b) vaginal cells and cervical cells
c) squamous epithelial cells and endocervical cells
d) leukocytes and RBCs

154

When assessing a patient suspected of having vertigo, which description provided by the patient is most consistent with the diagnosis?

a) a sensation of imbalance while walking
b) a sensation of spinning or rotating
c) a sensation of "passing out"
d) a sensation of lightheadedness when changing positions from reclining to standing

155

A 56-year-old man complains of episodes of lancinating pain that shoot up to his right cheek when he eats or drinks. He has stopped drinking cold drinks because of the pain. Which of the following is most likely?

a) trigeminal neuralgia
b) cluster headache
c) acute sinusitis
d) sinus headache

156

What does a KOH (potassium hydroxide) prep help the nurse practitioner diagnose?

a) herpes zoster infections
b) yeast infections
c) herpes simplex infections
d) viral infections

157

All of the following are considered as selective serotonin reuptake inhibitors (SSRIs) except?

a) imipramine (Elavil)
b) fluoxetine (Prozac)
c) sertraline (Zoloft)
d) paroxetine (Paxil CR)

158

All of the following tests require the patient's voice to perform correctly except?

a) egophony
b) tactile fremitus
c) whispered pectoriloquy
d) auscultation

159

While checking for the red reflex on a 3-year-old boy during a well child visit, a white reflection is seen on the child's left pupil. Which of the following conditions should be ruled out?

a) unilateral strabismus
b) unilateral cataracts

c) retinoblastoma of the left eye
d) color blindness of the left eye

160

All of the following infections are reportable diseases except?

a) Lyme disease
b) gonorrhea
c) nongonococcal urethritis
d) syphilis

161

A menopausal woman with osteopenia is attending a dietary education class. Which of the following foods are recommended?

a) yogurt and sardines
b) spinach and red meat
c) cheese and red meat
d) low-fat cheese and whole grain

162

A patient who is on warfarin sodium (Coumadin) is advised to avoid eating large amounts of leafy green vegetables because?

a) the high Vitamin K levels will increase her bleeding time
b) they have too much ascorbic acid, which can interact with the medicine
c) the high fiber content will decrease the absorption of the Coumadin
d) the vitamins in the vegetables will bind and inactivate Coumadin

163

You are following up a 65-year-old male who has been on a new prescription of fluvastatin (Lescol) for 6 weeks. During a follow-up visit, he reports feeling extremely fatigued and having dark-colored urine. He denies any generalized muscle soreness. Which of the following is the most appropriate treatment plan?

a) order a CBC with differential
b) order a liver function profile
c) recommend an increase in fluid intake and rest
d) order a urine for C&S test

164

Which of the following diagnoses is most likely in this patient?

a) rhabdomyolysis
b) acute drug-induced hepatitis
c) acute mononucleosis
d) a major depressive episode

165

What would you advise him regarding his fluvastatin (Lescol) prescription?

a) continue taking the medicine until the lab results are available
b) take half the usual daily dose until the lab results are available
c) take the medicine every other day instead of daily until the lab results are available
d) stop taking the medicine until the lab results are available

166

All of the following children are within the parameters of normal growth and development for their age group except?

a) a 2-month-old who coos and smiles
b) a 14-month-old who understands complex commands
c) a 20-month-old who can walk without support
d) a 3-year-old who can speak in three-to-four word sentences

167

You are reviewing the bilirubin level on a 3-day-old full-term neonate. You note that it is 10 mg/dL. The infant has a slight yellow color to his skin, mucous membranes, and sclera. The infant is feeding well, is not irritable, and has 8 to 10 wet diapers per day. Which of the following is a true statement?

a) keep on monitoring the infant's bilirubin level until it returns back to normal in about 1 week
b) recommend that the infant be treated with phototherapy 10 minutes a day until the bilirubin level is back down to a normal range
c) refer the infant to a neonatologist as soon as possible
d) refer the infant to the neonatal intensive care unit

168

All of the following statements are correct regarding the Td vaccine except?

a) fever occurs in up to 80% of the patients
b) a possible side effect is induration on the injection site
c) the Td is given every 10 years
d) the DPT and DT should not be given beyond the 7th birthday

169

Which of the following is recommended by JNC 7 as first line treatment for hypertension in patients with microalbuminuria?

a) angiotensin-converting enzyme (ACE) inhibitors
b) diuretics
c) calcium channel blockers
d) beta blockers

170

A woman is being evaluated by the nurse practitioner for complaints of dyspareunia. A microscopy slide reveals a large number of atrophic squamous epithelial cells. The vaginal pH is 4.0. There are very few leukocytes and no RBCs are seen on the wet smear. Which of the following is most likely?

a) atrophic vaginitis
b) bacterial vaginosis
c) trichomoniasis
d) this is a normal finding

171

A test called the visual fields by confrontation is used to evaluate for?

a) peripheral vision
b) central distance vision
c) narrow angle glaucoma
d) accommodation

172

The following skin findings are considered macules except?

a) a freckle
b) petechia
c) acne
d) a flat 0.5-cm brown birthmark

173

Clara is a 20-year-old college student who reports to the student health clinic with a laceration in her left hand. She tells the nurse practitioner that she cut her hand while working in her garden. Her last Td booster was 5.5 years ago. Which of the following is correct?

a) administer a booster dose of the Td vaccine
b) administer the Td vaccine and the Td immunoglobulin (HyperTet)
c) administer Td immunoglobulin (HyperTet) only
d) she does not need any Td immunoglobulin (Hypertet) or a Td booster

174

The apex of the heart is located at?

a) second ICS (intercostal space) to the right of the sternal border
b) second ICS to the left of the sternal border
c) the left lower sternal border
d) the left side of the sternum at the fifth ICS by the midclavicular line

175

Which of the following statements is false regarding jaundice in breast-fed infants?

a) breast-fed infants have a higher incidence of hyperbilirubinemia compared with formula-fed infants
b) the mechanism of breast milk jaundice is still not known
c) phytotherapy is usually not indicated for these infants
d) it usually starts in the first week of life

176

Koilonychia is associated with which of the following conditions?

a) lead poisoning
b) beta thalassemia trait
c) B12 deficiency anemia
d) iron deficiency anemia

177

Which of the following laboratory tests is positive in a large number of patients with systemic lupus erythematosus?

a) antinuclear antibody (ANA)
b) rheumatoid factor
c) antiparietal antibody
d) immunoglobulin

178

All of the following are correct statements regarding the S3 component of the heart sound except?

a) it occurs very early in diastole and is sometimes called an opening snap
b) it is a normal finding in some children, healthy young adults, and athletes
c) it can be a normal variant if heard on a person age 40 or older
d) it signifies CHF (congestive heart failure)

179

A positive straight leg raising test is indicative of which of the following?

a) myasthenia gravis
b) inflammation of the sciatic nerve
c) multiple sclerosis
d) Parkinson's disease

180

Which of the following would you recommend on an annual basis for an elderly type 2 diabetic?

a) eye exam with an ophthalmologist
b) follow-up visit with a urologist
c) periodic visits to an optometrist
d) colonoscopy

181

A 72-year-old female complains to you of a crusty and nonhealing small ulcer on her upper lip that she has had for several years. Which of the following would you recommend?

a) triamcinolone acetonide (Kenalog) cream BID for 2 weeks
b) triple antibiotic ointment BID × 2 weeks
c) hydrocortisone 1% cream BID for 2 weeks
d) the patient needs to be evaluated by a dermatologist

182

All of the following statements about phototherapy are correct except?

a) light from the blue to white spectrum is used
b) it is not always necessary to use a shield for the infant's eyes
c) unconjugated bilirubin in the skin is converted to a water-soluble nontoxic substance that is excreted in the bile
d) the infant's eyes should be shielded

183

Heberden's nodules are commonly found in which of the following diseases?

a) rheumatoid arthritis
b) degenerative joint disease
c) psoriatic arthritis
d) septic arthritis

184

The red blood cells in pernicious anemia will show?

a) microcytic and hypochromic cells
b) microcytic and normochromic cells
c) macrocytic and normochromic cells
d) macrocytic and hypochromic cells

185

You notice a medium-pitched harsh systolic murmur during an episodic exam. It is best heard at the right upper border of the sternum. What is most likely?

a) mitral stenosis
b) aortic stenosis
c) pulmonic stenosis
d) tricuspid regurgitation

186

A small abscess on a hair follicle on the eyelid is called?

a) hordeolum

b) ptyregium
c) pinguecula
d) ptosis

187

Which of the following is indicated for the prophylactic treatment of migraine headache?

a) ibuprofen (Motrin)
b) naproxen sodium (Anaprox)
c) propranolol (Inderal)
d) sumatriptan (Imitrex)

188

A 40-year-old male complains to the nurse practitioner of severe stabbing pains behind his left eye for the past 2 days. It is accompanied by some nasal congestion and rhinorrhea, which is clear in color. The patient denies pharyngitis and fever. Which of the following conditions is most likely?

a) migraine headache with aura
b) cluster headache
c) tic douloureux
d) cranial neuralgia

189

Ken has type 2 diabetes mellitus and a "sensitive stomach." Which medication is least likely to cause him gastrointestinal distress?

a) naproxen sodium (Anaprox)
b) aspirin (Bayer's aspirin)
c) erythromycin (E-mycin)
d) sucralfate (Carafate)

190

All of the following statements are true regarding domestic abuse except?

a) there is no delay in seeking medical treatment
b) the pattern of injuries is inconsistent with the history reported
c) injuries are usually in the "central" area of the body instead of the extremities
d) pregnant women have a higher risk of domestic abuse

191

A new mother is breastfeeding her full-term 4-week-old infant. She wants to know whether she should give the infant vitamin supplements. The best advice is?

a) since she is breastfeeding, the infant does not need any vitamin supplements until he is at least 6 months of age
b) breast milk gives the infant all the vitamins he needs until 12 months of age

c) breast-fed infants require iron and vitamin D supplementation right away
d) breast-fed infants require iron and vitamin E supplementation at 3 months of age

192

Beta thalassemia minor is considered a?

a) macrocytic anemia
b) normocytic anemia
c) microcytic anemia
d) hemolytic anemia

193

Potential complications of mitral valve prolapse (MVP) include all of the following except?

a) severe mitral regurgitation
b) endocarditis
c) increased risk of stroke and TIA
d) mitral stenosis

194

A new patient is complaining of severe pruritus that is worse at night. Several family members also have the same symptoms. Upon examination, areas of excoriated papules are noted on some of the interdigital webs of both hands and on the axillae. This finding is most consistent with?

a) contact dermatitis
b) impetigo
c) larva migrans
d) scabies

195

An elderly woman with a history of rheumatoid arthritis reports to the nurse practitioner that she had been taking ibuprofen BID for many years. Which of the following organ systems has the highest risk of damage from chronic nonsteroidal anti-inflammatory drug (NSAIDs) use?

a) cardiovascular system
b) neurological system
c) gastrointestinal system
d) renal system

196

Ted, who is 15 years old, has just moved into the community and is staying in a foster home temporarily. There is no record of his immunizations. His foster mother wants him to be checked before he enters the local high school. Which of the following does this patient need?

a) Mantoux test
b) MMR
c) Td
d) All of the above

197

Which cranial nerve (CN) is being evaluated when patients are instructed to shrug their shoulders?

a) CN IX
b) CN X
c) CN XI
d) CN XII

198

A lab technician has a 10.5-mm area of redness and induration in his left forearm after getting a Mantoux test 72 hours ago. The last test, which was done 12 months ago, was negative. He denies cough, night sweats, and weight loss. What is the next best intervention?

a) obtain a sputum culture and a chest X-ray
b) obtain a chest X-ray
c) obtain a sputum for C&S and an acid fast stain
d) obtain a CBC and chest X-ray

199

Swim therapy for a 13-year-old with cerebral palsy is an example of?

a) primary prevention
b) secondary prevention
c) tertiary prevention
d) health prevention

200

Which of the following individuals is most likely to be at higher risk for osteoporosis?

a) 70-year-old female of African ancestry who walks daily for exercise
b) 42-year-old obese woman from Cuba who has been taking prednisone 10 mg daily for the last 12 years to control her severe asthma
c) 55-year-old Caucasian female who is an aerobics instructor
d) 4-year-old Asian female who has been on high-dose steroids for 1 week

SECTION E

201

What is the primary carbohydrate found in breast milk and commercial infant formulas?

a) fructose
b) lactose
c) glucose
d) sucrose

202

Which of the following patients is least likely to become an alcoholic?

a) A patient whose father has a history of alcoholism
b) A patient whose wife complains that he drinks too much
c) A patient who drinks one cup of wine nightly with dinner
d) A patient who feels he drinks all the time

203

The following conditions are absolute contraindications for the use of oral contraceptives except?

a) hepatomas
b) history of emboli that resolved with heparin therapy 15 years ago
c) muscle tension headaches
d) a history of gallbladder disease during pregnancy

204

The most common cause of cancer deaths in males is?

a) lung cancer
b) prostate cancer
c) colon cancer
d) skin cancer

205

Which of the following findings are seen on a patient with folate deficiency anemia?

a) microcytic and hypochromic RBCs
b) microcytic and normochromic RBCs
c) normal size and color of the RBCs
d) macrocytic and normocytic RBCs

206

When confirming a case of temporal arteritis, the erythrocyte sedimentation rate (ESR) is expected to be?

a) normal
b) lower than normal
c) elevated
d) indeterminate result

207

Mrs. Green, age 45, is complaining of generalized morning stiffness especially in both her wrist and hands. It is much worse in the morning and lasts for a few hours. She also complains of fatigue and generalized body aches that have been present for the past few months. Which of the following is most likely?

a) osteoporosis
b) rheumatoid arthritis
c) osteoarthritis
d) gout

208

During a well child visit, a new father wants to know if he can give fresh whole milk to his 6-month-old son. The nurse practitioner would recommend that?

a) he can start giving whole milk but not skim milk by 6 months of age
b) he should not give whole milk to his son until he is at least 12 months of age
c) he can give whole milk to his son at anytime
d) he should not give whole milk to his son without diluting it with water

209

Which of the following drugs is effective therapy for treating pain in patients who are having an acute exacerbation of gout?

a) acetaminophen (Tylenol)
b) systemic steroids
c) indomethacin (Indocin)
d) allopurinol (Zyloprim)

210

The complications of untreated gout include?

a) loss of joint mobility and renal failure
b) loss of joint mobility and liver failure
c) an increased risk of urinary tract infections
d) bladder cancer

211

A 21-year-old female who is complaining of random palpitations is diagnosed with mitral valve prolapse (MVP). Her echocardiogram (EKG) reveals redundant and thickened leaflets. You note a Grade III/VI systolic murmur with an ejection click during physical examination. You would recommend?

a) endocarditis prophylaxis for most dental and urologic procedures
b) endocarditis prophylaxis is not necessary
c) lifetime anticoagulation therapy with warfarin sodium
d) endocarditis prophylaxis for dental procedures only

212

You note bony nodules located at the proximal interphalangeal joints on both the hands of your 65-year-old female patient. Which of the following is most likely?

a) Bouchard's node
b) Heberden's node
c) osteoarthritic nodules
d) Tophi deposits

213

Which chronic illness disproportionately affects the Hispanic population?

a) diabetes mellitus
b) hypertension
c) alcohol abuse
d) skin cancer

214

A lipid profile done on a newly diagnosed hypertensive patient shows a triglyceride level of 650 mg/dL, total cholesterol 240 mg/dL, LDL 145 mg/dL, and an HDL of 35 mg/dL. What is the best intervention for this patient?

a) educate the patient about lifestyle changes that will help lower cholesterol levels
b) initiate a prescription of pravastatin (Pravachol)
c) recommend that the patient exercise at least every other day and avoid eating fatty or fried foods
d) initiate a prescription of nicotinic acid (Niacin, Niaspan)

215

Cullen's sign is most commonly associated with which of the following?

a) acute pancreatitis
b) myocardial infarction
c) acute pyelonephritis
d) preeclampsia

216

The "gold standard" for the diagnosis of active Helicobacter pylori infection of the stomach or duodenum is?

a) a Helicobacter pylori titer
b) an endoscopy with tissue biopsy
c) an upper GI series
d) a urea breath test

217

Which of the following foods would you advise a new mother to introduce to her 6-month-old infant first?

a) iron-fortified rice cereal
b) plain rice cereal
c) iron-fortified pureed chicken meat
d) plain pureed carrots

218

Jim Wheeler is obese (BMI of 33), fatigued, and complaining of excessive thirst and hunger. You suspect type 2 diabetes mellitus. Initial testing to confirm diagnosis can include all except?

a) fasting plasma glucose level
b) glycosylated hemoglobin level (HbA1c)
c) random plasma glucose level
d) glucose tolerance testing

219

A bulla is defined as?

a) a solid nodule less than 1 cm in size
b) a superficial vesicle filled with serous fluid greater than 1 cm in size
c) a maculopapular lesion
d) a shallow ulcer

220

A newborn's mother is discovered to be HBsAg (hepatitis B surface antigen) positive. Which of the following would you recommend for this infant?

a) give the baby hepatitis B immunoglobulin
b) give the baby both Hepatitis B vaccine and hepatitis B immunoglobulin
c) give the baby Hepatitis B vaccine only
d) send the baby home because he is not infected

221

Which of the following is the confirmatory test for the HIV screening test?

a) ELISA test for HIV
b) Western blot
c) HIV polymerase chain reaction test
d) HIV antibody

222

All of the following findings are associated with the secondary stage of an infection by the organism treponema pallidum except?

a) condyloma acuminata
b) maculopapular rash of the palms and soles
c) lymphadenopathy
d) condyloma lata

223

The following are acceptable methods of birth control for breast-feeding mothers except?

a) diaphragm with spermicidal gel
b) progesterone-only pills (Micronor)
c) condoms
d) low-dose oral contraceptives with at least 20 μg of estradiol (Alesse, Lo-estrin)

224

Women with a history of pelvic inflammatory disease (PID) have an increased risk for all of the following complication(s) except?

a) ectopic pregnancy
b) scarring of the fallopian tube(s)
c) infertility
d) ovarian cysts

225

The differential diagnosis for genital ulceration includes all of the following except?

a) syphilis
b) genital herpes
c) chancroid
d) molluscum contagiosum

226

Lead poisoning can cause which type of anemia?

a) a mild macrocytic anemia

b) normocytic anemia
c) microcytic anemia
d) a mild hemolytic anemia

227

Hypovolemic shock would most likely occur with fractures of the?

a) spine
b) pelvis
c) femur
d) humerus

228

Podagra is associated with which of the following?

a) rheumatoid arthritis
b) gout
c) osteoarthritis
d) septic arthritis

229

While assessing for a cardiac murmur, the first time that a thrill can be palpated is at?

a) Grade II
b) Grade III
c) Grade IV
d) Grade V

230

A medium-pitched harsh mid-systolic murmur is best heard at the right second ICS of the chest. It radiates into the neck. Which of the following is the correct diagnosis?

a) aortic stenosis
b) pulmonic stenosis
c) aortic regurgitation
d) mitral stenosis

231

Which type of hepatitis virus infection is more likely to result in chronic hepatitis and increased risk of developing hepatocellular carcinoma?

a) Hepatitis A virus
b) Hepatitis B virus
c) Hepatitis C virus
d) Hepatitis D virus

232

What is the caloric content of infant formula and breast milk?

a) 10 kcal/30 mL
b) 15 kcal/30 mL
c) 20 kcal/30 mL
d) 25 kcal/30 mL

233

A 19-year-old female has recently been diagnosed with acute Hepatitis B. She is sexually active and is monogamous. She reports using condoms inconsistently. What would you recommend for her male sexual partner who was also tested for hepatitis with the following results: HBsAg (−), anti-HBs (−), anti-HCV (−), anti-HAV (+)?

a) a hepatitis B vaccination
b) hepatitis B immunoglobulin
c) hepatitis B vaccination and hepatitis B immunoglobulin
d) no vaccination is needed at this time

234

All of the following conditions are associated with an increased risk for normocytic anemia except?

a) rheumatoid arthritis
b) lupus
c) chronic autoimmune disorders
d) pregnancy

235

You can determine a pulse deficit by counting the?

a) apical and radial pulses at the same time, then subtracting the difference between the two
b) apical pulse first, then the radial pulse, and subtracting the difference between the two
c) apical pulse and the femoral pulse at the same time and subtracting the difference between the two
d) radial pulse first, then counting the femoral pulse, and subtracting the difference between the two

236

An infant who does not have a history of reactive airway disease and allergy has both inspiratory and expiratory wheezing accompanied by fever and profuse clear nasal discharge. Which of the following is most likely?

a) tracheobronchitis
b) bronchiolitis

c) croup

d) a small foreign body that is lodged on the left main bronchus

237

Patients who are being screened for TB and are immunocompromised should be evaluated for anergy. Which of the following is the best description of anergy testing?

a) apply candida or mumps antigen to the right forearm and the PPD on the left forearm and read results in 48 to 72 hours

b) apply candida or mumps antigen and PPD on left forearm only and check for a reaction in 24 hours

c) mix the candida or mumps antigen with the PPD and apply it to both forearms

d) apply the candida or mumps antigen 24 hours before the PPD on the left forearm

238

A nurse practitioner is evaluating an 80-year-old woman from a nursing home. She is instructing the patient to remember the words "orange," "house," and "world." A few minutes later, the patient is told to recall these three words. Which of the following is being described?

a) the Lachman test

b) a neurologic exam

c) the Romberg test

d) the Mini Mental Exam

239

In most states, patients younger than age 18 years may consent to health care without parental or legal guardian consent except for which of the following?

a) contraception

b) pregnancy

c) school physicals

d) STD evaluation and treatment

240

A hypertensive middle-aged man who is Native American has recently been diagnosed with mild renal insufficiency. He has been on lisinopril (Accupril) for many years. Which of the following laboratory values should be carefully monitored?

a) hemoglobin, hematocrit, and the MCV (mean corpuscular volume)

b) serum creatinine and potassium levels

c) aspartate aminotransferase and alanine aminotransferase

d) serum sodium, potassium, and magnesium

241

You suspect an enterobiasis infection in a 6-year-old girl. Which of the following tests would you recommend?

a) stool culture and sensitivity
b) stool for ova and parasites
c) the scotch tape test
d) a Hemoccult test

242

What is the most common cause of left ventricular hypertrophy in the United States?

a) chronic atrial fibrillation
b) chronic hypertension
c) mitral valve prolapse
d) pulmonary hypertension

243

Asthmatics may have all of the following symptoms during an exacerbation except?

a) rapid pulse
b) wheezing
c) chronic coughing
d) tachypnea

244

Laws governing nurse practitioner authority are determined by the?

a) Board of Nursing
b) State Legislature
c) American Nursing Association
d) State Medical Association

245

A 10-year-old male who recently became accepted into his school's soccer team has a history of exercise-induced asthma. The child wants to know when he should take his albuterol inhaler. The nurse practitioner would advise the patient?

a) premedicate himself 20 minutes prior to starting exercise
b) wait until he starts to exercise before using the inhaler
c) premedicate 60 minutes before starting exercise
d) wait until he finishes his exercises before using his inhaler

246

Atrophic macular degeneration of the aged (AMD) is the leading cause of blindness in the elderly in the U.S. Which of the following statements is correct?

a) it is a slow or sudden painless loss of central vision
b) it is a slow or sudden painless loss of peripheral vision
c) it is an occlusion of the central retinal vein causing degeneration of the macular area
d) it is commonly caused by diabetic retinopathy

247

A 12 year-old girl is complaining of a 2-week history of facial pressure that worsens when she bends over. She complains of tooth pain in her upper molars on the right side of her face. On physical exam, her lung and heart sounds are normal. Which of the following is the most likely diagnosis?

a) an acute dental abscess
b) chronic sinusitis
c) acute sinusitis
d) severe allergic rhinitis

248

Which of the following findings is associated with thyroid hypofunction?

a) Graves Disease
b) eye disorder
c) thyroid storm
d) myxedema

249

What is the best procedure for evaluating a corneal abrasion?

a) tonometry
b) fluorescein stain
c) visual field test
d) funduscopy

SECTION F

250

You are examining a patient who has just been diagnosed with Bell's palsy. Bell's palsy is characterized by all of the following except?

a) drooling
b) inability to swallow
c) inability to close the eye on the affected side
d) drooping of the corner of the mouth on the affected side

251

A new mother who is on her 4th day of breastfeeding complains to the nurse practitioner of very sore breasts. The nurse practitioner would?

a) recommend a decrease in the number of times she breastfeeds her infant per day
b) recommend that she stop breastfeeding and use infant formula for the next 48 hours
c) educate the mother that this is normal during the 1st week or 2 of breastfeeding and the soreness will eventually go away
d) recommend that she purchase plastic nipple pads for her nursing bra and use them daily

252

A 12-year-old male's peak expiratory flow results indicate 60 to 80% predicted range. How would you classify his asthma?

a) mild intermittent asthma
b) mild persistent asthma
c) moderate persistent asthma
d) severe asthma

253

Which of the following conditions is associated with a positive Auspitz sign?

a) contact dermatitis
b) seborrheic dermatitis
c) systemic lupus erythematosus
d) psoriasis

254

Which of the following is used to confirm a diagnosis of Hashimoto's thyroiditis?

a) thyroid needle biopsy
b) TSH
c) antimicrosomal antibody test
d) complement-fixation test

255

A first grader presents to a school nurse practitioner with a few blisters on one arm and on the face. The child keeps scratching the affected areas. Some of the lesions have ruptured with yellow serous fluid that crusts easily. This best describes?

a) acute cellulitis
b) herpes zoster
c) bullous impetigo
d) erysipelas

256

All of the following statements reflect inadequate breast milk production except?

a) full-term infant is at birth weight by the 2nd week of life
b) less than six wet diapers per day or less than four stools per day
c) infant is nursing fewer than eight times per 24-hour period
d) weight loss of >10% of birth weight

257

The best screening test for detecting and monitoring both hyperthyroidism and hypothyroidism is?

a) the total T3–4
b) thyroid stimulating hormone (TSH)
c) thyroid profile
d) palpation of the thyroid gland

258

A patient who recently returned from a vacation in Latin America complains of a severe headache and stiff neck that are accompanied by a high fever for the past 12 hours. While examining the patient, the nurse practitioner flexes both the patient's hips and legs and then tells the patient to straighten them against resistance. The name of this test is?

a) Kernig's maneuver
b) Brudzinski's maneuver
c) Murphy's sign
d) Homan's sign

259

Which of the following groups has been recommended to be screened for thyroid disease?

a) women 50 years or older
b) adolescent females
c) elderly males
d) school-age children

260

A 65-year-old Hispanic woman has a history of type 2 diabetes. A routine urinalysis reveals a few epithelial cells and is negative for leukocytes, nitrites, and protein. Which of the following would you recommend next?

a) order a urine for C&S
b) order a 24-hour urine for microalbumin
c) because it is negative, no further tests are necessary
d) recommend a screening IVP (intravenous pyelogram)

261

Rhogam's mechanism of action is?

a) the destruction of Rh-positive fetal RBCs that are present in the mother's circulatory system
b) the destruction of maternal antibodies against Rh-positive fetal RBCs
c) the stimulation of maternal antibodies so that there is a decreased risk of hemolysis
d) the destruction of maternal antibodies against fetal RBCs

262

A chest radiograph shows an area of consolidation on the lower lobe. Which of the following conditions is most likely?

a) bacterial pneumonia
b) acute bronchitis
c) COPD
d) atypical pneumonia

263

What type of breath sounds are best heard over the base of the lungs?

a) fine breath sounds
b) vesicular breath sounds
c) bronchial sounds
d) tracheal breath sounds

264

The Joint National Commission on the Evaluation and Treatment of High Blood Pressure in Adults' (JNC 7) most current recommendation for the blood pressure goal in diabetics is?

a) <140/90
b) <130/85
c) <130/80
d) <125/75

265

All of the following pharmacologic agents are used to treat inflammation in the lungs of asthmatics except?

a) nedocromil sodium (Tilade) two sprays QID
b) cromolyn sodium inhaler (Intal) two puffs QID
c) a long-acting oral theophylline (Theo-Dur) 200 mg every 12 hours
d) fluticasone inhaler (Flovent) two puffs BID

266

All of the following clinical findings are considered benign oral findings except?

a) a patch of leukoplakia
b) Fordyce spots
c) torus palatinus
d) fishtail uvula

267

The nurse practitioner examines a 4-week-old boy whose mother reports that he cries for at least 3 hours a day at the same time of the day since birth. What is the main goal in the clinical evaluation of this infant?

a) rule out any physiologic cause for the crying spells
b) make sure that the infant is well clothed
c) evaluate the environment
d) order laboratory and diagnostic testing

268

During a routine physical exam of a 90-year-old woman, a low-pitched diastolic murmur Grade II/VI is auscultated. It is located on the fifth ICS on the left side of the midclavicular line. Which of the following is correct?

a) aortic regurgitation
b) mitral stenosis
c) mitral regurgitation
d) tricuspid regurgitation

269

Which of the following situations is considered emergent?

a) a laceration on the lower leg of a patient on aspirin (Bayer) 81 mg every other day
b) rapid breathing and tachycardia in a patient with a fever
c) an elderly man with abdominal pain whose vital signs appear stable
d) 37-year-old male biker with a concussion due to a fall who appears slightly agitated and does not appear to understand instructions given by the medical assistant checking his vital signs

270

Which of the following is considered an objective finding in patients who have a case of suppurative otitis media?

a) erythema of the tympanic membrane
b) decreased mobility of the tympanic membrane as measured by tympanogram
c) displacement of the light reflex
d) bulging of the tympanic membrane

271

Pulsus paradoxus is more likely to be associated with?

a) sarcoidosis
b) acute bronchitis
c) status asthmaticus
d) bacterial pneumonia

272

A 17-year-old boy reports feeling something on his left scrotum. On palpation, soft and moveable blood vessels that feel like a "bag of worms" are noted underneath the scrotal skin. It is not swollen or reddened. The most likely diagnosis is?

a) chronic orchitis
b) chronic epididymitis
c) testicular torsion
d) varicocele

273

All of the following are true statements regarding elderly abuse except?

a) those age 80 years or older are at the highest risk for abuse
b) a delay in medical care is a common finding
c) a new onset of an STD in an elderly patient may signal sexual abuse
d) decreased anxiety and depression are common symptoms of abuse in the elderly

274

The S1 heart sound is caused by?

a) closure of the atrioventricular valves
b) closure of the semilunar valves
c) opening of the atrioventricular valves
d) opening of the semilunar valves

275

Patients with Down syndrome are at higher risk for all of the following except?

a) atlantoaxial instability
b) congenital heart disease
c) early onset of Alzheimer's disease
d) melanoma

276

Duvall and Miller used developmental theory to describe the family. Which of the following statements is true?

a) each family is developmentally unique in comparison to another family

b) families demonstrate common forms of membership across developmental stages
c) families complete each developmental task separately
d) families change over time because of the influence of environmental factors

277

The following abnormal lab results may be seen in patients with acute mononucleosis except?

a) lymphocytosis and/or atypical lymphocytes
b) positive EBV titers for immunoglobulin (Ig) M and Ig G
c) elevated liver function tests
d) elevated creatinine and BUN

278

Which of the following is considered an abnormal result on a Weber test?

a) lateralization to one ear
b) no lateralization in either ear
c) air conduction lasts longer than bone conduction
d) bone conduction lasts longer than air conduction

279

All of the following are considered benign physiologic variants except?

a) internal tibial torsion
b) supernumerary nipples
c) split uvula
d) cheilosis

280

A 65-year-old woman's bone density result shows severe demineralization of cortical bone. All of the following pharmacologic agents are useful in treating this condition except?

a) raloxifene (Evista)
b) calcitonin (Miacalcin)
c) medroxyprogesterone (Depo-Provera)
d) calcium with Vitamin D

281

A fracture on the navicular area of the wrist is usually caused by falling forward and landing with the hands. The affected wrist is hyperextended to break the fall. The nurse practitioner is aware that all of the following statements are true except:

a) it has higher rate of nonunion compared with the other bones on the wrist when it is fractured
b) the fracture frequently does not show up on an X-ray film when it is taken immediately after the injury

325

c) the X-ray film will show the fracture if the film is repeated in 2 weeks

d) these fractures always need surgical intervention to stabilize the joint

282

John, a 10-year-old boy, has type 1 diabetes. His late afternoon blood sugars over the past 2 weeks have ranged between 210 mg/dL and 230 mg/ldL. He is currently on 10 units of regular insulin and 25 units of NPH in the morning and 15 units of regular insulin and 10 units of NPH insulin in the evening. Which of the following is the best treatment plan for this patient?

a) increase both types of the morning dose

b) increase only the NPH insulin in the morning

c) decrease the afternoon dose of NPH insulin

d) decrease both NPH and regular insulin doses in the morning

283

The mother of a 13-year-old male with Down's syndrome is in the family nurse practitioner's office and wants a sports physical done for her son. She reports that he wants to join the football team in his school. You would tell the mother that her son?

a) can play a regular football game as long as he wears maximum protective football gear

b) cannot play some contact sports because of an increased risk of cervical spine injury

c) can play certain contact sports after he has been check for cervical instability

d) none of the above

284

The mother of an 8-year-old boy reports the presence of a round red rash on the child's left lower leg. It appeared 1 week after the child returned from visiting his grandparents, who live in Massachusetts. During the skin exam, the maculopapular rash is noted to have areas of central clearing making it resemble a round target. Which of the following is best described?

a) erythema migrans

b) Rocky Mountain spotted fever

c) meningococcemia

d) larva migrans

285

Some pharmacologic agents may cause confusion in the elderly. Which of the following pharmacologic agents is most likely to cause confusion in this population?

a) cimetidine (Tagamet), Lanoxin (digoxin), diphenhydramine (Benadryl)

b) acetaminophen (Tylenol), aspirin (Bayer), indomethacin (Indocin)

c) sucralfate (Carafate), docusate sodium (Surfak), psyllium (Metamucil)

d) cephalexin (Keflex), amoxicillin (Amoxil), clarithromycin (Biaxin)

286

A 55-year-old female with a history of migraine headaches has recently been diagnosed with Stage II hypertension. Her EKG strips reveal second degree heart block. The chest X-ray is normal. Which of the following drugs should this patient avoid?

a) ACE inhibitors
b) angiotensin receptor blockers
c) diuretics
d) calcium channel blockers

287

Which of the following cranial nerves is evaluated when a wisp of cotton is lightly brushed against the corner of the eye?

a) CN II
b) CN III
c) CN IV
d) CN V

288

When a patient is suspected of having acute pancreatitis, initial testing should include all of the following except?

a) electrolyte panel
b) serum amylase level
c) serum lipase level
d) a barium swallow

289

Which of the following is a true statement regarding pes planus in an infant?

a) pes planus should be evaluated by a pediatric orthopedist if it does not spontaneously correct itself by the age of 12 months
b) the fat pads on an infant's feet can mimic pes planus
c) it is always corrected by wearing special orthotic shoes
d) it is also called talipes equinovarus

290

All of the following statements are not true regarding the rehabilitation of alcoholics except?

a) Al Anon is not designed for family members of alcoholics
b) disulfiram (Antabuse) is always effective
c) Alcoholics Anonymous is not an effective method for treating this condition
d) avoid foods or drinks that contain alcohol such as cough syrups

291

A mother of a 7-year-old boy tells the family nurse practitioner that his teacher has complained to her of her son's frequent episodes of daydreaming. While the child is at home, the mother reports that sometimes her son seems not to hear her. The child "blanks out" for a short period of time. Which of the following is most likely?

a) a partial seizure
b) an absence seizure (petit mal seizure)
c) a grand mal seizure
d) a jacksonian seizure

292

All of the following are incorrect statements regarding the Healthy People 2010 objectives except?

a) the document's objectives are not only applicable nationally, but also internationally
b) one of the objectives of the document is help people achieve not only physical health
c) the document's objectives are applicable only to people of the United States of America
d) the document is formulated by a special committee formed by an alliance of all the state health departments

293

The pap smear result of a 20-year-old sexually active college student who used condoms inconsistently reveals a large number of white blood cells and blood along with inflammatory changes. During the speculum exam, the nurse practitioner who had examined the patient noticed that the patient's cervix bled very easily (friable) and a small amount of purulent discharge was present on the cervical surface. There was no cervical motion tenderness noted during the bimanual vaginal exam. What is the next step in the management of this patient?

a) call the patient and tell her to return for further testing with a Gen-Probe to rule out infection by chlamydia and gonorrhea
b) treat the patient with metronidazole vaginal cream over the phone
c) call the patient and tell her she needs a repeat pap smear in 6 months
d) advise her to use a Betadine douche at bedtime × 3 days

294

A 30-year-old female complains of having no period for the last 12 weeks. She is sexually active and has been using condoms inconsistently. The patient has a history of irregular menstrual cycles and severe dysmenorrhea. The urine pregnancy test result is positive. Which of the following is a true statement regarding this pregnancy?

a) the fundus of the uterus should be at the level of the symphysis pubis
b) the cervix should be dilated about 0.5 in. at this time of gestation

c) "quickening" starts during this period
d) Hegar's sign is present during this period of pregnancy

295

A newborn infant who is small for gestational age is noted to have shortened palpebral fissures and microcephaly with a small jaw. This infant is most likely to be diagnosed with the following?

a) Down's syndrome
b) fetal alcohol syndrome
c) growth retardation
d) avoid alcoholic drinks permanently

296

Which of the following is the most common cause of cancer deaths for women in the United States?

a) breast cancer
b) lung cancer
c) colon cancer
d) heart disease

297

Human papilloma virus infection in women has been associated with the development of?

a) ectopic pregnancy
b) infertility
c) cervical cancer
d) pelvic inflammatory disease

298

All of the following are included in the criteria used to diagnose patients with AIDS except?

a) profound fatigue
b) thrush
c) Kaposi's sarcoma
d) hairy leukoplakia of the tongue

299

Which of the following conditions is the most common cause of sudden death among athletes?

a) brain aneurysm
b) hypertrophic cardiomyopathy
c) left ventricular hypertrophy
d) aortic stenosis

SECTION G

300

The span of the normal adult liver is?

a) 6 to 12 cm in the right midclavicular line
b) 12 to 16 cm in the right midclavicular line
c) 2 to 6 cm in the midsternal line
d) 4 to 8 cm in the midsternal line

301

A patient who is complaining of a new onset of severe headache is being examined. The patient is instructed to lie down on the examining table while the nurse practitioner flexes his head and neck forward to his chest. The patient reacts by quickly flexing his hip and knee. What is the name of this positive finding?

a) Kernig's sign
b) Brudzinski's sign
c) Rovsing's sign
d) Drawer's sign

302

A neighbor's 14-year-old son, who is active in basketball, complains of pain and swelling on both knees. On physical exam, there is tenderness over the tibial tuberosity of both knees. Which of the following is most likely?

a) chondromalacia patella
b) left knee sprain
c) Osgood-Schlatter disease
d) tear of the medial ligament

303

A woman at 32 weeks gestation has a positive throat culture for strep pyogenes. She denies allergies but gets very nauseous with erythromycin. Which of the following is the best choice for this pregnant patient?

a) clarithromycin (Biaxin)
b) trimethoprim /sulfamethizole (Bactrim DS)
c) ofloxacin (Floxin)
d) penicillin (Pen VK)

304

During a sports physical exam, a 16-year-old patient is noted to have a few beats of horizontal nystagmus on extreme lateral gaze that disappeared when the eyes moved back toward midline. Which statement below best describes this clinical finding?

a) it is caused by occult bleeding of the retinal artery

b) this is a normal finding

c) it is a sign of a possible brain mass

d) this is a borderline result and needs further evaluation

305

An urgent care nurse practitioner is assessing a 45-year-old White woman with a BMI of 32 for complaints of intermittent right upper quadrant abdominal pain over the past few weeks that is precipitated by eating fried foods and peanut butter. On exam, the patient's heart and lungs are normal. There is no pain over the costovertebral angle. During abdominal exam, the bowel sounds are present on all quadrants. While palpating deeply on the right upper quadrant during deep inspiration, the patient complains of severe sharp pain to the nurse practitioner. Which of the following is best described?

a) acute cholecystitis

b) acute appendicitis

c) acute gastroenteritis

d) acute diverticulitis

306

Which of the following drugs is recommended by the Centers for Disease Control and Prevention (CDC) as first line treatment for treating infections by the organism Bacillus anthracis (anthrax)?

a) clindamycin (Cleocin)

b) fluconazole (Diflucan)

c) penicillin G injection

d) ciprofloxacin (Cipro)

307

A major risk factor for a Down syndrome infant is?

a) maternal age younger than 16 years

b) maternal age older than 35 years

c) a positive family history of Down syndrome

d) a positive family history of genetic disease

308

A new patient who is a 40-year-old female postal worker is being evaluated for complaints of a new onset of an erythematous rash on both her cheeks and on the bridge of the nose that is accompanied by fatigue. She reports a history of Hashimoto's thyroiditis and is currently being treated with Synthroid 1.25 mg daily. Which of the following conditions is most likely?

a) atopic dermatitis

b) thyroid disease

c) lupus erythematosus

d) rosacea

309

Mary, who is 65 years of age, comes into the clinic during the 1st week of November for her annual wellness visit. Her last Td booster was 9 years ago. Which immunization(s) would you recommend for this visit?

a) influenza vaccine
b) tetanus and influenza vaccine
c) pneumococcal (Pneumovax) and influenza vaccines
d) she does not need any vaccinations to be administered in this visit

310

Acute bronchitis is best characterized by?

a) fever and wheezing
b) purulent sputum and fever
c) paroxysms of coughing that is dry or productive of mucoid sputum
d) a gradual onset and fatigue

311

The nurse practitioner notices a gray ring on the edge of both irises of an 80-year-old female. She denies visual changes or pain. She reports that she has had the "ring" for many years. Which of the following is the most likely diagnosis?

a) arcus senilis
b) pinguecula
c) peripheral cataracts
d) macular degeneration

312

What is the clinical significance of the above finding on a 35-year-old?

a) the patient has a higher risk of blindness
b) the patient should be evaluated for hyperlipidemia
c) the patient should be evaluated by an ophthalmologist
d) the patient should be evaluated for acute glaucoma

313

The cones in the retina of the eye are responsible for?

a) central vision
b) peripheral vision
c) night vision
d) double vision

314

The nurse practitioner would refer all of the following to a physician except?

a) severe facial burns
b) electrical burns

c) burns that involve the cartilage of the ear
d) second degree burns on the lower arm

315

On auscultation of the chest, a split S2 is best heard at?

a) second intercostal space, right sternal border
b) second intercostal space, left sternal border
c) fifth intercostal space, midclavicular line
d) fourth intercostal space, left sternal border

316

According to the guidelines outlined in JNC 7, the normal blood pressure should be?

a) <140/90
b) <130/85
c) <120/80
d) <110/75

317

Which of the following would be classified as a second degree burn?

a) a severe sunburn with blistering
b) burns that involve the subcutaneous layer of skin
c) a reddened finger after touching a hot iron
d) burns that involve eschar

318

The mother of a 16-year-old boy is concerned that her son is not developing normally. On physical exam, the patient is noted to have small testes with no pubic or facial hair. What is the most appropriate statement to say to the mother?

a) her son is developing normally
b) her son's physical development is delayed and needs to be evaluated by a pediatric endocrinologist
c) her son should be rechecked in 3 months; if he still does not have secondary sexual characteristics, a thorough hormonal workup should be initiated
d) her son's physiological development is slower than normal but is within the lower limit of normal for his age group

319

The most common type of skin malignancy is?

a) squamous cell cancer
b) basal skin cancer
c) melanoma
d) dysplastic nevi

320

The posterior fontanel should be completely closed by

a) 3 months
b) 4 months
c) 5 months
d) 6 months

321

Which cranial nerve is being evaluated when Rinne testing is done?

a) CN VII
b) CN VIII
c) CN IX and X
d) CN XI

322

Jane, a middle-aged nurse, complains of localized pain on the sole of her left foot that is located between the 3rd and 4th toes. The pain is aggravated by weight bearing and feels like "a pebble in my shoe." During the physical examination, the nurse practitioner palpates a tender nodule in the metatarsal interspace on the left foot. There is no redness or swelling noted. Which of the following conditions is being described:

a) plantar wart
b) foreign body
c) Morton's neuroma
d) Metatarsalgia

323

Laura, who is 18 years old, is being followed up for acne by the nurse practitioner. During the facial exam, papules and pustules are present mostly on the forehead and the chin areas. The patient has been using prescription topicals and OTC medicated soap daily for 6 months without much improvement. Which of the following would you recommend next?

a) isotretinoin (Accutane)
b) tetracycline (Sumycin)
c) clindamycin topical solution (Cleocin T)
d) minocycline (Minocin)

324

The following statements are all true regarding herpes zoster except?

a) it is due to reactivation of latent varicella virus
b) the typical lesions are bullae
c) it is usually more severe in immunocompromised individuals
d) infection of the trigeminal nerve ophthalmic branch can cause corneal blindness

325

A middle-aged Black male complains of a history of outbreaks of painful large nodules and pustules on both his axillae that resolve after treatment with antibiotics. On physical examination, the nurse practitioner notices large red nodules that are tender to palpation. In addition, several pustules are present along with multiple scars on the skin. The nurse practitioner advises the patient that the condition is caused by a bacterial infection of the sweat glands in the axillae. Which of the following conditions is being described?

a) hidradenitis suppurativa
b) severe nodular acne
c) granuloma inguinale
d) cat scratch fever

326

A possible side effect from the use of nifedipine (Procardia XL) is?

a) hyperuricemia and hypoglycemia
b) hyperkalemia and angioedema
c) edema of the ankles and headache
d) dry hacking cough

327

Which of the following maneuvers is contraindicated in patients with acute prostatitis?

a) massaging the infected prostate
b) serial urine samples
c) rectal exams
d) palpation of the epididymis

328

Erysipelas is an infection of the skin most commonly caused by which of the following class of organisms?

a) streptococci
b) staphylococi
c) gram-negative bacteria
d) fungi

329

What is the first line class of antibiotics recommended by the American Thoracic Society (ATS) for patients younger than 60 years of age who are diagnosed with community-acquired pneumonia with no comorbidity?

a) first generation cephalosporins
b) second generation cephalosporins
c) macrolides
d) beta-lactam antibiotics

330

All of the following are clinical eye findings found in some patients with chronic uncontrolled hypertension. Which of the following findings is not associated with this disorder?

a) AV nicking
b) copper wire arterioles
c) flame-shaped hemorrhages
d) microaneurysms

331

While reviewing some lab reports, the nurse practitioner notes that one of her teenage male patient's lab results is abnormal. The liver function tests are all normal except for a slight elevation in the alkaline phosphatase level. The patient is a member of a soccer team and denies any recent injury. What is the next step in this patient's evaluation?

a) order a liver ultrasound to rule out fatty liver
b) this is a normal finding for his age group
c) the patient needs to be evaluated further for pancreatic disease
d) refer the patient to a pediatric rheumatologist

332

Which of the following would be appropriate initial management of a second degree burn?

a) irrigate with hydrogen peroxide and apply Silvadene cream BID
b) irrigate with normal saline and apply Silvadene cream BID
c) irrigate with tap water and apply Neosporin ointment BID
d) unroof all intact blisters and apply antibiotic ointment BID

333

When molluscum contagiosum is found on the genital area of children, which of the following is the best explanation?

a) it should raise the suspicion of child sexual abuse
b) it is not considered a sexually transmitted disease
c) it is caused by atypical bacteria
d) it is caused by the poxvirus and will resolve on its own

334

An 80-year-old woman complains about her "thin" and dry skin. Which of the following is the best explanation for her complaint?

a) genetic predisposition
b) loss of subcutaneous fat and lower collagen content

c) loss of sebaceous glands
d) damage from severe sun exposure

335

All of the following statements are correct regarding licensure for nurse practitioners except?

a) it ensures a minimum level of professional competency
b) it grants permission for an individual to practice in a profession
c) it requires verification of educational training from an accredited graduate program
d) it reviews information via a nongovernmental agency

336

Which of the following is the correct statement regarding the size of the arterioles and veins on the fundi of the eye?

a) the veins are larger than the arterioles
b) the arterioles are larger than the veins
c) the arterioles are half the size of the veins
d) the veins and the arterioles are equal in size

337

All of the following factors have been found to increase the risk of atrial fibrillation in predisposed individuals except?

a) hypertension
b) excessive alcohol intake in susceptible individuals
c) theophylline (Theodur) and pseudoephedrine (Sudafed)
d) acute esophagitis

338

At what age can a child copy a cross and ride a bicycle?

a) 1 year
b) 2 years
c) 3 years
d) 4 years

339

You would associate a positive iliopsoas muscle test result with?

a) left cerebral vascular accident
b) urinary tract infection
c) heel fractures
d) acute abdomen

340

Which cranial nerve innervates the extraocular muscles of the eyes?

a) CN II, CN III, and CN VI
b) CN III, CN IV, and CN VI
c) CN IV, CN V, and CN VII
d) CN V, CN VI, and CN VIII

341

Which of the following tests would you recommend to patients diagnosed with beta thalassemia or sickle cell anemia?

a) hemoglobin electrophoresis
b) bone morrow biopsy
c) peripheral smear
d) reticulocyte count

342

All of the following patients have an increased risk of developing adverse effects from Metformin (Glucophage) except?

a) patients with renal disease
b) patients with hypoxia
c) obese patients
d) patients who are alcoholics

343

A middle-aged hypertensive male presents to a public health clinic with complaints of an acute onset of fever, chills, and cough that is productive of rusty colored sputum. The patient reports episodes of sharp pains on the left side of his back and chest whenever he is coughing. His temperature is 102.2 degrees Fahrenheit, the pulse is 100/min, and the BP is 130/80. The urinalysis does not show leukocytes, nitrites, or blood. This finding is most consistent with?

a) atypical pneumonia
b) an upper urinary tract infection
c) bacterial pneumonia
d) acute pyelonephritis

344

Lifestyle modifications are an important aspect in the treatment of hypertension. Which of the following statements is incorrect?

a) reduce intake of sodium, potassium, and calcium
b) reduce intake of sodium and saturated fats
c) exercise at least three to four times per week
d) maintain an adequate intake of potassium, magnesium, and calcium

345

Which of the following classes of antihypertensive drugs should a patient be weaned off slowly to avoid the risk of severe rebound hypertension?

a) diuretics
b) beta blockers
c) ACE inhibitors
d) calcium channel blockers

346

A 70-year-old male with open-angle glaucoma is prescribed Betimol (timolol) ophthalmic drops. All of the following are contraindications to Betimol ophthalmic drops except?

a) overt heart failure or sinus bradycardia
b) asthmatic patients
c) second or third degree AV block
d) migraine headaches

347

At what time of the day would you recommend a scotch tape test be done to evaluate for a suspected case of enterobiasis?

a) in the evening after dinner
b) at night before bed
c) early in the morning
d) it does not matter what time of the day the test is done

348

At what age can a child copy a circle and ride a tricycle?

a) 1 year
b) 2 years
c) 3 years
d) 4 years

349

A 30-year-old male patient refuses to take his afternoon dose of pills. The nurse tells him of the possible consequences of his action, but the patient still refuses to cooperate. Which of the following is the best course for the nurse to follow?

a) document in the patient's record his behaviors and the action taken by the nurse
b) reassure the patient that he will be fine after taking the medicine
c) document only the patient behavior
d) document only the nurse's action

SECTION H

350

While performing a sports physical on a 16-year-old girl, the nurse practitioner notes a split S2 during inspiration that disappears during expiration. The girl is active and her growth and development have been uneventful. What is the best recommendation for the child's mother?

a) her daughter needs to be referred to a pediatric cardiologist
b) her daughter needs to be referred for a stress EKG
c) advise the mother that this is a normal finding
d) the child should avoid strenuous physical exertion until further evaluation

351

Patients who are considered mentally competent have a right to consent or refuse medical treatment. What is the legal term for this right?

a) informed consent
b) durable power of attorney
c) competence
d) advanced directives

352

The following statements are true about Wilms tumor except?

a) the most frequent clinical sign is a palpable abdominal mass
b) it is a congenital tumor of the kidney
c) microscopic or gross hematuria is sometimes present
d) the tumor commonly crosses the midline of the abdomen when it is discovered

353

At what level of prevention would you classify screening for lung cancer?

a) primary prevention
b) secondary prevention
c) tertiary prevention
d) screening for lung cancer is not currently recommended

354

Which of the following T-scores is indicative of osteoporosis?

a) T-score of 0 to -1.0
b) T-score of -1.0 to -2.0
c) T-score of -2.5 or less
d) the diagnosis of osteoporosis is based on an X-ray series of the spine

355

Which of the following methods is used to diagnose gonorrheal pharyngitis or proctitis?

a) serum chlamydia titer
b) Gen-Probe
c) Thayer-Martin culture
d) culture and sensitivity of the purulent discharge

356

The first nurse practitioner program was started by?

a) Alfred Bandura
b) President John F. Kennedy
c) Federal government
d) Loretta Ford, PhD

357

Terazosin (Hytrin), an alpha blocker, is used to treat which of the following conditions?

a) benign prostatic hypertrophy and hypertension
b) chronic prostatitis and atrial fibrillation
c) urinary tract infections and arrhythmias
d) benign prostatic hypertrophy and chronic prostatitis

358

A concerned new mother reports to you that her son, who is 3 years of age, is not toilet trained yet. Which of the following is an appropriate reply?

a) recommend a referral to a pediatric urologist
b) advise the mother that her child is developing normally
c) recommend a bed-wetting alarm
d) recommend a voiding cystogram

359

Which of the following clinical findings can mimic a case of testicular torsion but is not considered an emergent condition?

a) the "blue dot" sign
b) one swollen testicle with yellow-colored penile discharge
c) an acute onset of dysuria and frequency
d) a varicocele

360

Which of the following classes of drugs is implicated with blunting the signs and symptoms of hypoglycemia in diabetics?

a) calcium channel blockers
b) diuretics
c) beta blockers
d) ARBs (angiotensin receptor blockers)

361

All of the following factors increase the risk of mortality for patients diagnosed with bacterial pneumonia except?

a) alcoholism
b) very young age or the elderly
c) multiple lobar involvement
d) hypertension

362

The bacteria responsible for the highest mortality in patients with community-acquired pneumonia is?

a) streptococcus pneumoniae
b) mycoplasma pneumoniae
c) moraxella catarrhalis
d) haemophilus influenzae

363

Mr. R. J. is a 40-year-old asthmatic male with hypertension. For the past 6 months, he has been following a low fat, low sodium diet and walking three times a week. His BP readings from the past two visits were 160/95 and 170/100. On this visit, it is 160/90. What is the most appropriate action for the nurse practitioner to follow at this visit?

a) continue the lifestyle modifications and recheck his blood pressure again in 4 weeks
b) initiate a prescription of hydrochlorothiazide 12.5 mg PO daily
c) initiate a prescription of atenolol (Tenormin) 25 mg PO daily
d) refer the patient to a cardiologist for a stress EKG

364

When initially treating an adult for acute bronchitis, which of the following should the nurse practitioner be least likely to order?

a) expectorants
b) antibiotics
c) bronchodilators
d) antitussives

365

All of the following describe normal behavior for a 3-year-old child except?

a) speaks in three- to four-word sentences that are understood by most strangers
b) can draw a cross
c) can draw a circle
d) can ride a tricycle

366

Mary, who has recently been diagnosed with lupus, complains that her hands and feet always feel cold even in the summertime. Sometimes her fingertips become numb and turn a blue color. The fingertips eventually turn to a dark red color. Which of the following is most likely?

a) chronic arterial insufficiency
b) this is a normal reaction when one feels very cold
c) peripheral vascular disease
d) Raynaud's syndrome

367

Mrs. Nottam, who has a BMI of 29, has a 20-year history of primary hypertension. She has been on hydrochlorothiazide 25 mg PO daily with excellent results. On this visit, she is complaining of feeling thirsty all the time even though she drinks more than 10 glasses of water per day. She reports to the nurse practitioner that she has been having this problem for about 6 months. Upon reading the chart, the nurse practitioner notes that the last two fasting blood glucose levels have been 140 mg/dL and 168 mg/dL. A random blood glucose is at 210 mg/dL. Which of the following is the best treatment plan to follow at this visit?

a) order another random blood sugar test in 2 weeks
b) initiate a prescription of metformin (Glucophage) 500 mg PO BID
c) order a 3-hour glucose tolerance test
d) order a HgbA1c level

368

A newly diagnosed middle-aged type 2 diabetic wants to start an exercise program. All of the following statements are true except?

a) if the patient is unable to eat due to illness, antidiabetic agents can be continued with frequent glucose monitoring
b) strenuous exercise is contraindicated for type 1 diabetics because of a higher risk of hypoglycemic episodes
c) exercise increases the body's ability to metabolize glucose
d) patients who exercise vigorously in the afternoon may have hypoglycemic episodes in the evening or at night if they don't eat

369

What is the most common pathogen found in community-acquired atypical pneumonia?

a) *Chlamydia pneumoniae*

b) Streptococcus pneumoniae
c) Moraxella catarrhalis
d) Mycoplasma pneumoniae

370

All of the following are true about strawberry hemangiomas found in infants except?

a) most will involute spontaneously by the age of 18 to 24 months
b) watchful waiting is the most useful strategy
c) hemangiomas should be treated with laser therapy if they have not resolved by the age of 12 months
d) strawberry hemangiomas are benign

371

A 56-year-old mechanic is brought to your office complaining of heavy pressure in the substernal area of his chest that is radiating to his jaw. The pain began while he was lifting up a tire. He now appears pale and is diaphoretic. His blood pressure is 100/60 mmHg, and his pulse rate 50. What is the most appropriate action?

a) perform a 12-lead EKG
b) dial 911
c) administer a morphine injection for pain
d) observe the patient in the office

372

Which of the following is indicated for initial treatment of an uncomplicated case of H. pylori negative peptic ulcer disease?

a) omeprazole (Prilosec)
b) metoclopramide (Reglan)
c) ranitadine (Zantac)
d) Pepto Bismol tablets

373

Erythromycin inhibits the cytochrome P-450 system. The following drugs should be avoided because of a potential for a drug interaction except?

a) theophylline (Theo-Dur)
b) warfarin (Coumadin)
c) diazepam (Valium)
d) furosemide (Lasix)

374

If left untreated, Zollinger-Ellison syndrome can cause which of the following?

a) severe ulceration of the stomach or duodenum
b) toxic megacolon

c) chronic diarrhea

d) malabsorption of fat-soluble vitamins

375

All of the following are considered Category X drugs except?

a) misoprostol (Cytotec)
b) isotretinoin (Accutane)
c) finasteride (Proscar)
d) meperidine (Demerol)

376

You note during a physical exam on a 6-year-old child some pitting on the finger-nails. This finding is correlated with?

a) iron deficiency anemia
b) psoriasis
c) onychomycosis
d) vitamin C deficiency

377

Which of the following is correct regarding the best site to listen for mitral regurgitation?

a) the apical area during S2
b) it is best heard at the base at S1
c) it is best heard at the apex at S1
d) it is best heard at the base at S2

378

Extreme tenderness and involuntary guarding at McBurney's point is a significant finding for possible?

a) acute cholecystitis
b) acute appendicitis
c) acute gastroenteritis
d) acute diverticulitis

379

All of the following may help relieve the symptom(s) of GERD except?

a) losing weight
b) stopping caffeine intake
c) chewing breath mints
d) stopping alcohol intake

380

An 18-year-old waitress is diagnosed with pelvic inflammatory disease (PID). The cervical Gen-Probe result is positive for neisseria gonorrhea and negative for *Chlamydia trachomatis*. All of the following statements are true regarding the management of this patient except?

a) this patient should be treated for chlamydia even though the Gen-Probe for chlamydia is negative
b) Ceftriaxone 250 mg IM and Doxycycline 100 mg PO BID x 14 days are appropriate treatment for this patient
c) advise the patient to return to the clinic for a repeat pelvic exam in 48 hours
d) repeat the Gen-Probe test for *Chlamydia trachomatis* to ensure that the previous test was not a false-negative result

381

What Tanner Stage is a girl at when her breasts form a secondary mound?

a) Tanner Stage II
b) Tanner Stage III
c) Tanner Stage IV
d) Tanner Stage V

382

A 35-year-old smoker is being evaluated for birth control choices. The patient has a history of PID along with an embolic episode after her last pregnancy. Which of the following methods of birth control would you recommend?

a) condoms and the vaginal sponge (Today Sponge)
b) estrogen patches
c) intrauterine device
d) Depo Provera (depot medroxyprogesterone)

383

A 21-year-old woman complains of left-sided pelvic pain accompanied by dyspareunia. During the gynecological exam, the nurse practitioner notices green cervical discharge. The patient mentions a new onset of a painful and swollen left knee and denies a history of trauma. This best describes?

a) septic arthritis
b) Reiter's syndrome
c) chondromalacia of the patella
d) disseminated gonorrheal infection

384

You would recommend the pneumococcal vaccine (Pneumovax) to patients with all of the following conditions except?

a) sickle cell anemia

b) splenectomy
c) patients infected with HIV
d) G6PD deficiency anemia

385

A 40-year-old cashier complains of periods of dizziness and palpitations that have a sudden onset. The EKG shows p waves before each QRS complex and a heart rate of 170 beats/minute. A carotid massage decreases the heart rate to 80 beats/min. These best describe?

a) ventricular tachycardia
b) paroxysmal atrial tachycardia
c) atrial fibrillation
d) ventricular fibrillation

386

A 25-year-old woman complains of dysuria, severe vaginal pruritis, and a malodorous vaginal discharge. Pelvic examination reveals a strawberry-colored cervix and frothy yellow discharge. Microscopic exam of the discharge reveals mobile organisms which have flagella. The correct pharmacologic therapy for the condition is?

a) metronidazole (Flagyl)
b) ceftriaxone sodium (Rocephin)
c) doxycycline hyclate (Vibramycin)
d) clotrimazole (Gyne-Lotrimin)

387

A new mother reports to you that her 6-month-old infant has a cold and has a fever of 99.8 degrees Fahrenheit. The infant is not irritable and is feeding well without problems. She wants to know whether it is okay for him to be immunized at this time. Which of the following statements is true?

a) the infant should not be immunized until he is afebrile
b) an infant with a cold can be immunized at any time
c) an infant with a cold can be immunized as long as his temperature is no higher than 100.4 degrees Fahrenheit
d) because immunization is so important, it should be given to the infant as scheduled

388

Metronidazole (Flagyl) produces the disulfiram (Antabuse) effect when combined with alcoholic drinks or medicine. You would educate the patient to avoid?

a) alcoholic drinks during the time she takes the medicine
b) alcoholic drinks 1 day before, during therapy, and a few days after therapy
c) alcoholic drinks after she takes the medicine
d) there is no need to avoid any food or drink.

389

The treatment plan of patients with AIDS who have CD4 counts of <200/mm should emphasize?

a) administering an MMR vaccine
b) preventative therapy for toxoplasmosis
c) preventative therapy for Pneumocystis carinii pneumonia
d) evaluation of the home environment

390

A positive obturator sign might signify which of the following conditions?

a) acute appendicitis
b) acute pancreatitis
c) acute cholecystitis
d) acute hepatitis

391

Spermatogenesis occurs at the?

a) vas deferens
b) seminal vesicles
c) testes
d) epididymis

392

Prophylaxis for Pneumocystis carinii pneumonia includes all of the following drugs except?

a) Trimethoprim-sulfamethoxazole
b) Dapsone
c) Aerosolized pentamidine
d) Aerosolized albuterol sulfate (ventolin)

393

Mrs. Brands complains of dizziness when she moves her head. You suspect benign paroxysmal positional vertigo. The diagnosis is supported by the presence of?

a) tinnitus
b) horizontal nystagmus with rapid head movement
c) new onset of hearing loss
d) duration of greater than 2 years

394

While performing a routine physical exam on a 60-year-old male, the nurse practitioner notices a soft bruit over the carotid area on the left side of the neck. The patient has a history of hypertension. The patient is at higher risk for?

a) temporal arteritis and brain aneurysms
b) dizziness and headaches
c) abdominal aneurysm and congestive heart failure
d) stroke and coronary heart disease

395

A kindergarten teacher is diagnosed with acute pharyngitis. On exam, the throat is a bright red color with no tonsillar exudate and clear mucus is seen on the lower nasal turbinates. The result of her urinalysis shows a large amount of white blood cells and is positive for nitrites. The patient has a sulfa allergy and thinks she is also allergic to penicillins. Which of the following is the best treatment choice?

a) amoxicillin/clavulanic acid (Augmentin) 500 mg PO BID
b) levoquinolone (Levaquin) 250 mg PO daily
c) trimethoprim sulfamethoxazole (Bactrim DS) 1 tablet PO BID
d) clarithromycin (Biaxin) 500 mg PO BID

396

All of the following drugs interfere with the metabolism of oral contraceptives except?

a) tetracycline
b) rifampin
c) phenytoin (Dilantin)
d) ciprofloxacin (Cipro)

397

When starting an elderly patient on a new prescription of levothyroxine (Synthroid), the nurse practitioner should keep in mind that the rationale for starting an elderly patient on a lower dose is which of the following?

a) due to its central nervous system effects
b) due to its cardiac effects
c) due to its renal effects
d) due to its hepatic effects

398

Women who are pregnant during the winter months are recommended to have which of the following?

a) increased intake of vitamin C and folate
b) vaccination against the influenza virus
c) increased caloric intake of fruits and vegetables
d) heavier winter clothes to avoid chilling the fetus

399

The earliest age that an MMR can be administered is at?

a) 4 months
b) 6 months
c) 8 months
d) 12 months

SECTION I

400

Which of the following is a recommended treatment by the CDC for a case of uncomplicated gonorrheal and chlamydial infection?

a) metronidazole (Flagyl) 250 mg PO TID × 7 days
b) valacyclovir (Valtrex) 500 mg PO BID × 10 days
c) ceftriaxone sodium (Rocephin) 125 mg IM and doxycycline 100 mg BID × 7 days
d) penicillin G procaine (Bicillin) 4.8 million Units IM plus doxycycline hyclate (Vibramycin) 100 mg BID

401

Which of the following factors is a relative contraindication for oral contraceptive pills?

a) active Hepatitis A infection
b) history of an embolic episode that resolved with treatment
c) smoking
d) migraine headache without focal aura

402

A nurse practitioner is taking part in a community outreach program for a local hospital. Most of her audience has a diagnosis of hypertension. They are all interested in learning more about a proper diet. When discussing potential sources of potassium and magnesium, which of the following is the best advice?

a) most fruits and vegetables
b) whole grains and sausages
c) processed corn beef and yogurt
d) mushrooms and sauerkraut

403

A 35-year-old sexually active male presents with a 1 week history of fever and pain over the left scrotum. It is accompanied by frequency and dysuria. The scrotum is edematous and tender to touch. He denies flank pain, nausea, and vomiting. He reports that the pain is lessened when he uses scrotal support briefs. His urinalysis shows 2+ blood and a large number of leukocytes. What is the most likely diagnosis?

a) acute urinary tract infection
b) acute pyelonephritis
c) acute orchitis
d) acute epididymitis

404

Julia M., a 13-year-old patient, is being treated for her first urinary tract infection. Which of the following antibiotics would be contraindicated?

a) cephalexin (Keflex)
b) ampicillin (Amoxil)
c) ofloxacin (Floxin)
d) nitrofurantoin crystals (MacroBid)

405

The mother of a 4-month-old calls your office and reports that the infant has a fever of 101.4 degrees Fahrenheit. The infant received her immunizations yesterday. Which of the following is correct?

a) the fever is most likely due to the combination of the MMR and polio vaccines
b) the fever is most likely due to the pertussis component of the DTP vaccine
c) the infant is probably starting a viral upper respiratory infection
d) the infant had an allergic reaction to one of the vaccines given and should be brought to the emergency room

406

The following statements about benign prostatic hypertrophy are correct except?

a) it is seen in up to 50% of males older than 50
b) dribbling and nocturia are common patient complaints
c) saw palmetto is always effective in reducing symptoms
d) the PSA value is usually slightly elevated

407

Precocious puberty is defined as the onset of secondary sexual characteristics before the age of?

a) age 7 in girls and age 8 in boys
b) age 8 in girls and age 9 in boys
c) age 9 in girls and age 10 in boys
d) age 9 for both girls and boys

408

At what Tanner Stage does puberty start?

a) Tanner Stage I

b) Tanner Stage II
c) Tanner Stage III
d) Tanner Stage IV

409

Orchitis is caused by which of the following?

a) mumps virus
b) measles virus
c) *Chlamydia trachomatis*
d) chronic urinary tract infections that are not treated adequately

410

Acute prostatitis can present with all of the following signs and symptoms except?

a) fever and chills
b) tenderness of the scrotum on the affected side
c) perineal pain
d) slow onset of symptoms

411

Which of the following is the most common cause of nongonococcal urethritis?

a) escherichia coli
b) *Chlamydia trachomatis*
c) neisseria gonorrhea
d) mycoplasma

412

Which of the following is considered a relative contraindication for combined oral contraceptive pills?

a) undiagnosed vaginal bleeding
b) a hepatoma of the liver
c) suspected history of TIAs
d) depression

413

Joe, a 20-year-old Asian male, reports of pain in his right knee after twisting it playing soccer. The injured knee locks up when he attempts to straighten his leg. Which of the following is most likely?

a) injury to the meniscus of the right knee
b) injury to the patella of the right knee
c) injury to the ligaments of the right knee
d) rupture of the quadriceps tendon

414

Which of the following is the best course of treatment for this patient?

a) refer him to an orthopedic specialist
b) refer him to a chiropractor
c) advise him that the clicking noise will resolve within 2 to 4 weeks
d) advise him to use an ACE bandage wrap during the first 2 weeks for knee support and to see you again for reevaluation

415

All of the following are correct statements regarding oral contraceptives except?

a) the actual failure rate of oral contraceptives is 3%
b) desogestrel belongs to the progesterone family of drugs
c) the newer low-dose birth control pills don't require back-up during the first 2 weeks of use
d) oral contraceptives are contraindicated for women 35 years of age or older who smoke

416

A 15-year-old basketball player who is 6 ft tall is seen for complaints of painful lumps on his knees. Upon inspection, the nurse practitioner notes a bonelike growth on the upper tibia midline below the kneecap on both knees. The patient has full range of motion with no joint tenderness, redness, or swelling. Which of the following conditions is best described?

a) osteosarcoma of the tibia
b) juvenile rheumatoid arthritis
c) Osgood-Schlatter disease
d) Paget's disease of the bone

417

A cauliflower-like growth with foul smelling discharge is seen during an otoscopic exam of the left ear of an 8-year-old boy with a history of chronic otitis media. No tympanic membrane or ossicles are visible and the patient seems to have difficulty hearing the nurse practitioner's instructions. Which of the following conditions is best described?

a) chronic perforation of the tympanic membrane with secondary bacterial infection
b) chronic mastoiditis
c) cholesteatoma
d) cancer of the middle ear

418

Sources of legal risk for the nurse practitioner would include all of the following except?

a) invasive procedures

b) electronic medical record entries
c) prescribing medication
d) inservice training

419

The best form of aerobic exercise for a patient with severe rheumatoid arthritis is?

a) walking
b) swimming
c) riding a bicycle
d) passive range of motion

420

The first line treatment consideration for managing acute alcohol withdrawal delirium includes?

a) intubation
b) benzodiazepines
c) avoidance of physical restraints to decrease agitation
d) antipsychotics

421

A 15-month-old infant is in your office for a well baby check. The mother denies history of chickenpox infection. Which of the following immunizations is indicated at this visit?

a) DTaP, Hib, IPV, Hepatitis B
b) DTaP, Hib, PCV, IPV, MMR
c) MMR, Hepatitis B, varicella
d) DTaP, IPV, MMR, varicella

422

All of the following are considered emancipated minors except?

a) 15-year-old male who is married
b) 14-year-old female who is a single parent
c) 17-year-old male who is enlisted in the U.S. army
d) 13-year-old being treated for a sexually transmitted disease

423

All of the following factors are not associated with an increased risk of osteopenia in teenage girls except?

a) drinking one glass of low-fat milk daily
b) anorexia nervosa
c) participation in sports
d) a normal BMI (basal metabolic index)

424

A 28-year-old male nurse tells the employee health nurse practitioner that he was treated for a UTI twice the previous year. The patient denies fever, flank pain, or urethral discharge during the visit. Which of the following is the best follow-up for this patient?

a) refer the patient to a urologist
b) prescribe the patient ofloxacin (Floxin) for 2 weeks instead of 1 week
c) advise the patient that he needs to void every 2 hours when awake
d) refer the patient to the local ER because he has a very high risk of sepsis

425

Henry, a 50-year-old male, complains of marked scalp tenderness accompanied by a bad headache on his left temple. He reports a sudden loss of vision in the left eye for the past several hours. The neurologic exam is normal except for the loss of vision in the left eye. Which of the following is most likely?

a) cluster headache
b) migraine headache with aura
c) migraine headache without aura
d) giant cell arteritis

426

Which of the following diagnostic tests would be most helpful in the diagnosis of this illness?

a) CT scan of the brain
b) cranial nerve exam
c) sedimentation rate
d) CBC with differential

427

A postmenopausal female complains of random episodes of vaginal bleeding for the past 6 months. Which of the following is recommended management for this condition?

a) cervical biopsy
b) pap smear
c) colposcopy
d) endometrial biopsy

428

Which of the following is not a characteristic of delirium?

a) sudden onset
b) patient is coherent
c) worse in the evenings
d) it has a brief duration

429

The signs and symptoms of dementia may include all of the following except?

a) personality changes
b) difficulty in verbalizing
c) difficulty in recognizing familiar objects
d) abstract thinking ability is increased

430

A 4-year-old boy is brought in by his mother for a wellness visit. His mother tells the family nurse practitioner that he had a bad case of chickenpox 1 year ago. Which of the following immunizations are indicated?

a) IPV, Hib (hemophilus influenzae type B), Hepatitis B
b) IPV, Hib, MMR
c) DTaP, IPV, MMR, Hepatitis B
d) DTaP, IPV

431

You are performing a pelvic exam on a 25-year-old sexually active woman. You palpate a tender and warm cystic mass on the lower edge of the left labia majora, which is red. The most likely diagnosis is?

a) Skene's gland cyst
b) cystocele
c) Lymphogranuloma venereum
d) Bartholin's gland abscess

432

Mary Walker is a 16-year-old who presents in the clinic for a physical exam. She tells the triage nurse that she would like contraception as well. How should the nurse practitioner proceed?

a) refuse to see the patient until consent can be obtained from her parent or legal guardian
b) perform a physical exam and discuss contraceptive options
c) speak with the patient about contraception and have her obtain parental consent for the physical exam
d) have the nurse discuss contraception with the patient

433

A patient diagnosed with bacterial vaginosis should be advised that her sexual partner be treated with?

a) ceftriaxone (Rocephin) 250 mg IM with doxycycline 100 mg BID for 14 days
b) metronidazole (Flagyl) 500 mg PO BID for 7 days and one dose of azithromax (Zithromax)

c) her partner does not need treatment

d) clotrimazole cream (Lotrimin) on his penis BID for 1 to 2 weeks

434

All of the following are correct statements regarding physiologic changes found in the elderly with the exception of?

a) there is an increase in the fat-to-lean body ratio

b) there is a decrease in the ability of the liver to metabolize drugs

c) there is an increase in renal function

d) loss of hearing to sounds on the high-frequency range (presbycusis)

435

The following clinical signs are seen in Parkinson's disease except?

a) pill-rolling tremor

b) difficulty initiating involuntary movement

c) shuffling gait with cogwheel rigidity

d) increased facial movements due to tics

436

Which of the following conditions is a possible complication of severe eclampsia?

a) placenta previa

b) placenta abruptio

c) erythroblastosis fetalis

d) uterine rupture

437

A possible complication from Bell's Palsy is?

a) corneal ulceration

b) acute glaucoma

c) inability to swallow

d) loss of sensation in the affected side

438

Which of the following is most likely to cause delirium?

a) dehydration

b) multiple brain infarcts

c) malnutrition

d) acute infection

439

A 25-year-old female presents with an onset of severe right-sided pelvic pain for the past 48 hours. She reports small amounts of vaginal bleeding. The pain is aggravated by jumping or any movement that jars her pelvis. The best initial intervention is which of the following?

a) follicle-stimulating hormone (FSH)
b) serum quantitative pregnancy test
c) pelvic ultrasound
d) CBC with white cell differentials

440

Which of the following laboratory findings may be found elevated alone on the liver function panel of patients who are alcohol abusers?

a) serum GGT (gamma glutamyl transaminase)
b) serum ALT (alanine aminotransferase)
c) serum bilirubin
d) blood urea nitrogen

441

Which of the following effects is seen in every woman using Depo-Provera (medroxyprogesterone injection) for more than 5 years?

a) melasma
b) amenorrhea
c) weight loss
d) headaches

442

The following are treatment plans related to migraine headaches. Which one of the following would not be considered effective therapy?

a) propalanol (Inderal)
b) cold packs to the forehead
c) trimethobenzamide (Tigan)
d) moderate sodium restriction

443

Precocious puberty is defined as?

a) onset of puberty before age 8 in girls and age 9 in boys
b) onset of puberty before age 9 in girls and age 10 in boys
c) onset of puberty before age 10 in girls and age 11 in boys
d) onset of puberty at an earlier age than the child's parent(s)

444

A 19-year-old male athlete complains of acute knee pain after a football game. The nurse practitioner elicits the McMurray's sign, which is positive on the patient's injured knee. This is a test for?

a) meniscal injury

b) inflammation of the knee joint

c) osteophytes of the knee joint

d) tenosynovitis

445

A 35-year-old male has a history of an upper respiratory viral infection 4 weeks ago. He reports that he started feeling short of breath and now complains of sharp pain in the middle of his chest that seems to worsen when he lies down. The patient's physical exam is within normal limits with the exception of a precordial rub on auscultation. The most likely diagnosis would be?

a) pulmonary embolism

b) dissecting aneurysm

c) pericarditis

d) esophageal reflux

446

Which type of exercise would you recommend to a 65-year-old arthritic patient who complains of a new onset of a painful, swollen left knee caused by gardening for 2 days?

a) quadriceps strengthening exercises of the left knee followed by the application of cold packs for 20 minutes four times a day

b) rest the joint and apply cold packs intermittently for the next 48 hours

c) passive range of motion and cold packs

d) a cool tub bath with warm packs on the knee to avoid stiffening of the joint

447

Symptoms suggestive of ulcerative colitis include all the following except?

a) bloody diarrhea mixed with mucus

b) nausea and vomiting

c) weight gain

d) abdominal pain

448

Peak expiratory flow (PEF) meters are used to monitor asthma by using personal best measurements. All of the following factors are used to determine the PEF except?

a) age

b) gender

c) height

d) weight

449

A red, raised serpiginous-shaped rash is noted by the nurse practitioner on the right foot of a 4-year-old child brought in for a preschool physical by the mother.

The child complains of severe itch and keeps scratching the lesion. The mother reports that the child frequently played in the yard without shoes or sandals on. Which of the following is most likely?

a) larva migrans
b) erythema migrans
c) tinea pedis
d) insect bites

450

All of the following are considered risk factors for UTIs in women except?

a) diabetes mellitus
b) diaphragms and spermicide use
c) pregnancy
d) intrauterine device

SECTION J

451

The sentinel nodes (Virchow's nodes) are found at the?

a) right axillary area
b) left supraclavicular area
c) posterior cervical chain
d) submandibular chain

452

Pete J., a 20-year-old White male, is being seen for a physical exam by the nurse practitioner. He complains of pruritic macerated areas in his groin for the past 2 weeks. Which of the following is the most likely?

a) tinea cruris
b) tinea corporis
c) tinea capitis
d) tinea pedis

453

Cluster headaches are most often seen in?

a) adolescent females
b) middle-aged men
c) elderly men
d) postmenopausal women

454

An 18-year-old male is found to have a 47, XXY karyotype and is diagnosed with Klinefelter's syndrome. The patient is most likely to have all of the following physical characteristics except?

a) gynecomastia
b) long limbs
c) lack of secondary sexual characteristics
d) large testes

455

Which of the following drugs can increase the risk of bleeding in patients who are on anticoagulation therapy with warfarin sodium (Coumadin):

a) trimethoprim/sulfamethazole (Bactrim DS)
b) carafate (Sucralfate)
c) losartan (Cozaar)
d) furosemide (Lasix)

456

The mother of a 16-year-old boy is concerned that her son is not developing normally. On exam, you note that he has small testes with no pubic or facial hair. You would advise her?

a) that her son is developing normally
b) that her son is delayed and needs to be evaluated by a pediatric endocrinologist
c) that her son should be rechecked in 3 months
d) her son is developing slowly but is within normal limits

457

Mary, who is 65 years old, comes into the public health clinic for her annual visit. Her last Td booster was 9 years ago. Which immunization(s) would you recommend?

a) influenza vaccine only
b) Td and influenza vaccine
c) pneumococcal and influenza vaccine
d) Td, influenza, and pneumococcal vaccine

458

The cremasteric reflex is elicited by?

a) asking the patient to open his or her mouth and touching the back of the pharynx with a tongue blade

b) hitting the biceps tendon briskly with a reflex hammer and watching the lower arm for movement
c) hitting the patellar tendon briskly with a reflex hammer and watching the lower leg for movement
d) stroking the inner thigh of a male client and watching the testicle on the ipsilateral side rise up toward the body

459

You have diagnosed Tom J., a 30-year-old male, with contact dermatitis on the left side of the face secondary to poison ivy. You would recommend?

a) washing with antibacterial soap BID to reduce risk of secondary bacterial infection until it is healed
b) hydrocortisone cream 1% BID until it is healed
c) clotrimazole (Lotrimin) cream BID for 2 weeks
d) halcinonide (Halog) 1% ointment BID for 2 weeks

460

Pulsus paradoxus is best described as?

a) an increase in systolic blood pressure on inspiration
b) a decrease in diastolic blood pressure on exhalation
c) a decrease in systolic blood pressure on inspiration
d) an increase in diastolic blood pressure on expiration

461

A 10-year-old boy complains of a sudden onset of scrotal pain when he woke up that morning. He is also complaining of severe nausea and vomiting. During the physical examination, the nurse practitioner finds a tender, warm, and swollen left scrotum. The cremasteric reflex is negative and the urine dipstick is negative for leukocytes, nitrites, and blood. The most likely diagnosis is?

a) acute epididymitis
b) a severe salmonella infection
c) testicular torsion
d) acute orchitis

462

What type of follow-up should this patient receive?

a) refer him within 48 hours to a urologist
b) refer him to the emergency room as soon as possible
c) prescribe ibuprofen (Advil) 600 mg QID for pain
d) order a testicular ultrasound for further evaluation

463

Which of the following conditions are possible causes for secondary hypertension?

a) leukemia and thalassemia major
b) Hashimoto's thyroiditis and polycystic ovaries
c) renal stenosis and adrenal tumors
d) myocardial infarction and coronary artery disease

464

What cholesterol level is classified as borderline?

a) 180 to199 mg/dL
b) 200 to 239 mg/dL
c) >240 mg/dL
d) >300 mg/dL

465

You note that your 11-year-old female patient is at Tanner Stage II. You would advise her mother that menarche will probably start in?

a) 1 to 2 years
b) 2.5 to 3 years
c) 4 years
d) it is dependent on the girl's genetic makeup

466

All of the following do not require parental consent to be obtained by the nurse practitioner except?

a) a 17-year-old who wants to be treated for a sexually transmitted infection
b) a 12-year-old who wants a serum pregnancy test
c) a 15-year-old who wants birth control pills
d) a 14-year-old who wants to be treated for dysmenorrhea

467

There is a higher risk of balanitis in which of the following conditions?

a) renal insufficiency
b) diabetes mellitus
c) Graves disease
d) asthma

468

Which of the following is useful in the primary care area when evaluating a patient for possible acute sinusitis or hydrocele?

a) check for the cremasteric reflex
b) transillumination
c) ultrasound
d) CT scan

469

All of the following are associated with emphysema except?

a) a barrel-shaped chest
b) purse-lipped breathing
c) a chest radiograph result with infiltrates and flattening of the costovertebral angle
d) dyspnea when at rest

470

A split S2 is best heard at which of the following areas?

a) the aortic area
b) the pulmonic area
c) the tricuspid area
d) the mitral area

471

Balanitis is caused by?

a) staphyloccocus aureus
b) streptococcus pyogenes
c) candida albicans
d) trichomonads

472

A 22-year-old male is brought to an urgent care center by his anxious mother. She reports that her son returned from a camping trip 2 days ago with a high fever and bad headache. Apparently, the patient had complained to her of a painful and stiff neck along with nausea shortly after he had arrived. According to the mother, her son started breaking out in a rash the day before, some of which is turning a dark red to purple color. During the physical exam, the nurse practitioner evaluates the patient for Kernig's sign, which is positive. Which of the following conditions is most likely?

a) Stevens-Johnson syndrome
b) meningococcemia
c) Rocky Mountain spotted fever
d) erythema multiforme

473

Your newly diagnosed diabetic patient reports to you that she had severe hives and swollen lips when she took Bactrim for a bladder infection 2 months ago. Which of the following statements is correct?

a) she cannot take any pills in the sulfonylurea class
b) she can take some of the pills in the sulfonylurea class
c) she can take any of the pills in the sulfonylurea class
d) none of the above

474

Which of the following is responsible for the symptoms of dysmenorrhea?

a) estrogen
b) human chorionic gonadotropin
c) prostaglandins
d) progesterone

475

Which of the following tests would you order for an older diabetic male with the following CBC results? Hb 11 g/dL, Hct 38%, and an MCV 105 fl. His reticulocyte count is normal:

a) serum ferritin and a peripheral smear
b) hemoglobin electrophoresis
c) serum folate acid and B12 level
d) Schilling Test

476

Auscultation of normal breath sounds of the chest will reveal?

a) bronchial breath sounds heard at the lower bases
b) high-pitched vesicular breath sounds heard over the upper lobes
c) vesicular breath sounds heard over the trachea
d) vesicular breath sounds in the lower lobe

477

The bell of the stethoscope is best used for auscultation of which of the following?

a) S3 and S4 and low-pitched tones
b) S3 and S4 only
c) S1 and S2 and high-pitched tones
d) S1 and S2 only

478

Which of the following is the best method for diagnosing candidiasis in the primary care setting?

a) wet smear
b) Tzanck smear
c) KOH (potassium hydroxide) smear
d) clinical findings only

479

During a sports physical of a 14-year-old female, you note her breast development. The areola and the breast tissue are all in one mound. In which Tanner Stage is this patient?

a) Tanner Stage I
b) Tanner Stage II
c) Tanner Stage III
d) Tanner Stage IV

480

A 13-year-old boy wants to be treated for his acne. He has a large number of closed and open comedones on his face. The patient has been treating himself with OTC benzoyl peroxide and salicylic acid topical products. Which of the following would be recommended next?

a) retinoic acid (Accutane)
b) tetracycline
c) Retin A 0.25% gel
d) wash face carefully with medicated soap at bedtime

481

The Romberg test is done to check for problems with balance. Which area of the brain is responsible for balance?

a) frontal lobe
b) temporal lobe
c) the midbrain
d) the cerebellum

482

All of the following vaccines are contraindicated in pregnant women except?

a) influenza
b) mumps
c) varicella
d) rubella

483

Females with polycystic ovarian syndrome are at higher risk for?

a) heart disease and breast cancer
b) uterine fibroids and ovarian cancer
c) premature menopause
d) PID (pelvic inflammatory disease)

484

A 16-year-old complains of a severe sore throat for 3 days along with a generalized rash and fever. The skin has the texture of fine sandpaper. This best describes?

a) Kawasaki's disease
b) scarlet fever

c) German measles

d) rubeola

485

A college freshman who is on oral contraceptives calls the nurse practitioner's office asking for advice. She forgot to take her pills 2 days in a row during the 2nd week of the pill cycle and wants to know what to do. What is the best advice?

a) start a new pack of pills and dispose of the old one

b) take two pills today and two pills the next day; use condoms for the rest of the cycle

c) stop taking the pills right away and start a new pill cycle in 2 weeks.

d) take one pill now and two pills the next day and use condoms

486

All of the following patients should be screened for diabetes mellitus except?

a) an obese man of Hispanic descent

b) an overweight middle-aged Black woman whose mother has type 2 diabetes

c) a woman who delivered an infant weighing 9.5 lb

d) a 30-year-old White man with hypertension

487

A 40-year-old nurse complains of a new onset of back pain secondary to her job on the medical-surgical floor of a hospital. She reports lifting some obese patients while working the previous night shift. She reports to the workmen's compensation clinic where she was referred. She describes the pain as starting in her right buttocks area and radiating down the back of her thigh. It becomes worse when she sits down for long periods. You would suspect?

a) sciatica

b) acute muscle spasm

c) cauda equina syndrome

d) acute muscle strain

488

A sexually active 22-year-old man is asking to be screened for Hepatitis B because his new girlfriend has recently been diagnosed with Hepatitis B infection. His lab results are the following: anti-HBV is negative, HBsAg is positive, and HBeAg is negative. Which of the following is indicated?

a) the patient is immune to the Hepatitis B virus

b) the patient is not infected with Hepatitis B virus

c) the patient needs hepatitis B vaccine and Hepatitis B immunoglobulin

d) the patient needs only hepatitis B immunoglobulin

489

Three of the following are eye findings associated with chronic uncontrolled hypertension. Which one of the following is associated with diabetic retinopathy?

a) AV nicking
b) copper wire arterioles
c) flame hemorrhages
d) microaneurysms

490

You would advise a patient who is on a MAOI (monoamine oxidase inhibitor) prescription to avoid taking one of the following drugs because of increased potential for a serious reaction. Which of the following is this drug?

a) alprazolam (Xanax)
b) fluoxetine (Prozac)
c) erythromycin (E-mycin)
d) amoxicillin (Amoxil)

491

In the majority of children, the first permanent teeth start to erupt at the age of 6 years. Which of the following are the first permanent teeth to erupt in this time period?

a) first molars
b) second molars
c) lower or upper incisors
d) canines

492

Which of the following pathogenic bacteria are commonly found in the lungs of older children and adults with cystic fibrosis?

a) *streptoccocus pneumoniae*
b) *Chlamydia pneumoniae*
c) *pseudomonas aeruginosa*
d) *staphylococcus aureus*

493

All of the following are physiologic changes that occur in the body as we age. Which of the following is the false statement?

a) the half-life of some drugs is prolonged
b) there is an increase in cholesterol production by the liver
c) there is a mild increase in renal function
d) there is a slight decrease in the activity of the immune system

494

A 15-month-old child who is eating and behaving normally is found to have a high fever. After a few days, the fever resolves and the infant breaks out in a maculopapular rash. This is a description of which of the following conditions?

a) erythema infectiosum
b) roseola infantum
c) fifth disease
d) scarlet fever

495

Which of the following conditions is associated with three stages of rashes?

a) fifth disease
b) erythema infectiosum
c) varicella
d) Rocky Mountain spotted fever

496

Which of the following drug classes is recommended for the treatment of postherpetic neuralgia?

a) TCAs (tricyclic antidepressants)
b) SSRIs (selective serotonin reuptake inhibitors)
c) atypical antidepressants
d) benzodiazepines

497

A new patient who recently visited a relative in North Carolina complains of an onset of fever and red rashes that started 2 days ago. The rash first appeared on the wrist and the ankles and included the palms of the hands. The patient reports that it is spreading toward his trunk. The patient's eyes are not injected and no enlarged nodes are palpated on his neck. There is no desquamation of the skin. Which of the following is most likely?

a) Kawasaki's disease
b) meningococcemia
c) Rocky Mountain spotted fever
d) measles

498

Carpal tunnel syndrome is due to inflammation of the?

a) ulnar nerve
b) radial nerve
c) brachial nerve
d) median nerve

499

The Somogyi effect is characterized by which of the following?

a) it is a complication of high levels of growth hormone
b) it is the physiologic spike of serum blood glucose in the early morning
c) it is characterized by high fasting blood glucose in the morning
d) it is a rare phenomenon that only occurs in type 1 diabetic patients

500

The following findings are considered benign lesions of the skin except?

a) lentigo
b) seborrheic keratosis
c) actinic keratosis
d) rosacea

Answers

SECTION A (1–50)

[1]
b) it inhibits the effect of renal prostaglandins and blunts the effectiveness of the diuretic

[2]
d) *Chlamydia trachomatis*

[3]
b) acute appendicitis

[4]
d) a prescription of methyldopa (Aldomet) to control blood pressure

[5]
c) nursing home care

[6]
b) mycoplasma pneumonia

[7]
c) 10 mm

[8]
d) the patient's spouse has a right to override the durable power of attorney's decisions

[9]
b) the patient has a medical illness that causes an anxiety reaction and denial

[10]
c) beta blockers

[11]
a) perform a complete and thorough history

[12]
b) edema of the face and the upper extremities

[13]
d) tingling and numbness of both feet

[14]
a) order an ultrasound

[15]
c) most diverticula in the colon are infected with Gram-negative bacteria

[16]
b) *Chlamydia trachomatis*

[17]
c) osteoporosis

[18]
b) higher than normal

[19]
a) calcium channel blockers

[20]
a) knee instability

[21]
b) Tanner Stage III

[22]
a) *Toxoplasma gondii*, other infections, rubella, cytomegalovirus, and herpes

[23]
a) laryngeal neoplasia

[24]
c) degenerative joint disease

[25]
b) instability of the knee

[26]
a) advise the mother that her pregnancy is progressing well

[27]
c) from 33 to 35 cm

[28]
b) creatinine

[29]
c) the screening test for the disorder is the barium swallow test

[30]
d) apraxia and fatigue

[31]
a) upon deep inspiration by the patient, palpate firmly in the right upper quadrant of the abdomen below the costovertebral angle

[32]
b) placenta previa

[33]
a) middle-aged to older women

[34]
c) severe vaginal atrophic changes

[35]
b) hepatomegaly, AV nicking, bibasilar crackles

[36]
a) vaginal bleeding and cramping are present, but the cervix remains closed

[37]
b) bacterial vaginosis

[38]
a) call the patient to return to the clinic so she can get tested for a possible cervical infection

[39]
b) lichen sclerosus

[40]
b) closure of the semilunar valves

[41]
b) just rising above the suprapubic bone

[42]
d) anesthesiologist's services

[43]
d) a 17-year-old teen who has only one close friend in school

[44]
d) subconjunctival hemorrhage

[45]
c) advise the patient that it is a benign condition and will resolve spontaneously

[46]
a) urine for culture and sensitivity (C&S)

[47]
d) bedrest on the left side with bathroom priviledges

[48]
b) tonometry

[49]
b) tick

[50]
b) it does not have a linear distribution

SECTION B (51–100)

[51]
c) viral conjunctivitis

[52]
c) urine pregnancy test

[53]
b) S1, S2, and S3

[54]
b) elevation of the affected limb and intermittent applications of cold packs for the next 48 hours

[55]
a) G6PD deficiency anemia

[56]
d) recommend immediate referral to the emergency room (ER)

[57]
a) the mother has autoantibodies against Rh-positive red blood cells (RBCs)

[58]
b) prevent anencephaly

[59]
a) acute pyelonephritis

[60]
b) *Chlamydia trachomatis*

[61]
b) 5 mm

[62]
c) varicella

[63]
a) inevitable abortion

[64]
a) Td and Hepatitis B

[65]
d) during the postpartum period

[66]
d) eyeglasses and routine dental care

[67]
b) Ishihara chart

[68]
b) left-heart failure

[69]
c) furosemide (Lasix)

[70]
a) foods with aspartame (Equal) because they can trigger migraines

[71]
d) prophylaxis is not recommended for this patient

[72]
b) measles

[73]
a) mitral regurgitation

[74]
c) treponema pallidum

[75]
a) placenta

[76]
a) fetal liver

[77]
a) order an ELISA test as soon as possible

[78]
b) order a serum TSH, digoxin level, and an electrolyte panel

[79]
b) pregnancy-induced hypertension (preeclampsia)

[80]
c) elevated serum cortisol levels

[81]
c) incisors

[82]
a) palpation of the fetus and auscultation of the fetal heart tones by the nurse practitioner

[83]
b) blue coloration of the cervix and vagina

[84]
c) apply acetic acid to the penile shaft and look for acetowhite changes

[85]
d) all of the above

[86]
a) paroxetine (Paxil CR)

[87]
b) she should not get pregnant within the next 3 months

[88]
c) obtain a history from the patient and family members

[89]
a) recheck the patient's urine and order a urine for culture and sensitivity

[90]
d) spinach, liver, and whole wheat bread

[91]
b) it is a test to detect antibodies against the HIV

[92]
b) probable sign of pregnancy

[93]
c) at the level of the umbilicus

[94]
b) chronic obstructive pulmonary disease

[95]
b) it is a precancerous lesion and needs to be followed up with her dermatologist

[96]
a) medical information is given to a spouse

[97]
c) presumptive signs of pregnancy

[98]
a) angina pectoris

[99]
b) consult with a cardiologist for further evaluation

[100]
c) transient ischemic attack (TIA)

SECTION C (101–150)

[101]
a) drinking organic juice

[102]
a) acute sinusitis

[103]
b) placenta abruptio

[104]
a) an immune-mediated reaction precipitated by the destruction of a large number of spirochetes due to an antibiotic injection

[105]
b) tell her to return 1 week after her period so her breasts can be rechecked

[106]
a) the blood pressure is higher in the arms than in the legs

[107]
c) a large amount of bacteria coating the squamous cells and very few leukocytes

[108]
d) mitral valve prolapse

[109]
d) renal stenosis

[110]
b) pterygium

[111]
a) discontinue his Pravastatin and order a liver function profile

[112]
b) probable sign

[113]
a) breast buds and some straight pubic hair

[114]
a) inflammation of the median nerve

[115]
c) an increase of up to 50% of the plasma volume in pregnant women

[116]
c) acute viral upper respiratory infection

[117]
d) the effect on platelet function is irreversible and lasts 15 to 20 days

[118]
a) albuterol inhaler (Proventil)

[119]
a) an acute abdomen such as during a ruptured appendix

[120]
b) intravaginal ultrasound

[121]
b) order a hepatitis C PCR (polymerase chain reaction) lab test

[122]
c) cauda equina syndrome

[123]
b) Rovsing's sign

[124]
b) Epstein-Barr virus (EBV)

[125]
d) spina bifida

[126]
a) order a urinalysis and urine for culture and sensitivity (C&S) and treat the patient with antibiotics

[127]
a) they are associated with neurofibromatosis or von Recklinghausen's disease

[128]
c) papilledema

[129]
b) gastroesophageal reflux

[130]
a) cataracts

[131]
c) Alzheimer's disease

[132]
d) leukoplakia and oral cancer

[133]
a) doxycycline (Vibramycin) 100 mg PO BID × 21 days

[134]
a) the Nurse Practice Act of the state where they practice

[135]
b) order a mammogram and refer the patient to a breast surgeon

[136]
c) a child who was born in Japan

[137]
c) this is a normal finding in some young athletes

[138]
c) three risk factors

[139]
d) gastrointestinal problems

[140]
a) atrial fibrillation

[141]
c) a 21-year-old woman who is under treatment for two sexually transmitted infections

[142]
b) congestive heart failure (CHF)

[143]
a) advise the patient that she had a normal exam

[144]
a) the patient can see at 20 ft. what a person with normal vision can see at 30 ft.

[145]
a) Somogyi phenomenon

[146]
a) HCV RNA

[147]
c) check the ankle and brachial blood pressure before and after exercise

[148]
b) montelukast (Singulair)

[149]
c) mitral regurgitation

[150]
b) strabismus

SECTION D (151–200)

[151]
b) advise the mother that this is a normal finding in infants up to 2 months of age

[152]
a) weight

[153]
c) squamous epithelial cells and endocervical cells

[154]
b) a sensation of spinning or rotating

[155]
a) trigeminal neuralgia

[156]
b) yeast infections

[157]
a) imipramine (Elavil)

[158]
d) auscultation

[159]
c) retinoblastoma of the left eye

[160]
c) nongonococcal urethritis

[161]
a) yogurt and sardines

[162]
a) high Vitamin K levels will increase her bleeding time

[163]
b) order a liver function profile

[164]
b) acute drug-induced hepatitis

[165]
d) stop taking the medicine until the lab results are available

[166]
b) a 14-month-old who understands complex commands

[167]
a) keep on monitoring the infant's bilirubin level until it returns back to normal in about 1 week

[168]
a) fever occurs in up to 80% of the patients

[169]
a) angiotensin-converting enzyme (ACE) inhibitors

[170]
a) atrophic vaginitis

[171]
a) peripheral vision

[172]
c) acne

[173]
a) administer a booster dose of the Td vaccine

[174]
d) the left side of the sternum at the fifth ICS by the midclavicular line

[175]
b) the mechanism of breast milk jaundice is still not known

[176]
d) iron deficiency anemia

[177]
a) antinuclear antibody (ANA)

[178]
c) it can be a normal variant if heard on a person age 40 or older

[179]
b) inflammation of the sciatic nerve

[180]
a) eye exam with an ophthalmologist

[181]
d) the patient needs to be evaluated by a dermatologist

[182]
b) it is not always necessary to use a shield for the infant's eyes

[183]
b) degenerative joint disease

[184]
c) macrocytic and normochromic cells

[185]
b) aortic stenosis

[186]
a) hordeolum

[187]
c) propranolol (Inderal)

[188]
b) cluster headache

[189]
d) sucralfate (Carafate)

[190]
a) there is no delay in seeking medical treatment

[191]
a) since she is breastfeeding, the infant does not need any vitamin supplements until he is at least 6 months of age

[192]
c) microcytic anemia

[193]
d) mitral stenosis

[194]
d) scabies

[195]
d) renal system

[196]
d) all of the above

[197]
c) CN XI

[198]
b) obtain a chest X-ray

[199]
c) tertiary prevention

[200]
b) 42-year-old obese woman from Cuba who has been taking Prednisone 10 mg daily for the last 12 years to control her severe asthma

SECTION E (201–250)

[201]
b) lactose

[202]
c) a patient who drinks one cup of wine nightly with dinner

[203]
d) musle tension

[204]
a) lung cancer

[205]
d) macrocytic and normocytic red blood cells

[206]
c) elevated

[207]
b) rheumatoid arthritis

[208]
b) he should not give whole milk to his son until he is at least 12 months of age

[209]
c) indomethacin (Indocin)

[210]
a) loss of joint mobility and renal failure

[211]
b) endocarditis prophylaxis is not necessary

[212]
a) Bouchard's node

[213]
a) diabetes mellitus

[214]
d) initiate a prescription of nicotinic acid (Niacin, Niaspan)

[215]
a) acute pancreatitis

[216]
b) an endoscopy with tissue biopsy

[217]
a) iron-fortified rice cereal

[218]
b) glycosylated hemoglobin level (HbA1c)

[219]
b) a superficial vesicle filled with serous fluid greater than 1 cm in size

[220]
b) give the baby both Hepatitis B vaccine and hepatitis B immunoglobulin

[221]
b) Western blot

[222]
a) condyloma acuminata

[223]
d) low-dose oral contraceptives with at least 20 μg of estradiol (Alesse, Lo-estrin)

[224]
d) ovarian cysts

[225]
d) molluscum contagiosum

[226]
c) microcytic anemia

[227]
b) pelvis

[228]
b) gout

[229]
c) Grade IV

[230]
a) aortic stenosis

[231]
c) Hepatitis C virus

[232]
c) 20 kcal/30 mL

[233]
c) hepatitis B vaccination and hepatitis B immunoglobulin

[234]
d) pregnancy

[235]
a) apical and radial pulses at the same time, then subtracting the difference between the two

[236]
b) bronchiolitis

[237]
a) apply candida or mumps antigen to the right forearm and the PPD on the left forearm and read results in 48 to 72 hours

[238]
d) the Mini Mental Exam

[239]
c) school physicals

[240]
d) serum sodium, potassium, and magnesium

[241]
c) the scotch tape test

[242]
b) chronic hypertension

[243]
c) chronic coughing

[244]
a) Board of Nursing

[245]
a) premedicate himself 20 minutes prior to starting exercise

[246]
a) it is a slow or sudden painless loss of central vision

[247]
c) acute sinusitis

[248]
d) myxedema

[249]
b) fluorescein stain

SECTION F (251–300)

[250]
b) inability to swallow

[251]
c) educate the mother that this is normal during the 1st week or 2 of breastfeeding and the soreness will eventually go away

[252]
c) moderate persistent asthma

[253]
d) psoriasis

[254]
c) antimicrosomal antibody test

[255]
c) bullous impetigo

[256]
a) full-term infant is at birth weight by the 2nd week of life

[257]
b) thyroid stimulating hormone (TSH)

[258]
a) Kernig's maneuver

[259]
a) women 50 years or older

[260]
b) order a 24-hour urine for microalbumin

[261]
a) the destruction of Rh-positive fetal RBCs that are present in the mother's circulatory system

[262]
a) bacterial pneumonia

[263]
b) vesicular breath sounds

[264]
c) < 130/80

[265]
c) a long-acting oral theophylline (Theo-Dur) 200 mg every 12 hours

[266]
a) a patch of leukoplakia

[267]
a) rule out any physiologic cause for the crying spells

[268]
b) mitral stenosis

[269]
d) 37-year-old male biker with a concussion due to a fall who appears slightly agitated and does not appear to understand instructions given by the medical assistant checking his vital signs

[270]
b) decreased mobility of the tympanic membrane as measured by tympanogram

[271]
c) status asthmaticus

[272]
d) varicocele

[273]
d) decreased anxiety and depression are common symptoms of abuse in the elderly

[274]
a) closure of the atrioventricular valves

[275]
d) melanoma

[276]
b) families demonstrate common forms of membership across developmental stages

[277]
a) lymphocytosis and/or atypical lympho-cytes

[278]
a) lateralization to one ear

[279]
d) cheilosis

[280]
c) medroxyprogesterone (Depo-Provera)

[281]
d) these fractures always need surgical intervention to stabilize the joint

[282]
b) increase only the NPH insulin in the morning

[283]
b) cannot play some contact sports because of an increased risk of cervical spine injury

[284]
a) erythema migrans

[285]
a) cimetidine (Tagamet), Lanoxin (digoxin), diphenhydramine (Benadryl)

[286]
d) calcium channel blockers

[287]
d) CN V

[288]
d) barium swallow

[289]
b) the fat pads on an infant's feet can mimic pes planus

[290]
d) avoid foods or drinks that contain alcohol such as cough syrups

[291]
b) an absence seizure (petit mal seizure)

[292]
c) the document's objectives are applicable only to people of the United States of America

[293]
a) call the patient and tell her to return for further testing with a Gen-Probe to rule out infection by chlamydia and gonorrhea

[294]
a) the fundus of the uterus should be at the level of the symphysis pubis

[295]
b) fetal alcohol syndrome

[296]
b) lung cancer

[297]
c) cervical cancer

[298]
a) profound fatigue

[299]
b) hypertrophic cardiomyopathy

SECTION G (301–350)

[300]
a) 6 to 12 cm in the right midclavicular line

[301]
b) Brudzinski's sign

[302]
c) Osgood-Schlatter disease

[303]
d) penicillin (Pen VK)

[304]
b) this is a normal finding

[305]
a) acute cholecystitis

[306]
d) ciprofloxacin (Cipro)

[307]
b) maternal age older than 35 years

[308]
c) lupus erythematosus

[309]
c) pneumococcal (Pneumovax) and influenza vaccines

[310]
c) paroxysms of coughing that is dry or productive of mucoid sputum

[311]
a) arcus senilis

[312]
b) the patient should be evaluated for hyperlipidemia

[313]
a) central vision

[314]
d) second degree burns on the lower arm

[315]
a) second ICS, right sternal border

[316]
b) <130/85

[317]
a) a severe sunburn with blistering

[318]
b) her son's physical development is delayed and needs to be evaluated by a pediatric endocrinologist

[319]
a) squamous cell cancer

[320]
a) 3 months

[321]
b) CN VIII

[322]
c) Morton's neuroma

[323]
b) tetracycline (Sumycin)

[324]
b) the typical lesions are bullae

[325]
a) hidradenitis suppurativa

[326]
c) edema of the ankles and headache

[327]
a) massaging the infected prostate

[328]
a) streptococci

[329]
c) macrolides

[330]
d) microaneurysms

[331]
b) this is a normal finding for his age group

[332]
b) irrigate with normal saline and apply Silvadene cream BID

[333]
a) it should raise the suspicion of child sexual abuse

[334]
b) loss of subcutaneous fat and lower collagen content

[335]
d) it reviews information via a nongovernmental agency

[336]
a) the veins are larger than the arterioles

[337]
d) acute esophagitis

[338]
d) 4 years

[339]
d) acute abdomen

[340]
b) CN III, CN IV, and CN VI

[341]
a) hemoglobin electrophoresis

[342]
c) obese patients

[343]
c) bacterial pneumonia

[344]
a) reduce intake of sodium, potassium, and calcium

[345]
b) beta blockers

[346]
d) migraine headaches

[347]
c) early in the morning

[348]
c) 3 years

[349]
a) document in the patient's record his behaviors and the action taken by the nurse

SECTION H (351–400)

[350]
c) advise the mother that this is a normal finding

[351]
c) competence

[352]
d) the tumor commonly crosses the midline of the abdomen when it is discovered

[353]
d) screening for lung cancer is not currently recommended

[354]
c) T-score of -2.5 or less

[355]
c) Thayer-Martin culture

[356]
d) Loretta Ford, PhD

[357]
a) benign prostatic hypertrophy and hypertension

[358]
b) advise the mother that her child is developing normally

[359]
a) the "blue dot" sign

[360]
c) beta blockers

[361]
d) hypertension

[362]
a) *Streptococcus pneumoniae*

[363]
b) initiate a presciption of hydrochlorothiazide 12.5 mg PO daily

[364]
b) antibiotics

[365]
b) can draw a cross

[366]
d) Raynaud's syndrome

[367]
b) initiate a prescription of metformin (Glucophage) 500 mg PO BID

[368]
b) strenuous exercise is contraindicated for type 1 diabetics because of a higher risk of hypoglycemic episodes

[369]
d) Mycoplasma pneumoniae

[370]
c) hemangiomas should be treated with laser therapy if they have not resolved by the age of 12 months

[371]
b) dial 911

[372]
c) ranitadine (Zantac)

[373]
d) furosemide (Lasix)

[374]
a) severe ulceration of the stomach or duodenum

[375]
d) meperidine (Demerol)

[376]
b) psoriasis

[377]
c) it is best heard at the apex at S1

[378]
b) acute appendicitis

[379]
c) chewing breath mints

[380]
d) repeat the Gen-Probe test for *Chlamydia trachomatis* to ensure that the previous test was not a false-negative result

[381]
c) Tanner Stage IV

[382]
a) condoms and the vaginal sponge (Today Sponge)

[383]
d) disseminated gonorrheal infection

[384]
d) G6PD deficiency anemia

[385]
b) paroxysmal atrial tachycardia

[386]
a) metronidazole (Flagyl)

[387]
c) an infant with a cold can be immunized as long as his temperature is no higher than 100.4 degrees Fahrenheit

[388]
b) alcoholic drinks 1 day before, during therapy, and a few days after therapy

[389]
c) preventative therapy for Pneumocystis carinii pneumonia

[390]
a) acute appendicitis

[391]
c) testes

[392]
d) aerosolized albuterol sulfate (Ventolin)

[393]
b) horizontal nystagmus with rapid head movement

[394]
d) stroke and coronary heart disease

[395]
b) levoquinolone (Levaquin)

[396]
d) ciprofloxacin (Cipro)

[397]
b) due to its cardiac effects

[398]
b) vaccination against the influenza virus

[399]
d) 12 months

SECTION I (401–450)

[400]
c) ceftriaxone sodium (Rocephin) 125 mg IM and doxycycline 100 mg BID for 7 days

[401]
c) smoking

[402]
a) most fruits and vegetables

[403]
d) acute epididymitis

[404]
c) ofloxacin (Floxin)

[405]
b) the fever is most likely due to the pertussis component of the DTP vaccine

[406]
c) saw palmetto is always effective in reducing symptoms

[407]
b) age 8 in girls and age 9 in boys

[408]
b) Tanner Stage II

[409]
a) mumps virus

[410]
d) slow onset of symptoms

[411]
d) *Chlamydia trachomatis*

[412]
d) depression

[413]
a) injury to the meniscus of the right knee

[414]
a) refer him to an orthopedic specialist

[415]
c) The newer low-dose birth control pills do not require back-up during the first 2 weeks of use

[416]
c) Osgood-Schlatter disease

[417]
c) cholesteatoma

[418]
d) inservice training

[419]
b) swimming

[420]
b) benzodiazepines

[421]
d) DTaP, IPV, MMR, varicella

[422]
d) 13-year-old being treated for an STD

[423]
b) anorexia nervosa

[424]
a) refer the patient to a urologist

[425]
d) giant cell arteritis

[426]
c) sedimentation rate

[427]
d) endometrial biopsy

[428]
b) patient is coherent

[429]
d) abstract thinking ability is increased

[430]
d) DTaP, IPV

[431]
d) Bartholin's gland abscess

[432]
c) speak with the patient about contraception and have her obtain parental consent for the physical exam

[433]
c) her partner does not need treatment

[434]
c) there is an increase in renal function

[435]
d) increased facial movements due to tics

[436]
b) placenta abruptio

[437]
a) corneal ulceration

[438]
d) acute infection

[439]
b) serum quantitative pregnancy test

[440]
a) serum gamma glutamyl transaminase

[441]
b) amenorrhea

[442]
d) moderate sodium restriction

[443]
a) onset of puberty before age 8 in girls and age 9 in boys

[444]
a) meniscal injury

[445]
c) pericarditis

[446]
b) rest the joint and apply cold packs intermittently for the next 48 hours

[447]
c) weight gain

[448]
d) weight

[449]
a) larva migrans

[450]
d) intrauterine device

SECTION J (451–500)

[451]
b) left supraclavicular area

[452]
a) tinea cruris

[453]
b) middle-aged men

[454]
d) large testes

[455]
d) trimethoprim/sulfamethazole (Bactrim DS)

[456]
b) that her son is delayed and needs to be evaluated by a pediatric endocrinologist

[457]
c) pneumococcal and influenza vaccine

[458]
d) stroke the inner thigh of a male client and watch the testicle on the ipsilateral side rise up toward the body

[459]
b) hydrocortisone cream 1% BID until it is healed

[460]
c) a decrease in the systolic blood pressure on inspiration

[461]
c) testicular torsion

[462]
b) refer him to the ER as soon as possible

[463]
c) renal stenosis and adrenal tumors

[464]
b) 200 to 239 mg/dL

[465]
a) 1 to 2 years

[466]
d) a 14-year-old who wants to be treated for dysmenorrhea

[467]
b) diabetes mellitus

[468]
b) transillumination

[469]
c) a chest radiograph result with infiltrates and flattening of the costovertebral angle

[470]
b) the pulmonic area

[471]
c) *Candida albicans*

[472]
b) meningococcemia

[473]
a) she cannot take any pills of the sulfonylurea class

[474]
c) prostaglandins

[475]
c) serum folate acid and B12 level

[476]
d) vesicular breath sounds in the lower lobe

[477]
a) S3 and S4 and low-pitched tones

[478]
a) wet smear

[479]
c) Tanner Stage III

[480]
c) Retin A 0.25% gel

[481]
d) the cerebellum

[482]
a) influenza

[483]
a) heart disease and breast cancer

[484]
b) scarlet fever

[485]
b) take two pills today and two pills the next day; use condoms for the rest of the cycle

[486]
d) a 30-year-old White man with hypertension

[487]
a) sciatica

[488]
c) the patient needs Hepatitis B vaccine and Hepatitis B immunoglobulin

[489]
d) microaneurysms

[490]
b) fluoxetine (Prozac)

[491]
a) first molars

[492]
c) *pseudomonas aeruginosa*

[493]
c) there is a mild increase in renal function

[494]
b) roseola infantum

[495]
a) fifth disease

[496]
a) TCAs (tricyclic antidepressants)

[497]
c) Rocky Mountain spotted fever

[498]
d) median nerve

[499]
b) it is the physiologic spike of serum blood glucose in the early morning

[500]
c) actinic keratosis

References

American Diabetes Association. (2006). Standards of medical care in diabetes, 2006. *Diabetes Care, 29*, S4–S42.

American Psychiatric Association. (1994). Diagnostic and statistical manual of mental disorders (4th ed.). Washington, DC: Author.

Anderson, B. C. (1995). *Office orthopedics for primary care*. Philadelphia: W. B. Saunders.

Bates, B., Bickley, L. S., & Hoekelmann, R. A. (1995). *A pocket guide to physical examination and history taking* (2nd ed.). Philadelphia: J. B. Lippincott.

Beers, M. H., & Berkow, R. (Eds.). (1999). *The Merck manual of diagnosis and therapy* (Centennial ed.). Philadelphia: W. B. Saunders.

Behrman, R. E., & Kliegman, R. M. (1998). *Nelson essentials of pediatrics* (3rd ed.). Philadelphia: W. B. Saunders.

Bosker, G. (Ed.). (2000). *Textbook of adult and pediatric emergency medicine*. Atlanta, GA: American Health Consultants.

Brown, K. M. (2000). *Management guidelines for women's health nurse practitioners*. Philadelphia: F. A. Davis.

Centers for Disease Control and Prevention (2006). *Sexually transmitted disease treatment guidelines*. Atlanta, GA: Author.

Centers for Disease Control and Prevention. (2007, April 13) *CDC Rabies*. Retrieved April 27, 2007, from http://www.cdc.gov/ncidod/dvrd/rabies/html

Chernecky, C. C., & Berger, B. J. (2004). *Laboratory tests and diagnostic procedures* (4th ed.). Philadelphia: W.B. Saunders.

Colyar, M. R., & Ehrhardt, C. R. (1999). *Ambulatory care procedures for the nurse practitioner*. Philadelphia: F. A. Davis.

Dambro, M. R. (2006). *Griffith's 5-minute clinical consult*. Philadelphia: Lippincott Williams & Wilkins.

Dunphy, L. M., & Winland-Brown, J. E. (2001). *Primary care: The art and science of advanced practice nursing*. Philadelphia: F. A. Davis.

Family Practice notebook.com. *Vestibular neuritis*. Retrieved March 1, 2007, from http:www.fpnotebook.com/ENT228.htm

Ferri, F. F. (2004). *Ferri's clinical advisor. Instant diagnosis and treatment*. Philadelphia: Mosby.

Fishbach, F. (2000). *A manual of laboratory & diagnostic tests* (6th ed.). Philadelphia: Lippincott Williams & Wilkins.

Gilbert, D. N. (2003). *The Sanford guide to antimicrobial therapy* (33rd ed.). Hyde Park, VT: Antimicrobial Therapy, Inc.

Green, M. (1998). *Pediatric diagnosis. Interpretation of symptoms and signs in children & adolescents* (6th ed.). Philadelphia: W. B. Saunders.

Harruff, R. C. (1994). *Pathology facts.* Philadelphia: J. B. Lippincott.

Harvey, R. A., & Champe, P. C. (2000). Lippincott's Illustrated Reviews. Pharmacology (2nd ed.). Philadelphia: Lippincott Williams & Wilkins.

Hay, W. M. Jr., Hayward, A. R., Levin, M. J., & Sondheimer, J. M. (2001). *Current pediatric diagnosis & treatment* (15th ed.). New York: Lange Medical Books/McGraw-Hill.

Hill, L. N., & Sullivan, L. (1999). *Management guidelines for pediatric nurse practitioners.* Philadelphia: F. A. Davis.

Joint National Committee on Prevention, Detection, and Treatment of High Blood Pressure (JNC). 7th report. Washington, DC: National Heart, Lung, and Blood Institute.

Mayo-Smith, M. F., Beecher, L. H., Fischer, T. L, Gorelick, D. A., Guillaume, J. L., & Hill, A. (2004). Management of alcohol withdrawal delirium. An evidence-based practice guideline. *Archives of Internal Medicine, 164,* 1405–1412.

McGraw-Hill's Access Medicine Web Site (2006). *Disease Screening.* Retrieved March 9, 2007, from http://www.accessmedicine.com/htm

McMinn, R. M. H., Hutchings, R. T., Pegington, J., & Abrahams, P. (1993). *Color atlas of human anatomy* (3rd ed.). St. Louis, MO: Mosby Yearbook.

Mycek, M. J., Harvey, R. A., & Champe, P. C. (2000). *Pharmacology* (2nd ed.). Philadelphia: Lippincott Williams & Wilkins.

National Asthma Education and Prevention Program. (2003). *Expert panel report: Guidelines for the diagnosis and management of asthma.* Washington, DC: National Heart, Lung, and Blood Institute.

National Cholesterol Education Panel. (2002). *Third report of the expert panel on detection, evaluation, and treatment of high cholesterol in adults (Adult treatment panel III).* Washington, DC: National Heart, Lung, and Blood Institute.

Nicoll, D., McPhee, S. J., & Pignone, M. (2004). *Pocket guide to diagnostic tests.* (4th ed.). New York: Lange Medical Books/McGraw-Hill.

Papadakis, M. A., & McPhee, S. J. (Eds.) (2005). *Lange 2005 current clinical consult: Medicine.* New York: Lange Medical Books/McGraw-Hill.

Robbins, S. L., Cotran, R. S., Kumar, V., & Collins, T. (1999). *Robbins pathologic basis of disease* (6th ed.). Philadelphia: W. B. Saunders.

Schwartz, M.W. (Ed.) (2000). *The 5-minute pediatric consult.* (2nd ed.). Philadelphia: Lippincott Williams & Wilkins.

Seidel, H. (2003). *Mosby's guide to physical examination* (3rd ed.). St. Louis, MO: Mosby.

Sinclair, C. (2004). *A midwife's handbook.* St. Louis, MO: W. B. Saunders.

Tierney, L. M. Jr., McPhee, S. J., & Papadakis, M. A. (Eds.). (2005). *Current medical diagnosis & treatment* (44th ed.). New York: Lange Medical Books/McGraw-Hill.

Tierney, L. M. Jr., Saint, S., & Whooley, M. A. (2002). *Essentials of diagnosis & treatment.* New York: Lange Medical Books/McGraw-Hill.

United States Department of Health and Human Services. (2003). *OCR privacy brief: Summary of the HIPAA privacy rule.* Washington, DC: Author.

United States Preventative Task Force. (2002). *The guide to clinical preventative services: Report of the United States preventative task force* (3rd ed.). Washington, DC: International Medical Publishing.

United States Public Health Service. (2005). Updated guidelines for the management of occupational exposure to HIV and recommendations for postexposure prophylaxis. *Morbidity and Mortality Weekly Report, 54(RR09),* 1–17. (September 30) Retrieved March 23, 2006, from http://www.cdc.gov/mmwr/preview/mmwrhtml/tt5409a1.htm

Vennes, D. B., Biderman, A., Adler, E., Fenton, B. G., & Enright, A. D. (Eds.). (2005). *Taber's encyclopedic medical dictionary.* Philadelphia: F. A. Davis.

Willms, J. L., Scheiderman, H., & Algranati, P. S. (1994). *Physical diagnosis. Bedside evaluation of diagnosis and function.* Baltimore: Williams & Wilkins.

Index

abortion, spontaneous, 203–204
abuse-related topics, in the exam, 33–34, 324, 336
acne, 76–77
acquired immunodeficiency syndrome (AIDS), 281
actinic keratoses, 63
acute appendicitis, 135–137
acute asthmatic exacerbation, 113
acute bacterial meningitis, 158–159, 162
acute bronchitis, 118–119, 270
acute cellulitis, 68–69, 320
acute closed-angle glaucoma, 79
acute gastritis, 276
acute hemorrhage, 151
acute leukemia, 150
acute lymphocytic leukemia (ALL), 150–151
acute mononucleosis (infectious mononucleosis), 302, 326
acute musculoskeletal injuries, 253
acute otitis media (AOM), 87–89
acute pharyngitis, 348
acute prostatitis, 148, 172, 243, 336, 362
acute pyelonephritis, 144–149, 202, 281
acute sinusitis, 81, 87, 89, 280, 319, 363
Adam's Forward Bend test, 230–231
adolescence, 41, 43–46
    danger signals
        Legg-Calvé-Perthes disease (Perthe's disease), 224
        suicidal and/or homicidal teenager, 224–225
        testicular torsion, 224
    disease review
        delayed puberty, 229–230
        gynecomastia, 228–229, 361
        idiopathic scoliosis, 230
        Klinefelter's syndrome, 230, 361
        Osgood-Schlatter disease, 234–235
        Turner's syndrome, 230
    immunizations, 227, 282, 308–309
    laboratory tests, 227
    legal issues with treatment, 228, 363
    normal findings
        adolescence, 225
        boys, 226
        girls, 225–226
        puberty, 225
advance directives, 265
alcoholism, 312, 329
allergic rhinitis, 67, 81, 86, 88, 271, 293
alpha fetoprotein (AFP) values, 193, 272
Alzheimer's disease, 235, 237–238, 287
American Thoracic Society (ATS) Guidelines for bacterial pneumonia,116–117, 335
anaphylactic episodes, management of, 16
anemia, 77, 128, 272, 280, 287, 292–293, 306, 310, 314–316, 338, 346–347
anti-hepatitis C virus (HCV), 301
antihypertensive medications, 299
asthma, 67, 98, 113, 119, 122–124, 271, 283, 295, 309, 320
atopic dermatitis, 67, 78, 279
atrial fibrillation, risk of, 98–99, 109, 298
atrophic macular degeneration, of the aged (AMD), 318–319
atrophic vaginitis, 190–191
atypical pneumonia, 117–118
Auspitz sign, 66, 320

Bacillus anthracis (anthrax), 331
bacterial pneumonia, 115–117, 322
bacterial vaginosis (BV), 182, 191, 276
balanitis, 134, 363
Barlow's test, 22–221
B12 deficiency anemia, 155, 272

Bell's Palsy, 166–168, 319, 357
beta thalassemia minor, 280
bites: human and animal, 69–70
blue dot sign, 242, 244 , 341
Bouchard's nodes (PIP), 250
breast cancer, 179
breastfeeding mastitis, 205
Budget Reconciliation Act of 1989 (HR 3299), 264
bullae, 63, 71, 78, 313
burns, 77–79, 332–333

café au lait spots, 208, 295
CAGE test, 34–35, 257
candida vaginitis, 188
candidiasis, 68
cardiovascular system
  abnormal findings
    aortic area, 97
    mitral area, 96
    murmur timing and location, 96
    pathologic murmurs, 96
    pulmonic area, 96
  Basal Metabolic Index (BMI) criteria, 103
  benign variants
    benign S4 in the elderly, 95
    benign split S2, 95
    clinical tips, 95
    exam tips, 95
    grading system for murmurs, 95–96
    locations of the ausculatory areas, 95
  clinical tips
    congestive heart failure, 105–106
    deep vein thrombosis (DVT), 106
    locations of the ausculatory areas, 95
  danger signals
    acute abdominal aneurysm, 92
    acute MI (myocardial infarction), 92
    bacterial endocarditis, 93
    congestive heart failure (CHF), 92–93
  disease review
    atrial fibrillation, 98–99
    hypertension, 98–100
    pulsus paradoxus, 98
  exam tips, 95
    ACE inhibitors, 105
    American Heart Association: therapeutic lifestyle changes diet, 111
    atrial fibrillation, 109
    bacterial endocarditis, 108
    benign variants, 95
    bile acid sequestrants, 112
    BMI calculation factors, 102–103
    cholesterol level, 110
    compelling indicators, 101–102
    eye findings, 100–101
    fibrates, 112
    HMG CoA Reductase Inhibitors (statins), 111–112
    hyperlipidemia, 110

    infective endocarditis prophylaxis, 109–110
    list of cardiac arrhythmias, 109
    medications and patient education, 111
    mitral valve prolapse (MVP), 109–110
    mnemonic devices, 98
    nicotinic acid, 112
    paroxysmal atrial tachycardia (PAT), 109
    risk factors for heart disease, 110–111, 299–300
    treatment goals, 111
    treatment plan, 111
  Hypertension Diagnosis and Management: JNC 7 Treatment Guidelines, 101
  medications, 103–105
  mnemonic devices
    aortic stenosis, 97
    MR (mitral regurgitation), 97
    MR TRAS, 97
    MS. PRAR, 97
  normal findings
    anatomy, 93
    deoxygenated blood, 93
    normal heart sounds, 94
    oxygenated blood, 93
    stethoscope skills, 94
    systole and diastole, 93–94
carpal tunnel syndrome (CTS), 168–179
cataracts, 82
cauda equina syndrome, 253, 294
cavernous hemangiomas, 208
Chadwick's sign, 198, 286
chalazion, 84
cheilosis, 77
chest X-ray films/electrocardiogram strips, analysis of, 28
chlamydia trachomatis, 170–171, 272, 281, 346
chronic bronchitis, 295
chronic obstructive pulmonary disease (COPD), 114–115, 288
classic textbook presentation, of disease, 22–23, 48–49
clock drawing test, 236
cluster headache, 165, 307, 360
colon cancer, 135, 234
  screening, 60
common cold, 87–88
complex sentence analysis, 18–19
condyloma acuminata (genital warts), 174, 177–178, 314
congenital glaucoma, 278
congenital heart disease, 109, 227, 279–280
congenital hip dysplasia, 220
contact dermatitis, 67–68, 78, 362
Coombs test, 202, 280
corneal abrasion, 79, 83, 319
cover/uncover test, 300
Crohn's disease, 135
Cullen's sign, 141, 312
cutaneous larva migrans, 223

Dawn phenomenon, 134
degenerative joint disease (DJD or osteoarthritis), 250, 274, 306
delayed puberty, 225–226, 229–230
delirium, 235–237, 257
dementia, 155, 235–239, 257, 265, 356
dermatology
  benign variants
    lipoma, 64
    melasma (mask of pregnancy), 64
    nevi (moles), 64
    seborrheic keratoses, 65
    vitiligo, 65
    xanthelasma, 65
    xerosis, 65
  clinical tips, 79
  danger signals
    actinic keratoses, 63
    erythema migrans (early Lyme disease), 62
    erythema multiforme, 63
    melanoma, 63
    meningococcemia, 62
    Rocky Mountain spotted fever, 62
    shingles infection of the trigeminal nerve, 62
    Stevens-Johnson syndrome, 63
developmental theory, of family, 324–325
  disease review
    acne vulgaris (common acne), 76
    actinic keratosis, 66
    acute cellulitis, 68–69
    bites: human and animal, 69–70
    burns, 77–78
    candidiasis, 68
    cheilosis, 77
    contact dermatitis, 67–68
    eczema (atopic dermatitis), 67
    erysipelas, 69
    erythrema migrans (early Lyme disease), 72
    herpes zoster (shingles), 72–73
    hidradenitis suppurativa, 70
    impetigo, 71
    meningococcemia, 71–72
    mild acne, 76
    moderate acne, 76
    onychomycosis (nails), 76
    psoriasis, 66
    ptyiasis rosea, 73
    Rocky Mountain spotted fever, 72
    rosacea (acne rosacea), 77
    scabies, 73–74
    severe cystic acne, 77
    tinea barbae (beard area), 76
    tinea capitis (scalp), 75
    tinea corporis or tinea circinata (ringworm of the body), 75
    tinea cruris (jock itch), 75
    tinea infections (dermatophytoses), 75
    tinea manuum (hands), 76
    tinea pedis (athlete's foot), 75
    tinea versicolor, 67
  exam tips, 78–79
  normal findings
    anatomy of skin, 63
    skin lesion review, 64
    vitamin D synthesis, 63
  topical steroids, 65–66
diabetes mellitus, 68, 101, 363
  acarbose (precose), 133
  antidiabetic agents, 132
  biguanides, 133
  clinical tips, 134–135
  complications, 134
  Dawn phenomenon, 134
  diagnosis methods, 130–131
  dieting and illnesses, 131
  exam tips, 134
  exercise, 132
  eye findings, 132–133
  foot care, 132
  glycemic parameters, 130
  hypoglycemia, 131
  impaired glucose tolerance, 131
  lab tests, 132
  management, 134
  repaglinide (prandin), 133
  as risk factor, 147
  sulfonylureas, 132–133
  target organs, 130
  treatment goals, 131
  type 1 diabetes, 126, 130
  type 2 diabetes, 130, 313
diabetic retinopathy, 81, 134
differential diagnoses, 46–47, 156, 284, 291, 314
disseminated gonococcal disease (disseminated gonorrhea), 170
diverticulitis, 140
  related questions, 272
Down's syndrome, 296, 324, 326, 331
drawer sign, 248–249, 274
drugs, related questions, 23–25, 53–54, 283, 299, 302, 308, 311, 327, 331, 339, 341–342, 344–345, 348–349
dysmenorrhea, 328, 365

ectopic pregnancy, 136, 179–180
eczema (atopic dermatitis), 67–68
ELISA test, 175, 177, 284, 314
emphysema, 114, 366
endocrine system
  danger signals
    hyperprolactinemia, 126
    pheochromocytoma, 126
    severe hypoglycemia, 125
    thyroid cancer, 126
    type 1 diabetes mellitus, 126

endocrine system (*cont.*)
  disease review
    diabetes mellitus, 126–127
    Graves' disease, 128–129
    Somogyi effect (rebound hyperglycemia), 135
  normal findings
    hypothalamus (master gland), 126
    pituitary gland, 127
  screening tests, 127–128
epicondylitis, 254
epistaxis (nosebleeds), 87, 150
erysipelas, 69, 335
erythema migrans (early Lyme disease), 62
erythema multiforme, 63, 66
erythema toxicum "infant acne," 207
erythrema migrans (early Lyme disease), 72
exam tips
  for ANCC and AANP exams, 9–11
  calming technique, 13
  for the day of exam, 14
  emotional readiness, 13
  identification issues, 14
  for maximizing scores, 11–12
  for night before exam, 14
  testing center details, 13–14
  time management, 12–13
eyes, ears, nose and throat
  abnormal physical findings
    cataracts, 82
    diabetic retinopathy, 81
    evaluation and testing, 82–83
    hairy leukoplakia, 82
    hypertensive retinopathy, 81
    Koplik spots, 82
    leukoplakia of the tongue, 82
    papilledema, 81
    vocabulary, 82
  benign variants
    fishtail or split uvula, 81
    nystagmus, 81
    torus palatinus, 81
  danger signals, 79–80
  disease review
    acute mononucleosis (infectious mononucleosis),
      91–92
    acute otitis media (AOM), 88–89
    acute sinusitis (acute rhinosinusitis), 89–90
    allergic rhinitis, 86–87
    chalazion, 84
    common cold, 87–88
    epistaxis (nosebleeds), 87
    herpes keratitis, 83
    hordeolum (stye), 83–84
    macular degeneration, 86
    otitis externa (swimmer's ear), 90–91
    pinguecula, 84
    primary angle-closure glaucoma, 85–86
    primary open-angle glaucoma, 85
    pterygium, 84

      rhinitis medicamentosa, 90
      subconjunctival hemorrhage, 84–85
    exam tips, 92
    normal findings, 80–81
    practice questions, 278–279, 291, 295, 298–302,
      305–307, 325, 327, 330, 332, 336–338, 349, 355,
      366, 368

factoid questions, 36–37
Family Systems Theory, 267
faun tail nevus, 208
faun tail nevus sign, 208, 294
fibrocystic breast, 190
fifth disease (erythema infectiosum), 221, 223
fishtail or split uvula, 81
Fitz-Hugh-Curtis syndrome (perihepatitis), 173, 281
focal migraines, 163–164
folate deficiency anemia, 128, 152, 235, 310
folic acid deficiency anemia, 156–157
folic acid supplementation, 281
food-related questions, 51–52
Form E of ANCC, 3
fundal heights, 199, 274

gastroesophageal reflux disease (GERD), 139–140, 295
gastrointestinal system
  benign variants, 136
  danger signals
    acute appendicitis, 135
    colon cancer, 135
    Crohn's disease, 135–136
    intussusception, 136
    pyloric stenosis, 136
    Zollinger-Ellison syndrome, 135
  disease review
    acute hepatis, 143–144
    acute pancreatitis, 140–141
    diverticulitis, 140–141
    gastric ulcer and duodenal ulcer disease, 138
    gastroesophageal reflux (GERD), 139–140
    Helicobacter pylori-ulcers, 139
    irritable bowel syndrome (IBS), 137–138
    viral hepatitis, 141–142, 145
  exam tips
    acute hepatitis, 144
    gastroesophageal reflux (GERD), 140
    Helicobacter pylori-ulcers, 139
    viral hepatitis, 145
  normal findings, 136
geriatrics
  danger signals
    actinic keratosis (precursor of squamous cell
      carcinoma), 232
    cerebrovascular accident (CVA), 232
    fractures of the hip, 232–233
    temporal arteritis (giant cell arteritis), 232
  disease review
    Alzheimer's disease, 238
    delirium, 237

dementia, 237
Parkinson's disease, 238
normal findings
arcus senilis (corneal arcus), 233
cardiac, 233
clinical tips, 239
drug effects, 235
endocrine, 234
exam tips, 238
gastrointestinal system (GI), 234
hematology, 235
immune system, 235
lentigines, 233
liver, 234
lungs, 234
musculoskeletal system, 234
presbyacusis (sensorineural hearing loss),
233
renal function, 234
seborrheic keratoses, 233
senile purpura, 233
sex hormones, 235
skin, 233
practice questions, 291, 304, 319, 334, 338
screening for dementia
clock drawing test, 236
exam tips, 235
mini-mental exam (MME), 236
gestational diabetes, 202
gold standard tests, 28–30
gonadotropin, 194, 229, 272, 284
gonorrhea, 171–173, 243, 274, 328, 346, 352
gonorrheal pharyngitis or proctitis, 341
gout, 252, 311, 315
gram stain test, 116, 162, 173, 183
Graves' disease, 128–129, 286
gynecology
danger signals
breast cancer, 179
ectopic pregnancy, 179
ovarian cancer, 180
disease review
atrophic vaginitis, 190–191
bacteria vaginosis (BV), 189–190
candida vaginitis, 188–189
fibrocystic breast, 187–188
osteoporosis, 191–192
polycystic ovary syndrome (PCOS), 188
trichomonas vaginitis (Trichomoniasis), 190
vaginal infections, 192
hormone replacement therapy (HRT) or estrogen
replacement therapy (no uterus), 182
laboratory procedures
gram stain, 182
KOH (potassium hydroxide) slide, 182
Pap smears, 182
Tzanck smear, 182–183
menopausal body changes
labia and vagina, 181

ovaries, 181
urethra and bladder, 181–182
normal findings
breasts (specialized sweat glands),
182
cervix, 182
menarche, 182
menopause, 183
menstrual cycle, 182–183
ovaries, 182
perimenopause, 183
oral contraceptives, 316
absolute contraindications, 183
clinical tips, 190
contraindications, 188
decreased incidence, 186
depo provera (depot medroxyprogesterone) 0.03%
failure rate, 186
diaphram with contraceptive gel, 188
drug interactions, 187
emergency contraception, 188
exam tips, 186, 189
IUD (intrauterine device), 188
male/female condoms, 189
missing consecutive days, 187
mnemonic device "My CUPLETS," 186
new prescriptions, 187
pill danger signals, 187–188
pill problems, 187
relative contradictions, 186
risk factors, 188–189
Paget's Disease of the Breast (ductal carcinoma in
situ), 179
practice questions, 292, 298–299
supranumerary nipples, 187
gynecomastia, 228–229

hairy leukoplakia, 82
Hashimoto's disease, 275, 320, 331
Health Belief Model, 266
health care organizations, 267
health screening recommendations, 59–60
Healthy People 2010 objectives, 328
heart murmurs, grading of, 38, 93, 95–96, 291, 299–300,
306, 312, 315, 323
Heberden's nodes (DIP), 250, 276, 308, 313
Hegar's sign, 198, 287
Helicobacter pylori infection, 138–139, 313
HELLP syndrome (hemolysis, elevated liver enzymes,
and low platelets), 192
hematology/blood disorders
benign variants, 154
danger signals
acute hemorrhage, 151
acute leukemia, 150
acute lymphocytic leukemia (ALL), 150
hemolytic disease of the newborn, 150
Hodgkin's lymphoma/disease, 150
neutropenia, 150

hematology/blood disorders (*cont.*)
  non-Hodgkin's lymphoma, 150
  thrombocytopenia, 150
  vitamin B12 deficiency, 151
diagnostic lab anemia, 155
disease review
  folic acid deficiency anemia, 156–157
  iron deficiency anemia, 153–154
  macrocytic/megaloblastic anemias, 155–156
  microcytic anemias, 151
  thalassemia minor/trait, 154–155
exam tips, 156–158
laboratory testing, 152–153
practice questions, 293
hemoglobin and hematocrit screening, in infants,
  209–210, 313, 338
hemolytic disease, of the newborn, 150
hepatitis virus infection, 141–144, 315
herpes keratitis, 79, 83
herpes simplex: HSV1 and HSV 2, 167, 178–179
herpes zoster (shingles), 72–73, 161, 222, 334
hidradenitis suppurativa, 70
Hodgkin's lymphoma/disease, 117, 150
hordeolum (stye), 83–84
HPV (human papilloma virus) infection, 177–178, 273,
  286
human chorionic gonadotropin (hCG), 194, 272,
  284
human immunodeficiency virus (HIV), 68, 170,
  175–177
human papilloma virus infection, *see* HPV (human
  papilloma virus) infection
hydrochlorothiazide, therapeutic effects of, 269, 297,
  342
hypertensive patients, 276, 285, 295
hypertensive retinopathy, 81
hypovolemic shock, 315

idiopathic scoliosis, 230–231
iliopsoas muscle test, 337
illicit drugs, 260
impetigo, 64, 71–72, 74, 223, 308, 320
informed consent, 265
internal tibial torsion, 220, 325
intussusception, 136
iron deficiency anemia, 21–22, 77, 135, 151–155, 157,
  184, 210, 305, 345
isometric exercise, 247–248, 280

Jarisch-Herxheimer reaction, 173, 290
JNC 7 guidelines, 36, 101, 303, 322, 333
Jones criteria, for pelvic inflammatory disease (PID),
  172–173

Kawasaki disease, 222–223
Klinefelter's syndrome, 230, 361
KOH (potassium hydroxide) slide test, 182,
  286
Koilonychia, 153, 305

Koplik's spots, 224, 283
Kyphosis, 234, 272

laboratory and diagnostic tests, 25–27
Lachman maneuver, 273
Lachman sign, 248–249
lead screening test, for infants, 208–209
left ventricular hypertrophy, 94–95, 100, 102, 318,
  329
legal issues, related to health care, 46, 264–265
Legionnaire's disease, 270
leukoplakia of the tongue, 82, 170, 329
lipoma, 64
living will, 265
low back pain, 180, 240, 245, 252–253, 294
lyme disease, 62, 72, 74, 167, 296, 302
lymphogranuloma venereum (LGV), 179, 281

macrocytic/megaloblastic anemias, 155–156
macular degeneration, 86, 318, 332
major depression, 31–32, 256, 258
mammography, 59
McMurray's sign, 249, 358
Medicare services, 262, 264, 266, 270, 277,
  282
melanoma, 63–64, 324, 333
melasma (mask of pregnancy), 64
meningococcemia, 62, 71–72, 78, 326, 364, 369
meniscus tear (of knees), 254
menopause, 181, 187, 235, 276, 366
men's health
  danger signals
    priapism, 240
    prostate cancer, 240
    testicular cancer, 240
    testicular torsion, 239–240
  disease review
    acute bacterial epididymitis, 244
    acute prostatitis, 244–245
    benign prostatic hypertrophy (BPH), 242–243
    blue dot sign (testicular appendage torsion),
      242
    chronic prostatitis, 243
    erectile dysfunction (ED), 245
    prostate cancer, 242
    testicular cancer, 241
  normal findings
    cremasteric reflex, 241
    epididymis, 241
    prostate gland, 240
    spermatogenesis, 240
    testes, 241
    transillumination: scrotum, 241
mental health
  abuse
    child, 261
    exam tips, 262
    physical examination, 261
  danger signals, 255

disease review
  alcoholism, 256–257
  anorexia nervosa, 258
  delirium tremens, 257
  Korsakoff's syndrome, 257
  major depression, 256
psychotropic drugs
  acute serotonin syndrome, 259
  benzodiazepines, 259
  clinical tips, 260
  exam tips, 260
  illicit drugs, 260
  monoamine oxidase inhibitors (MAOI), 259
  nicotine patches, 259
  selective serotonin reuptake inhibitors (SSRIs), 258–259
  smoking cessation, 259
  tricyclic antidepressants (TCAs), 259
metformin (Glucophage) therapy, 297
microcytic anemias, 151, 153
microscopic hematuria, 291
migraine headaches (with or without aura), 162–163, 183
milia, miliaria or "prickly heat," 207
mini-mental exam (MME), 159, 236
mitral regurgitation, 94, 97, 284, 300, 308, 323, 345
mitral valve prolapse (MVP), 108–112, 283, 291, 308, 312, 318
mnemonic devices
  aortic stenosis, 97
  HEARS, 209
  MR (mitral regurgitation), 97
  MR TRAS, 97
  MS. PRAR, 97
  MS. SPAIN, 17
  My CUPLETS, 183
  RICE, 248, 254–255
  SOAPE, 19–20
molluscum contagiosum: poxvirus, 74, 223–224, 314, 336
Mongolian spots, 207–208
Munchausen's syndrome, 271, 290
Murphy's sign, 275, 294, 321
muscle tension headache, 165–166
musculoskeletal system
  benign variants, 247
  danger signal
    hip fracture, 246
    navicular fracture, 246
    pelvic fracture, 246
  disease review
    acute musculoskeletal injuries, 253
    Bouchard's nodes (PIP), 250
    cauda equina syndrome, 253
    degenerative joint disease (DJD or osteoarthritis), 250
    epicondylitis, 254
    gout, 252
    Heberden's nodes (DIP), 250
    low back pain, 252–253
    meniscus tear (of knees), 254
    rheumatoid arthritis (RA), 251
    ruptured baker's cyst (bursitis), 255
    sprains, 254
    tendonitis, 254
  exam tips, 247, 250–253, 255
  exercise and injuries, 247–248
  normal findings, 247
  orthopedic maneuvers, 248–249
mycoplasma pneumonia, 115, 117, 270, 284, 342,

negative polarity questions, 39–40
neisseria gonorrhea (GC), 171–173, 176, 183, 243, 346, 352
nervous system
  benign variants, 162
  danger signals, 158–159
  disease review
    abortive treatment, 163
    acute bacterial meningitis, 158–159, 162
    Bell's palsy, 166
    carpal tunnel syndrome (CTS), 168–169
    cluster headache, 166
    contraindications (vasoconstricting drugs), 163
    focal migraines, 163
    migraine headaches (with or without aura), 162–163
    muscle tension headache, 165–166
    prophylactic treatment, 163
    temporal arteritis (giant cell arteritis), 158, 164
    trigeminal neuralgia (tic douloureux), 164–165
  exam tips
    on cranial nerves, 161
    focal migraines, 164
    muscle tension headaches, 166
    temporal arteritis (giant cell arteritis), 164
    Tinel's or Phalen's sign, 169
  neurological testing
    Brudzinski sign, 160
    cranial nerve testing (CN), 160–161
    Kernig sign, 160
    neurological exam, 159
    neurological maneuvers, 159–160
  signs and symptoms of headaches, 166
  treatment of headaches, 167
neutropenia, 151
nevi (moles), 64, 333
nevus flammeus or "port wine" stain, 207
nongonococcal urethritis, 302, 352
non-Hodgkin's lymphoma, 150
Nurse Practice Act, 262
nurse practitioners, 262–265, 296, 337
nursing certification exams
  ANCC *vs* AANP exams, 3–8
  credentialing organizations, 1–2
  examination information, sources of, 2–3
  tips for exams, 9–14
nystagmus, 81, 330

obsessive-compulsive disorder, 258, 286
obstetrics
  danger signals
    abruptio placentae, 193
    HELLP syndrome (hemolysis, elevated liver
      enzymes, and low platelets), 192
    placenta previa, 192–193
    preeclampsia to eclampsia (pregnancy induced
      hypertension), 192
  drugs and vaccines in pregnancy
    antibiotics, 195
    anti-hypertensives, 195
    category A, 194
    category B, 195
    category C, 195–196
    category D, 196
    category X, 196–197
    contraindicated in the 3rd trimester, 196
    teratogens, 197
    vaccines, 197
  fundal heights, 199
  health education, 197–198
  laboratory tests
    amniocentesis, 194
    doubling time, 194
    human chorionic gonadotropin, 194
    serum alpha-fetoprotein (AFP), 193–194
    urinalysis, 193
    vaginal cultures, 197
  Naegele's rule (estimated date of delivery or EDD),
    201
  physiologic changes during pregnancy, 199–201
  signs of pregnancy, 198–199
onychomycosis (nails), 76, 345
oral contraceptives, 76, 172, 183–187, 310, 314, 349,
    353, 367
  clinical tips, 187
  contraindications, 185
  decreased incidence, 184
  depo provera (depot medroxyprogesterone) 0.03%
    failure rate, 186
  diaphram with contraceptive gel, 186
  drug interactions, 184
  emergency contraception, 185
  exam tips, 184, 187
  IUD (intrauterine device), 186
  male/female condoms, 186
  missing consecutive days, 185
  mnemonic device "My CUPLETS," 183
  new prescriptions, 184
  pill danger signals, 185
  pill problems, 184–185
  relative contradictions, 186
  risk factors, 18–18
orchitis, 176, 324
Ortolani test, 220
Osgood-Schlatter disease, 231–232, 330
osteopenia, 186, 191, 232, 234, 258, 272, 302,
    354

osteoporosis, 124, 129, 186, 191–192, 197, 232, 234, 246,
    248, 252–253, 258, 260, 272–274, 289, 309, 311,
    340
otitis externa (swimmer's ear), 90–91
ovarian cancer, 180–181, 184, 366

Paget's Disease of the Breast (ductal carcinoma in situ),
    179, 353
papilledema, 81, 100, 158, 295
pap smear test, 60, 177, 182, 276–277, 300, 328, 355
Parkinson's disease, 235, 237–238, 305
peak expiratory flow (PEF) meters, 359
peak expiratory flow volume, factors for, 300
pediatrics
  danger signals
    chlamydial pneumonia, 209
    cryptorchidism (undescended testicle), 205
    gonococcal ophthalmia, 206
    trachoma, 206
  disease review
    abdominal tumors: malignant tumors, 219
    coarctation of the aorta, 219
    congenital lacrimal duct obstruction, 218–219
    epiglottitis, 205
    infant colic (rule of #3's), 219
    orthopedics, 220
    physiologic anemia of infancy, 218
    physiologic jaundice, 218
    rashes, 220–221
  growth and development, 215–218
    6 months old, 215
    9 months old, 215
    12 months old, 216
    newborns, 215
    practice questions, 333, 361
    2 years old, 216
    3 years old, 216
  immunizations
    influenza vaccine, 212–213
    MMR (mumps, measles, and rubella), 212
    primary series of vaccination, 214–215
    schedule, 214
    varicella vaccine, 212
  normal findings
    newborns, 213–214
    reflex testing, 214–215, 284
  safety education, 220–221
  screening tests, 208–210
  skin lesions of infancy, 207–208
  vascular lesions, 208
pediculosis capitis (lice), 222–223
pelvic inflammatory disease (PID), 172, 176, 272
pernicious anemia, 155–157, 251, 306
Peyronie's disease, 246
Phalen test, 292
phimosis, 246
Pigeon-toe, 220
pinguecula, 84, 92, 292
PKU (Phenylketonuria) testing, 209–210

placenta abruptio, 204, 275
placenta previa, 192–193, 197, 275
pneumococcal vaccine (Pneumovax), 346–347,
    361
pneumonia, 117–118, 322, 338, 343, 348
Podagra, 252, 315
polycystic ovary syndrome (PCOS), 188, 366
positive straight leg raising test, 305
postherpetic neuralgia, 73, 78, 369
power of attorney, 264–265
precocious puberty, 225–226, 351
pregnancy, related questions, 42–43, 271, 274, 276,
    281–282, 285–289, 290, 292, 310, 328, 346,
    357–358, 360
pregnancy-induced hypertension, 193, 271
primary angle-closure glaucoma, 85–86
primary open-angle glaucoma, 85
prostate specific antigen (PSA) with digital rectal exam
    (DRE), 60
prostatic hypertrophy, 240, 341
psoriasis, 66
psychopharmacotherapy, 32–33
pterygium, 84, 92, 291
ptyiasis rosea, 73
public health care policy, 266
pulmonary emboli (PE), 112
pulmonary system
    clinical tips
        asthma, 124
        pneumonia, 118
    danger signals
        impending respiratory failure (asthmatic patient),
            113
        pulmonary emboli (PE), 112
        treatment, 113
    disease review
        acute bronchitis, 118
        asthma, 122
        atypical pneumonia, 117–118
        bacterial pneumonia, 115–116
        chronic obstructive pulmonary disease (COPD),
            114–115
        smallpox (variola virus), 124–125
        tuberculosis (TB), 119–121
    exam tips
        asthma, 122–123
        chronic obstructive pulmonary disease (COPD),
            115
        pneumonia, 118
        smallpox (variola virus), 125
        tuberculosis (TB), 121
    normal findings, 113–114
pulsus paradoxus, 98, 324
purified protein derivative (PPD) test, 60,
    270
pyloric stenosis, 136

questions and dissections, analysis of
    abuse-related situations, 33–34
    adolescence, 45
        legal issues, 46
    benign variants, 64–65
    CAGE screening tool, 236, 257
    classic presentation of disease, 48–49
    classic signs and symptoms of disease, 22–23
    clinical decision-making skills, 15, 21–22
    complex sentences, 18–19
    diagrams, 28
    differential diagnoses, 46–48
    diseases and alternate names, 30
    emergent cases
        anaphylactic episodes, 16
        mnemomic MS. SPAIN, 17
    ethnic background and genetic disorders, 50–51,
        157
    factoid questions, 36–37
    finding *vs* name, 54–55
    on food habits, 51–52
    gold standard tests, 28–30
    grading heart murmurs, 38
    laboratory and diagnostic tests, 25–27
    negatively worded questions, 39–40
    pediatric growth and development, 43–44
    pertaining to drugs, 23–24, 53–54
    physical exam findings, 37–38
    practice questions and answers, 269–390
    pregnancy, 42–43
    psychiatric disorders
        drug therapy, 32–33
        major depression/unipolar depression, 31–32
    relating to normal growth and development, 41–42
    repetition of questions with variations, 56–57
    SOAPE mnemonic guide, 19–21
    two-part questions, 40–41
    uncommon diseases, 49–50

rashes, classic presentation of, 23
Raynaud's phenomenon, 108, 299
recurrent cystitis (three or more per year for females),
    149
Reiter's syndrome, 173–174, 274
renal system, 276
    danger signals
        acute pyelonephritis, 144
        acute pyelonephritis (child), 145
        acute renal failure, 145
        recurrent urinary tract infections (child), 145
        Wilm's tumor (nephroblastoma), 145
    disease review
        acute pyelonephritis, 149
        recurrent cystitis (three or more per year for
            females), 149
        urinary tract infections (UTIs), 145–150
    laboratory testing, 145–146
    normal findings, 145
rheumatoid arthritis (RA), 108, 128, 250, 274, 292, 298,
    306, 308, 311, 315–316, 353–354
rhinitis medicamentosa, 90

Rh-negative women, 201–202
RhoGAM (Rh-negative immunoglobulin), 201–202, 322
Rhogam's mechanism, 322
Rinne testing, 334
Rocky Mountain spotted fever, 62, 72, 74
rosacea (acne rosacea), 77–78, 331
roseola infantum: herpes virus 6, 220–221
Rovsing's sign, 136, 293
ruptured baker's cyst (bursitis), 255

scabies, 73–74, 78–79, 223, 277
scarlet fever, 74, 222–223, 366, 369
scotch tape test, 318, 339
seborrheic dermatitis ("cradle cap"), 207, 320
seborrheic keratoses, 65, 78, 233,
seizure, 259, 328
selective serotonin reuptake inhibitors (SSRIs), 256, 258, 369
Self-Efficacy Theory, 267
sentinel nodes (Virchow's nodes), 360
sexually transmitted diseases (STDs)
    danger signals
        disseminated gonococcal disease (disseminated gonorrhea), 170
        human immunodeficiency virus (HIV), 170
        syphilis, 170
    disease review
        chlamydia trachomatis, 170–171
        condyloma acuminata (genital warts), 177–178
        Fitz-Hugh-Curtis syndrome (perihepatitis), 173
        herpes simplex: HSV1 and HSV 2, 178–179
        HIV infection (human immunodeficiency virus), 175
        Jarisch-Herxheimer reaction, 173
        lymphogranuloma venereum (LGV), 179
        neisseria gonorrhea (GC), 171
        Reiter's syndrome, 173
        syphilis, 174
    exam tips, 174, 177, 179
    risk factors, 170
    STD screening recommended by the CDC, 170
    testing, 60
    treatment guidelines, 176
shingles infection of the trigeminal nerve, 62
sickle cell anemia, 117, 240, 280, 338, 346
sinus headache, 301
skin tenting sign, 18
smallpox (variola virus), 124–125
Snellen chart, 82, 209, 282
Somogyi effect (rebound hyperglycemia), 135, 370
spermatogenesis, 240, 348
spontaneous abortions, 203–204
sprains, 247, 254
Stevens-Johnson syndrome, 63, 364
strawberry hemangiomas, 208, 344

streptococcal pneumonia, 270
subconjunctival hemorrhage, 84–85, 278
suicide risk, 255
suppurative otitis media, 323
supranumerary nipples, 187
Swim therapy, 309
syphilis, 73, 170, 173–174, 176, 261, 281
systemic lupus erythematosus, 305, 320
Systems Theory, 267

talipes equinovarus "clubfoot," 220, 328
Tanner stages, 225–226, 273
temporal arteritis (giant cell arteritis), 158, 164, 166–167, 232, 311
tendonitis, 254
testicular torsion, 224, 239–240, 242, 324
thalassemia diagnosis, standard tests, 27
thalassemia minor/trait, 154–155
Thomson Prometric Testing Centers, 3
thrombocytopenia, 151
thyroid dysfunctions, 100, 126–128, 319, 321
tinea barbae (beard area), 76
tinea capitis (scalp), 75
tinea corporis or tinea circinata (ringworm of the body), 75
tinea cruris (jock itch), 75, 360
tinea infections (dermatophytoses), 75
tinea manuum (hands), 76
tinea pedis (athlete's foot), 75, 360
tinea versicolor, 67
Title XIX of the Social Security Act (Medicaid), 266
TORCH infections, 273
torus palatinus, 81, 323
trichomonas vaginitis (Trichomoniasis), 190–191
trichomoniasis, 190, 269
trigeminal neuralgia (tic douloureux), 164–167, 301
T scores, 191, 340
tuberculosis (TB), 119–121, 281, 297
    screening, 60
Turner's syndrome, 230
two-part questions, 40–41
Tzanck smear, 182–183, 365

ulcerative colitis, 359
upper respiratory infection (URI), 87, 278, 290, 293, 351
urinary tract infections (UTIs), 145–150
    clinical tip, 148
    complications, 147
    exam tip, 148
    medication, 147
    risk factors, 147
    special categories, 148
    uncomplicated *vs* complicated, 147–148
U.S. health statistics, 61–62
U.S. Preventative Task Force screening recommendations, 59–60

vaginal infections, 191
varicella (chickenpox), 72, 206, 212, 214, 222, 281
varicocele, 246, 324
vertigo, 289, 300–301, 348
viral infections, 294, 301
visual fields by confrontation test, 82, 304
vitamin B12 deficiency, 151, 155
vitiligo, 65

Weber test, 83, 161, 325
Western Blot test, 287

xanthelasma, 65
xerosis, 65

Zollinger-Ellison syndrome, 135, 138, 344–345